Clinical Cases in Uveitis

FIRST EDITION

Clinical Cases in Uveitis

Differential Diagnosis and Management

Editors

HARPAL S. SANDHU, MD, FRCSC
Assistant Professor of Ophthalmology
Department of Ophthalmology and Visual Sciences
University of Louisville School of Medicine
Louisville, Kentucky

HENRY J. KAPLAN, MD, FACS
Professor of Ophthalmology
Research Director Department of Ophthalmology
Saint Louis University (SLU) School of Medicine
St. Louis, Missouri

ELSEVIER

Elsevier
1600 John F. Kennedy Blvd.
Ste 1800
Philadelphia, PA 19103-2899

CLINICAL CASES IN UVEITIS

ISBN: 978-0-323-69541-1

Notices

Knowledge and best practice in this field are constantly changing. As new research and experience broaden our understanding, changes in research methods, professional practices, or medical treatment may become necessary.

Practitioners and researchers must always rely on their own experience and knowledge in evaluating and using any information, methods, compounds or experiments described herein. Because of rapid advances in the medical sciences, in particular, independent verification of diagnoses and drug dosages should be made. To the fullest extent of the law, no responsibility is assumed by Elsevier, authors, editors or contributors for any injury and/or damage to persons or property as a matter of products liability, negligence or otherwise, or from any use or operation of any methods, products, instructions, or ideas contained in the material herein.

Library of Congress Control Number: 2020941982

Content Strategist: Kayla Wolfe
Content Development Manager: Ellen Wurm-Cutter
Content Development Specialist: Sara Watkins
Publishing Services Manager: Deepthi Unni
Project Manager: Janish Ashwin Paul
Design Direction: Maggie Reid

Printed in India

Last digit is the print number: 9 8 7 6 5 4 3 2 1

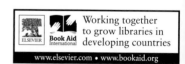

Working together
to grow libraries in
developing countries

www.elsevier.com • www.bookaid.org

DEDICATION

To my wife, Adele Lotner Kaplan, whose sacrifice and support throughout my professional career allowed me to pursue my dreams.

—HJK

To my grandparents. Somehow you knew we could come this far.

—HSS

LIST OF CONTRIBUTORS

Tomas S. Aleman, MD
Associate Professor
Scheie Eye Institute
Department of Ophthalmology
University of Pennsylvania
Philadelphia, PA

Sruthi Arepalli, MD
Uveitis Fellow
Casey Eye Institute
Oregon Health & Sciences University
Portland, OR

Rubens Belfort Jr., MD, PhD
Department of Ophthalmology and Visual
   Sciences
Paulista School of Medicine
Federal University of São Paulo
São Paulo, SP, Brazil

Frederick R. Blodi, MD
Department of Ophthalmology and Visual
   Sciences
University of Louisville
Louisville, KY

Bahram Bodaghi, MD, PhD, FEBO
Department of Ophthalmology
IHU FOReSIGHT
APHP-Sorbonne University
Paris, France

Weilin Chan
Department of Ophthalmology
Massachusetts Eye and Ear Infirmary
Harvard Medical School
Boston, MA

Peter Yuwel Chang, MD
Massachusetts Eye Research and Surgery
   Institution (MERSI)
Waltham, MA

Sarah Chorfi, MD
Department of Ophthalmology
Maisonneuve-Rosemont Hospital
University of Montreal
Montreal, Canada

Christopher Conrady, MD, PhD
Retina Fellow
Kellogg Eye Center
Department of Ophthalmology and Visual
   Sciences
University of Michigan
Ann Arbor, MI

Dean Eliott, MD
Associate Director, Retina Service
Retina Service
Massachusetts Eye and
   Ear Infirmary
Boston, MA

Stelios Evangelos Gragoudas Associate
   Professor
Harvard Medical School
Boston, MA

C. Stephen Foster, MD, FACS, FACR
President and Founder
Massachusetts Eye Research and Surgery
   Institution (MERSI)
Waltham, MA

Clinical Professor
Department of Opthalmology
Harvard Medical School
Boston, MA

Danielle Trief, MD, MSc
Assistant Professor
Department of Ophthalmology
Columbia University
New York, NY

Muhammad Hassan, MD
Byers Eye Institute
Stanford University School of Medicine
Palo Alto, CA

Swathi Kaliki, MD
LV Prasad Eye Institute
Hyderabad, India

Henry J. Kaplan, MD, FACS
Professor of Ophthalmology
Research Director Department of
    Ophthalmology
Saint Louis University (SLU) School of Medicine
St. Louis, Missouri

Jelena Karadzic, MD
University Eye Clinic
Faculty of Medicine
University of Belgrade
Belgrade, Serbia

Madison E. Kerley, BA
University of Louisville School of Medicine
Louisville, KY

Ashleigh L. Levison, MD
Colorado Retina Associates
Denver, CO

Aaron Lindeke-Myers, MD
Emory School of Medicine
Atlanta, GA

George Magrath, MD
Medical University of South Carolina
Charleston, SC

Albert M. Maguire, MD
Professor of Ophthalmology
Scheie Eye Institute
Department of Ophthalmology
University of Pennsylvania Perelman School
    of Medicine
Philadelphia, PA

Caroline L. Minkus, MD
Massachusetts Eye and Ear Infirmary/
    Harvard Medical School
Boston, MA

Bobeck S. Modjtahedi, MD
Department of Ophthalmology
Southern California Permanente Medical Group
Baldwin Park, CA

Eye Monitoring Center
Kaiser Permanente Southern California
Baldwin Park, CA

Department of Research and Evaluation
Southern California Permanente Medical Group
Pasadena, CA

Judith Mohay, MD
Associate Professor
Department of Ophthalmology and Visual
    Sciences
University of Louisville
Louisville, KY

Kareem Moussa, MD
Uveitis Fellow
F.I. Proctor Foundation
University of California, San Francisco
San Francisco, CA

Marion Ronit Munk, MD, PhD
Ophthalmology
Inselspital, University Clinic Bern
Bern, Switzerland
Ophthalmology
Northwestern University
Feinberg School of Medicine
Chicago, IL

Quan Dong Nguyen, MD, MSc
Professor of Ophthalmology
Byers Eye Institute
Stanford University School of Medicine
Palo Alto, CA

Neil Onghanseng, MD
Byers Eye Institute
Stanford University School of Medicine
Palo Alto, CA

George N. Papaliodis, MD
Associate Professor of Ophthalmology
Director of the Ocular Immunology and
    Uveitis Service

Department of Ophthalmology
Massachusetts Eye and Ear Infirmary/
Harvard Medical School
Boston, MA

Kathryn Pepple, MD, PhD
Assistant Professor
Ophthalmology
University of Washington
Seattle, WA

Aleksandra Radosavljevic, MD, PhD
University Eye Clinic
Faculty of Medicine
University of Belgrade
Belgrade, Serbia

Aparna Ramasubramanian, MD
Medical Director, Retinoblastoma Program
Phoenix Children's Hospital
Assistant Clinical Professor
Creighton University School of Medicine
Omaha, Nebraska

Sivakumar R. Rathinam, FAMS, PhD
Prof. of Ophthalmology and Head of uveitis
   service
Uveitis Service
Aravind Eye Hospital & PG. Institute of
   Ophthalmology
Madurai, Tamil Nadu, India

Clinician Scientist
Immunology
Aravind medical research foundation
Madurai, India

Mohammad Ali Sadiq, MD
Department of Ophthalmology and Visual
   Sciences
University of Louisville
Louisville, KY

Harpal S. Sandhu, MD, FRCSC
Assistant Professor of Ophthalmology
Department of Ophthalmology and Visual
   Sciences
University of Louisville School of
   Medicine
Louisville, Kentucky

Jessica G. Shantha, MD
Emory Eye Center
Atlanta, GA

Ryan A. Shields, MD
Byers Eye Institute
Stanford University School of
   Medicine
Palo Alto, CA

Lucia Sobrin, MD, MPH
Associate Professor
Department of Ophthalmology
Massachusetts Eye and Ear
   Infirmary
Harvard Medical School
Boston, MA

Dinu Stanescu, MD, PhD
Pitié Salpêtrière University Hospital
Département of Ophthalmolgy
Sorbonne University
Paris, France

Kim Anne Strässle, Dr. Med.
Inselspital, University Hospital Bern
Bern, Switzerland

Eric Suhler, MD, MPH
Chief of Ophthalmology
Eye Care/Operative Care Division
VA Portland Health Care System
Portland, OR

Professor
Ophthalmology and Public Health
Oregon Health & Science University
Portland, OR

Aristomenis Thanos, MD
Adult and Pediatric Vitreoretinal Surgery and
   Disease
Devers Eye Institute
Portland, OR

Sara Touhami, MD, PhD, FEBO
Sorbonne Université
Pitié Salpêtrière
University Hospital
Paris, France

Adelaide Toutee, MD, FEBO
Pitié Salpêtrière University Hospital
Département of Ophthalmolgy
Sorbonne University
Paris, France

Eduardo Uchiyama, MD
Retina Group of Florida
Fort Lauderdale, FL

Affiliate Assistant Professor of Clinical
  Biomedical Sciences
Charles E. Schmidt College of Medicine,
  Florida Atlantic University
Boca Raton, FL

Russell Neil Van Gelder, MD, PhD
Professor and Chair
Department of Ophthalmology
University of Washington
Seattle, WA

Camila V. Ventura, MD, PhD
Altino Ventura Foundation
HOPE Eye Hospital
Recife, Brazil

Liana O. Ventura, MD, PhD
Altino Ventura Foundation
HOPE Eye Hospital
Recife, Brazil

Albert Vitale, MD
Professor
Moran Eye Center
Department of Ophthalmology and Visual
  Sciences
University of Utah
Salt Lake City, UT

Steven Yeh, MD
M. Louise Simpson Professor
Director, Section of Uveitis and Vasculitis
Emory Eye Center
Ophthalmology
Emory University School of Medicine
Atlanta, GA

Faculty Fellow
Emory Global Health Institute
Emory University
Atlanta, GA

Manfred Zierhut, MD
Professor of Ophthalmology
Centre for Ophthalmology
University of Tübingen
Tubingen, Germany

Few presentations to the ophthalmologist provoke more anxiety and consternation than an unusual case of uveitis. The panoply of different presentations, etiologies, severities, and treatments of uveitis challenges even the experienced ophthalmologist, to say nothing of the novice. But for these very reasons, the intellectual and professional satisfaction of a case well managed offers immense rewards to the clinician. More importantly, it preserves or restores vision to patients with severe disease.

There are already many excellent texts in the field of uveitis, but to us something clearly was missing. The majority of works in the field are comprehensive in scope, essentially dense textbooks on different forms of uveitis. Other books have presented briefer and more targeted information, but the organizing principle remains the same. Much like most medical texts, they present information categorized by disease. This is of course a classic and time-tested way to learn. However, patients rarely present to us saying "I have syphilis", or tuberculosis, or sarcoidosis, or herpetic retinitis, or some other such disease entity. Rather, they frequently present with different constellations of symptoms, signs, and past medical history. Of particular note is the anatomical location of inflammation, morphology of lesions, and the demographic background of the patient. In the clinic, we go from identifying the important historical and exam features of a case to ordering tests, generating differential diagnoses, arriving at a working diagnosis, initiating treatment, and reassessing the patient in follow up. This is how patients actually present to clinicians, and it is precisely this sequence of events, and the clinician's concomitant thought process, that we seek to describe in this book.

Herein we present actual cases of uveitis from across the spectrum of the uveitic diseases (or uveitides). Infectious diseases, masquerade syndromes, idiopathic conditions, inflammatory diseases with systemic manifestations, and pediatric diseases all appear throughout the text. There are three goals: to cover the vast majority of uveitic diseases in a memorable and digestible case-based format, to describe typical, emblematic cases of most of these diseases, and to describe the thought process involved in managing complex cases. The last goal involves discussion of the important features of difficult cases that lead us in one direction versus another. A novel aspect of this book is a minority of more complex cases that do not progress as anticipated, prompting a reconsideration of diagnosis or management. After all, this happens to all of us no matter how experienced we are in the field.

This type of case-based approach is by no means unique in medical education, but it is a niche that has been largely ignored in ophthalmology, particularly in retina and uveitis. This is striking given the diagnostic and therapeutic complexity of the subject. In the genesis of this book, we both talked fondly of our days as medical students on internal medicine, pediatrics, and surgery, and the case-based texts we had each used that so memorably captured the essence of various diseases in a way that textbooks often had not. We hope the spirit and merit of those earlier books live on in this one. Enjoy.

—Harpal S. Sandhu and Hank J. Kaplan

ACKNOWLEDGMENTS

Many people are involved in a project of this breadth, both personally and professionally. First, we must thank our contributing authors. They are luminaries from around the globe. Some are our past teachers, others former collaborators, all are dedicated clinicians. Thank you for your effort, enthusiasm, and expertise.

HJK would like to foremost thank his wife, Adele, since his professional career would not have been possible without her many sacrifices and continual support over the past 54 years; as well as their family with children Wendi, Todd and Ariane, and grandchildren Noah, Emma, Lilah, Asher, Ava, and Rosie who are the greatest joy in his life. Many mentors have been responsible for his professional success and achievements, most notably two mentors and colleagues that have influenced him throughout his career, and still remain close friends, Thomas A. Weingeist and H. Dwight Cavanagh; additionally, his career would not have flourished without the mentorship of J. Wayne Streilein, Frederick C. Blodi, Thomas M. Aaberg Sr, and contributions of Tongalp H. Tezel and Lucian V. Del Priore. This textbook would not have been possible without the enormous contributions of his co-editor, Harpal Sandhu, whom it has been a privilege to work with and who has become a dear friend; Harpal's future contributions to ophthalmology will undoubtedly continue to be outstanding. Finally, HJK's contributions to this text would not have been possible without the assistance of Niloofar Piri, a vitreoretinal and uveitis specialist, who trained with him and is about to embark on a promising professional academic career.

HSS thanks above all his parents for their unconditional love and support. Everything they have done in their adult lives has been for their children, and he hopes he can be as selfless and strong as them some day. Sincere thanks also to his sisters Tej, Davinder, and Kiran, his nephews, and his extended family. He cannot imagine his life without them, and they should all take some credit for any of his success. He also would be nowhere without his many mentors and teachers in ophthalmology, particularly Frank Sutula, George Papaliodis, Dean Eliott, Demetrios Vavvas, John Kempen, Tomas Aleman, Joan O'Brien, Al Maguire, and Sandy Brucker. They never had to help him, but they always did, and years later they still do. Last, many thanks to his co-editor, teacher, and friend Hank Kaplan, whose insight and guidance made this and many other great things possible.

We would also like to thank Kayla Wolfe, without whose encouragement this book never would have happened, and Sara Watkins, who shepherded us through its creation, both of Elsevier.

Finally, no acknowledgment would be complete without mention of our patients. Some of you live within this book, your anonymized stories retold for the benefit of other physicians. You have taught us more than any book ever has. It is our unending quest to do more for you.

CONTENTS

CHAPTER 1

Introduction to Uveitis

Harpal S. Sandhu ▦ Henry J. Kaplan

Uveitis refers to inflammation in the uvea, a Latin word for *grape*, and specifically the vascular middle layer of the eye that involves the iris anteriorly, the ciliary body in the middle, and the choroid posteriorly (Fig. 1.1). It was recognized as a disease entity as early as 1500 BC during the era of Egyptian medicine, and several medicinal extracts were used for treatment of uveitis at that time.[1] Today, uveitis remains a major cause of ocular morbidity, causing approximately 10% of the cases of visual disability in the United States each year. It is estimated to cause 30,000 cases of new-onset legal blindness annually, with an annual prevalence of 58 to 115 per 100,000 population.[2]

Intraocular inflammation is frequently referred to as "uveitis," even when other structures of the eye are primarily involved—for example, the retina (i.e., retinitis) and sclera (i.e., scleritis). Many uveitic entities are caused by infection, trauma, or neoplasia, but the majority are of unknown etiology and thought to be autoimmune. Some autoimmune uveitic cases are associated with systemic immune-mediated diseases, such as HLA-B27−associated spondyloarthropathies, sarcoidosis, and Behçet disease, whereas others are limited only to the eye without any systemic manifestation—for example, pars planitis and serpiginous choroiditis. The patient's ocular complaints do not usually suggest a specific anatomic diagnosis; the exception is acute anterior uveitis, which is frequently associated with pain, redness, and photophobia. Most other uveitic entities present with blurred vision, floaters, a blind spot, or cloudiness.

Attempts have recently been made to standardize the nomenclature of uveitis, as well as its description and response to treatment. In 2005 the Standardization of Uveitis Nomenclature (SUN) Working Group (WG), consisting of 79 uveitis experts from 18 countries and 62 clinical centers, published a standardized and internationally accepted terminology for the uveitides, as well as recommendations for the grading of inflammation and development of disease outcomes.[3] Most recently (December 1, 2019), this group met again to adopt and confirm a set of classification criteria for specific uveitic entities, and the results of their work will be published in the near future.

It is important to understand the difference between classification and diagnostic criteria.[4] *Classification criteria* are standardized definitions that are primarily intended to enable *clinical studies* with uniform cohorts for research. Consequently, they need to define homogeneous groups that can be compared across studies and geographic areas. In contrast, *diagnostic criteria* are a set of signs, symptoms, and tests developed for use in *routine clinical care* to guide the treatment of individual patients. They need to be broad and reflect all the possible different features and sensitivity of a disease that is characteristically heterogeneous. Thus, testing specificity and sensitivity for diagnostic criteria need to be very high, approaching 100%, whereas classification criteria require very high specificity, even with some loss in sensitivity. A detailed discussion of this issue is provided by the American College of Rheumatology[3] and suggests that the difficulty in establishing uniform diagnostic criteria lends support to the proposals of the SUN WG for diagnostic criteria using standard nomenclature, terminology, and testing even though further refinements in diagnostic criteria will undoubtedly be forthcoming.

Because the eye is an extension of the central nervous system (CNS), it makes unique demands on the immune system; it cannot tolerate the full array of immune responses available to other

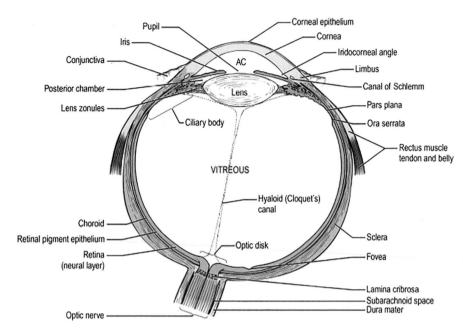

Fig. 1.1 Schematic diagram of the human eye in horizontal section revealing the major components and the arrangement of the three layers. *AC*, Anterior chamber. The corneoscleral envelope *(blue)*, the uveal tract *(orange/red)*, and the inner neural layer *(purple)*. (Forrester J, Dick A, McMenamin P, et al. *The Eye*. 4th ed. Saunders Ltd; 2015:14, Figure 1-10, by Elsevier.)

organs. The eye has only one function, to provide sight by the transmission of light to the photoreceptors of the retina, where the light is processed by a complex neural network, and from there, to the visual cortex. This remarkable neurologic function is critical to the survival of the host so that destructive inflammation, even in protection of the eye from infection, is not tolerable. Thus a complex immunoregulatory network to protect the eye from destructive inflammation evolved to prevent immune-mediated injury. This immunologic phenomenon is referred to as *immune privilege* and is a feature of the CNS and only a few other organs in the body. For example, destruction of a quarter of the liver combating infection would be harmful to the host but would not threaten functional survival of that organ or the host; in contrast, destruction of the fovea (300 to 500 μ) within the center of the retina will cause legal blindness.

A basic understanding of immune privilege is important to appreciate the presentation of intraocular inflammatory diseases such as uveitis. As ophthalmologic specialists, we have the unique ability to observe tissues within an organ (i.e., the eye) during active inflammation; consequently, our specialty has described many different clinical presentations of uveitic entities that are linked to the novel regulation of immunity. Both anatomic and functional factors contribute to the development of immune privilege within the eye, including the blood–retina barrier, absence of lymphatic drainage, soluble immunomodulatory factors, immunomodulatory ligands on the surface of ocular parenchymal cells, chronic activation of the complement system, and tolerogenic parenchymal antigen-presenting cells (APCs). The maintenance of immune privilege involves many different regulatory mechanisms, the details of which are too numerous to discuss in this chapter. Instead, we will briefly mention just three major strategies used by the eye to modify innate and adaptive immune responses within the organ: (1) *tissue-associated immunologic ignorance* (e.g., the decreased immunogenicity of retinal photoreceptors compared with retinal pigment epithelium [RPE] because of reduced expression of major histocompatibility complex [MHC] antigens on photoreceptors); (2) *peripheral tolerance to ocular antigens* (e.g., microglia, perivascular macrophages, and dendritic cells within the retina and uvea that can act as tolerogenic APCs); and (3) *immunosuppressive microenvironment* (e.g., maintained by multiple immunosuppressive soluble factors, surface immune modulators on parenchymal cells, and complement regulatory components). Excellent reviews of ocular immune privilege have recently been published for those interested in further reading on this subject.[5,6]

Each of the following book chapters present and discuss a different uveitis case. The incidence and prevalence of uveitis differs based on age, sex, anatomic location within the eye, gender, genetic factors, and etiology. Fortunately, although the etiology of a specific uveitic entity is frequently unknown, the characteristic clinical presentation allows a specific diagnosis, frequently confirmed by diagnostic testing, which is important because it provides insight into the likely course of the disease and response to treatment. The large number of idiopathic uveitic entities is partly the result of the fragile nature of ocular tissue, which has hindered the aggressiveness of tissue biopsy, and the value patients place on preservation of sight. However, interventional diagnostic techniques into the anterior chamber, vitreous cavity, and fine needle aspiration biopsy of intraocular tumors are now routinely available, although the limited quantity of fluid or tissue removed limits extensive studies. The recent advances in diagnostic imaging of the eye using optical coherence tomography (OCT) and the advent of new diagnostic laboratory techniques like polymerase chain reaction (PCR), genetic profiling (DNA), and single-cell transcriptomics (RNA) hold promise in providing understanding of the cause of many cases of uveitis that are now considered idiopathic.

The incidence and prevalence of uveitis differ based on age, gender, anatomic location of the inflammatory process (anterior, intermediate, posterior uveitis, panuveitis), type of inflammatory process (acute, chronic, recurrent), geographic location, and etiology (infectious, noninfectious). Anterior uveitis is the most common form, and the underlying cause is usually not identified (30% to 60%), with the disease referred to as *idiopathic anterior uveitis*. With our newer diagnostic techniques, the etiology of many cases will be determined in the future.[7]

It is our hope that you will find the subsequent case chapters both informative and interesting. They are designed to provide the reader with insight into the fascinating diagnostic and therapeutic field of uveitis.

References

1. Foster CS, Vitale AT. *Diagnosis and Treatment of Uveitis*. 2nd ed. New Delhi, India: Jaypee Brothers Medical Publishers; 2013:3–4.
2. Gritiz DC, Schwaber EJ, Wong IG. Complications of uveitis: The Northern California Epidemiology of Uveitis Study. *Ocul Immunol Inflamm.* 2018;26(4):584–594.
3. Trusko B, Thorne J, Jabs D, et al. The Standardization of Uveitis Nomenclature (SUN) project. Development of a clinical evidence base utilizing informatics tools and techniques. *Methods Inf Med.* 2013;52(3). 2592–65, S1–S6.
4. Aggarwal R, Ringold S, Khanna D, et al. Distinctions between diagnostic and classification criteria? *Arthritis Care Res.* 2015;67(7):891–897.
5. Taylor AW. Ocular immune privilege and transplantation. *Front Immunol.* 2016;7:37.
6. Xu H, Chen M. Targeting the complement system for the management of retinal inflammatory and degenerative diseases. *Eur J Pharmacol.* 2016;787:94–104.
7. Tsirouki T, Dastiridou A, Symeonidis C, et al. A focus on the epidemiology of uveitis. *Ocul Immunol Inflamm.* 2018;26(1):2–16.

CHAPTER 2

Approach to Diagnostic Testing

Harpal S. Sandhu ▓ Henry J. Kaplan

Introduction

Patients are often preoccupied with the "cause" of their affliction. Although this is understandable, the etiology of a given uveitis syndrome is often elusive, and about half of cases are labeled idiopathic or undifferentiated. In contrast, for the clinician, the first goal of any diagnostic testing is to differentiate between infectious and noninfectious/inflammatory etiologies. A third important but rare category is ocular neoplasm masquerading as uveitis (e.g., retinoblastoma, primary vitreoretinal lymphoma), and a fourth is nonneoplastic masquerade syndromes, such as inherited retinal degenerations or intraocular foreign bodies. The distinction between these four groups is critical because management is so radically different, at times even diametrically opposed.

Once a diagnosis of noninfectious uveitis (NIU) has been made, it is less important to make the diagnosis of a specific uveitis syndrome. The critical determination—that the disease should be treated with antiinflammatory therapy—has already been established. However, it can still be helpful to make a more specific diagnosis for three purposes: first, it informs prognosis; second, it may help guide therapy; and third, it may shed light on other systemic symptoms of heretofore unknown origin. For instance, a patient in her 20s with new-onset, acute unilateral anterior uveitis with a 1-year history of low back pain that she has been ignoring tests positive for HLA-B27. This result raises the diagnosis of ankylosing spondylitis as the origin of her back pain, prompting referral to a rheumatologist and radiographs that confirm the diagnosis. Moreover, HLA-B27 disease is typically recurrent and carries a fairly good prognosis if managed correctly.

The goal of this chapter is to briefly review the appropriate use of laboratory tests based on the uveitic entity determined predominantly by the anatomic site of inflammation. Other common historical or examination features will occasionally be included to help narrow testing. Although uveitis specialists have struggled to decide on a standard set of tests for a given presentation, there is a general consensus that targeted testing, based on key historical or examination features, is strongly preferred over broad "shotgun testing" for every case of intraocular inflammation. Recall that based on Bayes' theorem, a diagnostic test is most helpful when one's pretest probability of the diagnosis is closest to 50%. As clinical suspicion of a diagnosis decreases (i.e., pretest probability approaches zero), the positive predictive value (i.e., the probability that a patient truly has the diagnosis given a positive test for it) declines precipitously, such that even highly sensitive and specific tests become nearly useless when positive. Lyme testing is an excellent example of this theorem. As such, each of the following sections outlines essentially a first line of testing with the knowledge that specific features of a case often lead to more targeted and sometimes esoteric testing. The point that specific cases, based on their features, can warrant other tests beyond the ones included here cannot be overemphasized, and the proceeding case chapters serve to illustrate that very concept.

Anterior Uveitis

Most cases of anterior uveitis are noninfectious in etiology. First-time episodes without any other ocular or systemic features do not mandate testing. In repeated or severe episodes, HLA-B27 is an excellent first test. If this is negative, then testing for the great intraocular imitators—syphilis, sarcoidosis, and tuberculosis—is warranted: rapid plasma reagin (RPR) and fluorescent treponemal antibody absorption (FTA-ABS) (or other treponemal test, such as *Treponema pallidum* particle agglutination assay [TP-PA]) for syphilis; a chest x-ray (CXR), angiotensin-converting enzyme (ACE), and lysozyme for sarcoidosis; and a QuantiFERON or purified protein derivative (PPD) for tuberculosis (Fig. 2.1). In cases where the clinical suspicion for sarcoidosis is high or when the CXR (probably the most useful of the three tests) is negative but ACE and/or lysozyme is positive, a computed tomography (CT) scan of the chest is indicated.

Several other common settings in which anterior uveitis occurs warrant additional investigations. If intraocular pressure (IOP) is elevated and/or there is sectoral iris atrophy, an anterior chamber (AC) tap to perform polymerase chain reaction (PCR) for Herpesviridae is reasonable and indicated in refractory cases. For pediatric patients, antinuclear antibody (ANA), rheumatoid factor (Rf), urinary and serum beta-2 microglobulin, a basic metabolic panel, and urinalysis are indicated to look for juvenile idiopathic arthritis and tubulointerstitial nephritis with uveitis syndrome. Finally, for patients of advanced age and chronic anterior uveitis, a complete blood count (CBC) should be performed and AC tap for cytology and/or flow cytometry should be strongly considered, given concerns for leukemia/lymphoma.

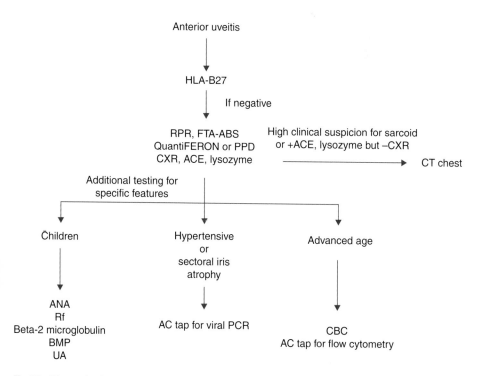

Fig. 2.1 Diagnostic algorithm for first-line testing for recurrent or chronic unilateral anterior uveitis or bilateral uveitis.

Intermediate Uveitis

Intermediate uveitis is the most narrowly defined uveitic syndrome with a more limited set of causes. Patients meeting the classic description of pars planitis (i.e., snowballs, snowbanks, and vitreal inflammation in a child) require no immediate testing. However, testing is indicated in two specific instances. If the patient has a positive neurologic review of systems, magnetic resonance imaging (MRI) of the brain is indicated to rule out demyelinating disease. Second, if the patient requires immunomodulatory therapy (IMT), then baseline testing is also indicated (Fig. 2.2).

Patients with intermediate uveitis atypical for pars planitis or who have a poor response to anti-inflammatory treatment warrant testing, namely again for syphilis, sarcoidosis, and tuberculosis (RPR, FTA-ABS, CXR, ACE, lysozyme, QuantiFERON or PPD), but also this time for Lyme disease with serologies and reflex Western blot. In patients of advanced age with chronic or recurrent intermediate uveitis, one must be concerned for intraocular lymphoma (primary or secondary vitreoretinal lymphoma), and a vitreous biopsy via pars plana vitrectomy (PPV) sent for flow cytometry, cytology, IL-10/Il-6 ratio, and MyD88 genetic mutation.

Panuveitis

Panuveitis is a highly heterogeneous entity with many different associations and causes. Exhaustive testing is costly, impractical, and prone to false positives. Again, first-line diagnostic tests are

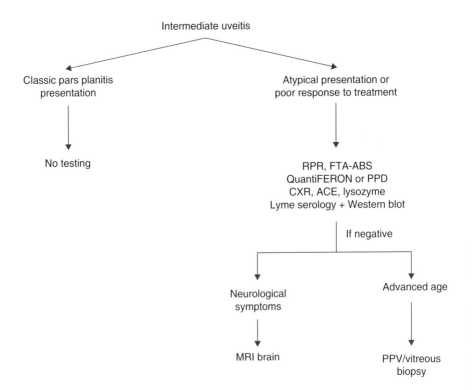

Fig. 2.2   Diagnostic algorithm for first-line testing for intermediate uveitis.

directed towards syphilis, sarcoidosis, and tuberculosis (RPR, FTA-ABS, CXR, ACE, lysozyme, QuantiFERON or PPD). If the history is suggestive of Lyme disease (endemic region, tick bite, bull's-eye rash, migratory arthralgias, facial nerve palsy, etc.), then Lyme serologies plus reflex Western blot are ordered. A history of recent blisters or sores raises concern for Behçet's disease, for which there is no good test, but also for Herpesviridae, in which case their serologies and an AC tap for PCR are reasonable tests. If the first-line tests are negative and there is a poor response to anti-inflammatory therapy, a vitreous tap or PPV to rule out infection before escalating therapy to IMT, for instance, is indicated (Fig. 2.3).

Retinal Vasculitis

Much like panuveitis, there are again many causes of retinal vasculitis. Several important diseases include retinal vasculitis as one sign among many, such as acute retinal necrosis and birdshot chorioretinopathy, and can be readily diagnosed by other characteristic clinical features. However, a presentation of predominantly retinal vascular inflammation presents a different set of considerations. In addition to testing for syphilis, sarcoidosis, and tuberculosis (RPR, FTA-ABS, CXR, ACE, lysozyme, QuantiFERON or PPD), antineutrophil cytoplasmic antibodies (ANCA) testing is very important, and a CBC and basic metabolic panel (BMP) are also warranted, as systemic vasculitides commonly cause glomerulonephritis. Human immunodeficiency virus (HIV) testing is also very helpful because cytomegalovirus (CMV) infection can uncommonly present as a florid retinal vasculitis, mimicking frosted branch angiitis. When retinal arteriolar occlusions are present, antiphospholipid antibody testing is indicated, and with retinal venous occlusions, broad hypercoagulability testing should be considered if in an unusual clinical presentation (e.g., young age). Again, Lyme testing, replete with so many false positives and consequent overdiagnoses, is indicated only with suggestive features (Fig. 2.4).

Scleritis

Although not strictly a uveitis, scleritis can present to almost any eye care provider because of its ability to involve not only the ocular surface but also occasionally the anterior or posterior segment of the eye. Rheumatoid arthritis, ANCA-associated vasculitis, and HLA-B27 are common associations. First-line testing includes RPR, FTA-ABS, CXR, ACE, lysozyme, HLA-B27, QuantiFERON or PPD, ANCA, ANA, BMP, and uric acid. If testing is negative and there is poor response to treatment, one should consider a scleral and conjunctival biopsy to assess for infectious organisms or neoplasia (Fig. 2.5).

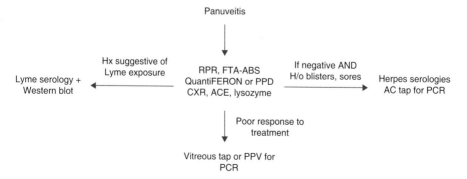

Fig. 2.3 Diagnostic algorithm for first-line testing for panuveitis.

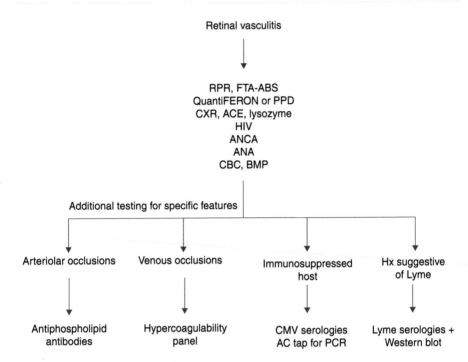

Fig. 2.4 Diagnostic algorithm for first-line testing for retinal vasculitis.

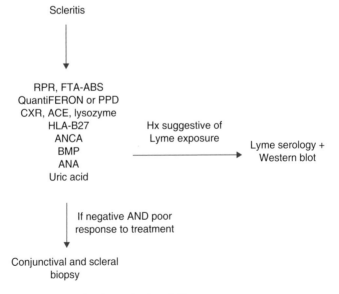

Fig. 2.5 Diagnostic algorithm for first-line testing for scleritis.

CHAPTER 3

Approach to Therapy

Harpal S. Sandhu ■ Henry J. Kaplan

Introduction

The goal of uveitis therapy is to suppress intraocular inflammation to zero or minimal activity and then maintain quiescence. In other words, excellent, enduring control is the goal. If we can achieve this, then patients are spared the multiple structural complications of uveitis that ultimately lead to vision loss, be they mild or severe: band keratopathy, synechiae, glaucoma, cyclitic membranes, hypotony, macular edema, epiretinal membranes, chorioretinal scarring or atrophy, and optic neuropathy, to name a few.

The field has indeed come a long way in just a half-century. As recently as the 1960s, the only systemic therapies available to ophthalmologists were systemic corticosteroids and methotrexate. The latter was used sparingly because of the bugaboo of the label "chemotherapy," terrifying patients and perhaps even doctors alike. Before that, fever chambers were used to induce pyrexia in uveitis patients, sometimes treating the disease but also sometimes killing the patient. We now know that low-dose antimetabolites and other systemic immunomodulatory therapies (IMTs), although possessing the potential for serious adverse effects, are preferred compared with the ravages of under-treated severe, chronic uveitic diseases. Today, we have a plethora of systemic IMT agents, biologic agents, and local drugs and implants with which to treat these diseases. There are still many challenging and refractory cases, but we have come a long way from the 1960s, and longer still from the days of the fever chamber.

This chapter will briefly review the standard systemic and local therapies for noninfectious uveitis (NIU) and, more importantly, will discuss the approach to therapy. When is local therapy sufficient? When should one consider systemic therapy and systemic IMT and, if so, how does one combine the various agents we now have at our disposal?

General Guidelines: Local Versus Systemic Therapy

Assuming one has identified active uveitis with the potential to cause structural damage, the first decision is whether to treat locally or systemically. There are several broad rules to guide the initial route of therapy in many cases. Like all guidelines, there will be many exceptions, but they should bring a measure of order to one's thinking, especially for the novice. Recalling the Standardization of Uveitis Nomenclature's (SUN) variables for categorizing uveitis (anatomy, course, laterality) is particularly helpful here.

First, anterior uveitis can typically be treated with topical therapy, whereas NIU involving the posterior segment (NIU-PS) typically requires locally injected or systemic therapy. Second, unilateral disease can often be treated locally, whereas bilateral disease is more often treated systemically. Third, chronic disease warrants chronic therapy, be it chronic (or frequently repeated) local therapy or chronic systemic therapy. Because ocular adverse effects with chronic local corticosteroid therapy are serious (glaucoma being usually the most concerning), the authors generally prefer systemic therapy in these cases, particularly for aggressive disease.

Exceptions immediately come to mind. For instance, acute posterior multifocal placoid pigment epitheliopathy (APMPPE) is a bilateral NIU involving the posterior segment but is generally self-limited and requires no treatment. Then there are other cases where some variables favor systemic therapy and others favor local. For instance, bilateral, chronic, anterior uveitis associated with juvenile idiopathic arthritis (JIA) has two variables in favor of systemic treatment (bilaterality and chronicity) but one variable in favor of topical therapy (anterior anatomic location). In this case, the specific systemic disease association has added key information. It has been well established by multiple studies that JIA-associated anterior uveitis is generally best treated with aggressive systemic therapy. Similarly, a patient with biopsy-proven sarcoidosis could also have chronic, bilateral anterior uveitis. Again, the systemic disease association provides valuable information. Sarcoidosis is usually highly corticosteroid responsive. In a mild case, a patient could be maintained on one drop of topical corticosteroids daily with good control, sparing her the potentially adverse effects of systemic IMT. If the patient is already pseudophakic and/or has shown little sign of corticosteroid response with increased intraocular pressure (IOP), this becomes an even more sensible treatment plan.

Thus knowledge of the individual patient and of the specific uveitic entity are critical. One of the goals of this book is to familiarize the reader with the latter via its case-based format.

Systemic Therapy: Corticosteroids and Systemic Immunomodulatory Therapy

CORTICOSTEROIDS

The fourth general rule is that acute episodes of inflammation should be treated with corticosteroids, whereas chronic inflammation is better treated with corticosteroid-sparing therapy. Corticosteroids have a plethora of effects on the immune response, a full discussion of which is beyond the scope of this book. For acute, systemic treatment, the authors will typically use prednisone 0.75 to 1 mg/kg up to 80 mg PO daily. There are exceptions to this dosing. Vogt–Koyanagi–Harada syndrome and sympathetic ophthalmia may require very large doses of systemic corticosteroids (e.g., prednisone 100 mg PO daily) to gain adequate initial control. Intravenous (IV) methylprednisolone can also be used if particularly large doses are required to control intraocular inflammation. Once quiescence has been established, the prednisone is tapered. The author uses the following tapering schedule: 70 mg PO daily × 1 week, then 60 mg PO daily × 1 week, 50 mg PO daily × 1 week, 40 mg PO daily × 1 week, 30 mg PO daily × 1 week, 20 mg PO daily × 2 weeks, 15 mg PO daily × 2 weeks, 10 mg PO daily × 2 weeks, then hold at 5 to 7.5 mg PO daily × 3 months before resuming the taper (Box 3.1).

Other uveitis specialists endorse other tapering regimens, but the authors feel this program strikes a good balance between the competing goals of efficacious therapy tapered slowly and the many adverse effects of systemic corticosteroid therapy, which usually become much more tolerable at a dose of approximately 10 mg PO daily. Holding prednisone at a low dose before resuming the taper is helpful to prevent recurrences, but there is no high-level evidence for this recommendation.

SYSTEMIC IMMUNOMODULATORY THERAPY: WHEN TO START

The decision to start IMT is driven by an understanding of the severity, laterality, and chronicity of the patient's intraocular inflammation; the status of the patient's fellow eye in cases of unilateral uveitis; the adverse effects incurred by local and/or systemic treatment with corticosteroids; and the patient's ability to adhere to the frequent laboratory and clinical follow-up necessary for all patients on IMT. If this sounds complex, it can be. However, a few straightforward guidelines can help to make the decision (Box 3.2).

BOX 3.1 ■ **Suggested Tapering Regimen for Oral Prednisone**

- 0.75–1 mg/kg up to 80 mg daily × 2 weeks, then
- 70 mg daily × 1 week
- 60 mg daily × 1 week
- 50 mg daily × 1 week
- 40 mg daily × 1 week
- 30 mg daily × 1 week
- 20 mg daily × 2 weeks
- 15 mg daily × 2 weeks
- 10 mg daily × 2 weeks
- Hold at 5 or 7.5 mg × 3 months before resuming taper
- ≤5 mg, taper by 1 mg every 2–4 weeks

BOX 3.2 ■ **Relative Indications for Chronic Systemic IMT Based on Course and Laterality**

1. Chronic bilateral uveitis
2. Chronic unilateral uveitis, particularly in a monocular patient
   AND
   A. Inability to control inflammation with local and/or systemic corticosteroids, or
   B. Unacceptable adverse effects of local and/or systemic corticosteroids
3. Acute, recurrent, or chronic uveitis with highly damaging inflammation, unilateral or bilateral

---

First, any patient with active, bilateral, chronic uveitis despite prednisone 10 mg or greater should typically be on IMT. Chronic doses of 10 mg or more have been shown to significantly increase the risk of osteoporosis and cardiac disease with long-term treatment. Chronic unilateral uveitis requiring ≥10 mg is a different situation, as local therapies, detailed later, may allow for disease quiescence with an acceptable level of local adverse effects and for tapering of prednisone to <10 mg PO daily.

Second, and in a similar vein, some patients with either chronic unilateral or bilateral uveitis may achieve quiescence with a combination of low doses of systemic prednisone (<10 mg PO daily) and local therapies (e.g., intravitreal or periocular triamcinolone, fluocinolone implants, etc.) but incur unacceptable adverse effects. Whereas a cataract is easily managed with a safe and effective surgical procedure, glaucoma can be more difficult to control in certain patients. Patients with severe and prolonged increases in IOP with local corticosteroid therapy are also candidates for IMT.

In a monocular patient, one has a heightened sensitivity both to ocular adverse effects and the damaging impact of uveitis flares that may arise as the effects of local therapy wane. Thus in monocular patients with chronic unilateral uveitis, the authors have a lower threshold (though not absolute indication) to start IMT.

Finally, an understanding of the severity of a patient's disease and the potential for irreversible damage with any flare is critical, not simply in monocular patients but in all patients. Certain uveitic syndromes are highly vision-threatening and present strong indications for nearly immediate initiation of IMT (Box 3.3), almost simultaneous with high-dose corticosteroid therapy. Other cases are less clear-cut and highly specific to the individual patient. These can present a challenging and somewhat subjective assessment for the clinician. For instance, some patients with recurrent HLA-B27–associated anterior uveitis experience severe flares, albeit in one eye, causing profound inflammation and hypotony from which it can take many months to recover. Every flare is a

---

BOX 3.3 ■ Indications for Chronic Systemic IMT Based on Uveitic Syndrome

1. Behçet disease
2. Sympathetic ophthalmia
3. Serpiginous or ampiginous choroiditis
4. ANCA-positive scleritis or retinal vasculitides
5. Necrotizing scleritis

_____

ANCA, Antineutrophil cytoplasmic antibodies.

---

prolonged physical and psychological ordeal for these patients. Moreover, one worries about the potential for cyclitic membranes to develop with multiple severe flares, a condition that portends a poor prognosis. Thus even if the patient only flares once a year, for instance, IMT may be a reasonable management plan based on the history of extremely severe flares.

SYSTEMIC IMMUNOMODULATORY THERAPY: TYPES

Broadly speaking, there are four classes of IMT agents: antimetabolites, T-cell inhibitors, alkylating agents, and biologics. Each of these will be briefly reviewed to shed light on their strengths and weaknesses. An adverse effect common to all systemic IMT agents is that they increase susceptibility to infection, although to varying degrees, particularly with regard to certain pathogens. This will be detailed later. Another is increased incidence of cancer, particularly nonmelanoma skin cancer. Therefore all patients on any of these agents should avoid sunbathing and must not receive vaccinations using live organisms.

ANTIMETABOLITES

Methotrexate and mycophenolic acid are two of the mainstays of steroid-sparing IMT and are commonly used as first-line steroid-sparing agents. Azathioprine has also shown efficacy in uveitis, though it is now less commonly employed.

Methotrexate has been used for decades and is a familiar drug to uveitis specialists. It is the antimetabolite of choice in children, but is also readily used in adults. Although it is an antimetabolite, it has multiple different mechanisms of action, including inhibition of folate metabolism, which reduces T-cell proliferation and induces activated T-cell apoptosis; an increase in adenosine signaling, which has antiinflammatory effects; and changes to the cytokine profile of helper T cells. The contribution of each to the control of ocular inflammation remains unclear. The authors commonly start the drug at the very low dose of 5 mg PO every week (the subcutaneous route is also readily available) and add 2.5 mg per week (typically 2.5 mg in a tablet) to a minimum dose of 15 mg every week in the effort to improve gastrointestinal (GI) tolerability of the drug. Other initial dosing regimens are used by other specialists. In general, uveitis requires higher doses than rheumatologic diseases. Methotrexate is no exception, as the minimum efficacious dose in adults is 15 mg in contrast to rheumatoid arthritis, for instance, where 7.5 mg is a common dose. The maximum dose is 25 mg every week (Table 3.1). Folic acid supplementation (1–2 mg PO daily or folinic acid 5–7.5 mg PO every week) is essential. Adverse effects include hepatotoxicity, stomatitis, GI distress and ulcers, hair loss, cytopenias, and, less commonly, pneumonitis. Patients should not drink any alcohol while on the drug.

Mycophenolate mofetil (CellCept) or mycophenolate sodium (Myfortic) was originally approved for suppression of allograft rejection in organ transplant recipients. It is an inosine monophosphate inhibitor. This enzyme is critical in the purine salvage pathway, upon which leukocytes are heavily dependent but other cells are not. It also reduces expression of integrins on endothelial cells, thus reducing transmigration of inflammatory cells from the vasculature into target tissues, and inhibits nitric oxide. A common dose is 1000 mg PO BID, with a maximum dose of 1500 mg

TABLE 3.1 ■ Systemic Therapies

	Class	Mechanism of Action	Dosing
Methotrexate	Antimetabolite	Dihydrofolate reductase inhibitor	15–25 mg PO or SC every week
Mycophenolate mofetil	Antimetabolite	Inosine monophosphate dehydrogenase inhibitor	1000–1500 mg PO BID
Azathioprine	Antimetabolite	Purine synthesis inhibitor	1–3 mg/kg/day PO
Cyclosporine	T-cell inhibitor	Calcineurin inhibitor	2.5–5.0 mg/kg/day
Tacrolimus	T-cell inhibitor	Calcineurin inhibitor	Treat to therapeutic trough ≈5–12 ng, typically 0.03–0.1 mg/kg/day divided BID
Adalimumab	Biologic	TNF-α inhibitor	40 mg SC q2 weeks
Infliximab	Biologic	TNF-α inhibitor	5–10 mg/kg IV q4 weeks
Rituximab	Biologic	Anti-CD20	1000 mg IV × 2 (given 2 weeks apart), then q4–6 months; or 375 mg/m^2 IV × 1, repeated PRN
Tocilizumab	Biologic	IL-6 inhibitor	4–8 mg/kg IV q4 weeks
Cyclophosphamide	Alkylating agent	DNA alkylating and cross-linking	Treat to WBC 3000–4000, multiple regimens, including 1.5–3 mg/kg/day PO, 1 g/m^2 IV every month
Chlorambucil	Alkylating agent	DNA alkylating and cross linking	Treat to WBC 3000–4000, multiple regimens, including 0.1–0.2 mg/kg/day PO or short-term, high-dose therapy

BID, Twice a day; DNA, deoxyribonucleic acid; IL, interleukin; IV, intravenously; PO, by mouth; SC, subcutaneously; TNF, tumor necrosis factor; WBC, white blood cell.
*All agents associated with increased susceptibility to infection and increased risk of nonmelanoma skin cancers.

PO BID. Adverse effects include diarrhea, nausea, cytopenia, and hepatotoxicity, though to a lesser degree than methotrexate.

Azathioprine is a third antimetabolite that has historically been used for uveitis. Like mycophenolate, it is also an inhibitor of purine synthesis. With the advent of mycophenolate, its use has probably declined, but it can be particularly useful in patients with both uveitis and inflammatory bowel disease (IBD), for which it is still commonly used, starting at 50 to 100 mg daily.

Methotrexate and mycophenolate both have their advantages and disadvantages. Methotrexate has an excellent safety record in children, hence its use for pediatric uveitis, rheumatologic diseases, and cancers. The weekly dosing is convenient and simple for patients as well. On the other hand, patients cannot drink any alcohol while on the drug, and this is an issue for some. Hepatotoxicity is a legitimate concern, and even mild liver disease (e.g., nonalcoholic fatty liver disease) is a relative contraindication. Methotrexate takes at least 3 months to take effect; mycophenolate may be faster. Both have approximately the same efficacy. Although there was some feeling in the uveitis community that mycophenolate was perhaps slightly more efficacious than methotrexate, a recent clinical trial directly comparing the two found similar efficacy and onset of effect for the two (FAST Trial).

T-CELL INHIBITORS

Cyclosporine and tacrolimus are both calcineurin inhibitors that have been widely used for uveitis. Calcineurin forms a complex in the cytoplasm of T cells that enables the transcription factor nuclear factor of activated T cells (NFAT) to translocate to the nucleus. This cascade of events culminates in the expression of genes that activate T lymphocytes; thus inhibiting the translocation of NFAT family members into the nucleus inhibits T-cell activation. Other T-cell inhibitors, like sirolimus (formerly rapamycin), a mammalian target of rapamycin inhibitor (MToR), have been used both systemically and locally, but with less of a proven track record.

Cyclosporine is started at 2.5 mg/kg/day and can be increased to 5 mg/kg/day or even more in cases of low bioavailability. Cyclosporine, like tacrolimus, can have highly variable serum concentrations for any given dose. Tacrolimus is generally started at 0.03 mg/kg/day and titrated up to achieve a serum drug trough level of about 5 to 12 ng/μl.

They are generally thought to have lower efficacy than the antimetabolites and are thus second-line agents. They share many of the same adverse effects, which are numerous and at times very serious: electrolyte disturbances (hypomagnesemia, hyperkalemia), hypertension, hyperglycemia, nephrotoxicity, adrenal dysregulation, gingival hyperplasia, hirsutism, headache, malaise, and, in the case of tacrolimus, tremor. The many adverse effects seriously limit their utility, as even patients who clinically respond to the drug and have no serious laboratory abnormalities may strongly dislike the concomitant malaise, headache, or other ailments that greatly reduce quality of life.

With the emergence of biologics, the authors have generally moved away from employing these agents.

BIOLOGICS

Biologics are a class of immunomodulatory drugs that commonly take the form of monoclonal antibodies. At present, the single most important biologic target in uveitis is tumor necrosis factor-alpha (TNF-α). Anti−TNF-α therapy has revolutionized the treatment of multiple autoimmune diseases, including rheumatoid arthritis, JIA, psoriasis, inflammatory spondyloarthropathy, sarcoidosis, and IBD. It also has considerable efficacy in uveitis. Some uveitic entities are particularly sensitive to these drugs. Behçet disease, which is bilateral and can be highly aggressive and potentially blinding, shows sometimes exquisite sensitivity to the drug, to the point where it can be considered first-line IMT in this disease. Similarly, the drug has substantial effect against JIA-associated uveitis and its systemic manifestations.

There are multiple anti−TNF-α agents. Adalimumab (Humira) is a subcutaneously delivered, fully human monoclonal antibody that has been Food and Drug Administration (FDA)−approved for uveitis, thus making it more accessible to ophthalmologists and our patients without systemic manifestations of inflammatory disease. In fact, as of this writing, it is the only drug in existence with such approval. Initial therapy involves a loading dose of 80 mg subcutaneously, then 40 mg subcutaneously 1 week later, followed by maintenance therapy of 40 mg subcutaneously q2 weeks. There is some evidence that weekly therapy improves efficacy in refractory cases, but data are limited. Initial response and remission of chronic uveitis followed by recurrence while on the drug are sometimes due to the development of antiadalimumab antibodies (AAAs), and such a clinical scenario warrants checking for these. Once AAAs develop, there is unlikely to be continued efficacy with this agent.

Infliximab (Remicade) is an intravenously delivered anti−TNF-α monoclonal antibody. It is conveniently dosed only every 4 weeks, and retrospective data show that its efficacy is comparable to that of adalimumab. Etanercept, a soluble TNF-α receptor, is the oldest such agent but has no efficacy in uveitis. In fact, it may even provoke uveitis in some instances. Golimumab (Simponi) and certolizumab (Cimzia) are two other monoclonal antibodies against TNF-α whose efficacy in uveitis is still unclear, and thus the authors do not use them. Biosimilars of adalimumab and infliximab are now available but have not been well studied in uveitis.

There are three significant advantages to anti−TNF-α therapy. The first is its substantial (though certainly not universal) efficacy. The second is its relatively rapid clinical effect, about 1 month, compared with other IMT agents. The third is that, unlike conventional IMT, the common side effects are mild, sometimes even nonexistent. The variable stomach upset, anorexia, and malaise of other IMTs are infrequent or absent. But this comes at a cost: the risk of lymphoma and reactivation of latent infections is higher. Tuberculosis and latent viral infection, such as hepatitis B and C, are particular concerns. Demyelinating disease is an absolute contraindication, and these drugs should be used with caution in anyone with intermediate uveitis. A thorough neurologic review of systems is absolutely necessary, and any concern for white matter disease should prompt magnetic resonance imaging (MRI) before initiation. These drugs also weakly reduce cardiac inotropy, so a history of congestive heart failure is a relative contraindication.

Although there are many other biologics, two others bear mentioning in this brief survey. The first is rituximab (Rituxan), an anti-CD20 agent that reduces the number and effect of B lymphocytes. It is not used routinely for most uveitic entities, but it has shown particular efficacy in antineutrophil cytoplasmic antibodies (ANCA)−positive systemic and ocular disease. Although these diseases are rare, this development was important, as it allowed for reduced reliance on cyclophosphamide, a highly toxic drug (see later). Rituximab, like all IMTs, increases susceptibility to infection, but a particular concern is the JC virus, which causes progressive multifocal leukoencephalopathy. The second is tocilizumab (Actemra), a humanized monoclonal antibody against the interleukin-6 receptor (IL-6R). Its use in uveitis is still in its infancy, and thus data are limited. However, smaller studies, mostly retrospective data, have shown notable effect for uveitic macular edema, including in some refractory cases.

ALKYLATING AGENTS

Chlorambucil and cyclophosphamide are cytotoxic agents that kill rapidly dividing cells. Their mechanism of action involves the addition of alkyl groups to DNA, as well as cross-linking of DNA, thereby inhibiting mitosis and ultimately resulting in cell death. They can be highly toxic, have a plethora of adverse effects, and, most concerningly, are carcinogenic. Both drugs cause myelosuppression, and indeed they achieve their therapeutic effect when white blood cell (WBC) counts fall to between 3000 and 4000 cells/μl. Thus very close laboratory monitoring is absolutely required. WBC counts must generally be kept above 3000, neutrophils above 1500, and platelets above 75,000. Clinical outcomes using the drugs have been mixed, but cyclophosphamide was particularly important for treating ANCA-positive vasculitides before the advent of rituximab, and still has a role.

Interestingly, there is evidence that both cyclophosphamide and chlorambucil can induce long-term remission of uveitis. Dosing regimens are highly variable and involve titrating the drug to a therapeutic WBC count. A short-term, high-dose regimen for chlorambucil has been employed in an effort to reduce long-term exposure to the drug and cancer risk. This involves starting at 2 mg PO daily and increasing the dose by 2 mg every week until the desired WBC count and clinical effect are reached, then maintaining therapy for 3 months before discontinuing the drug. These drugs are seldom used, and thus comanagement with an experienced hematologist-oncologist or rheumatologist is highly recommended.

INITIATING AND ESCALATING THERAPY

Once the decision to initiate IMT has been made, an antimetabolite is the usual first-line option. The authors tend to use mycophenolate for adults and methotrexate for children, although the latter is a reasonable choice in adults as well. If a suboptimal response is seen with initial doses, then one titrates up to the maximum dose. Because patients starting IMT have typically failed prednisone or are only adequately controlled on an excessively high dose of prednisone ($\geq$10 mg daily), a patient in such a situation may be on prednisone 10 mg daily and methotrexate 25 mg PO every week.

If inflammation is still inadequately controlled at the maximum dose of antimetabolite, several options are available. Of course, one can, and should, temporarily increase the prednisone dose and/ or treat locally (see local treatment options later), but these are only temporizing measures. Classically, the next step is to add a T-cell inhibitor to the antimetabolite and low-dose prednisone because these two classes of agents affect different proinflammatory pathways. Adding a second antimetabolite is highly atypical, and the authors discourage this. A second option is to switch one antimetabolite for a second, as sometimes patients who do not respond to mycophenolate will respond to methotrexate and vice versa. This suffers from the disadvantage of again having to wait 3+ months before efficacy is known. A third option, preferred by the authors, is to add a TNF-α inhibitor as the next step (Fig. 3.1). These agents have established efficacy and can take effect in as little as 1 month.

DE-ESCALATING THERAPY

All of these agents carry significant risks, and patients who are well controlled deserve a trial off all therapy. Typically, one should wait for at least 2 years of quiescence on IMT and off systemic corticosteroids before discontinuing all therapy. Before this time, the patient should have been slowly tapered off prednisone and IMT continued or even escalated to allow for a complete taper off prednisone. Patients who continue to require prednisone in addition to IMT to maintain quiescence are not good candidates for discontinuing therapy.

Local Injectable Therapies

PERIOCULAR CORTICOSTEROIDS

For a time the only local means of delivering corticosteroid to the posterior segment was via periocular injections. Its main indications are inflammation involving the posterior segment and uveitic macular

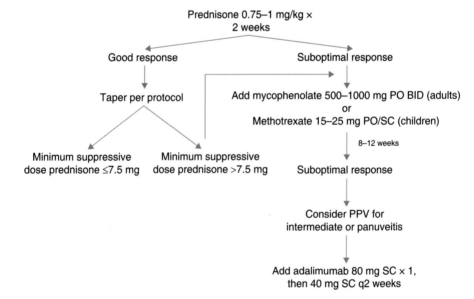

Fig. 3.1 Management algorithm for escalating immunomodulatory therapy.

edema. The drug can either be administered via an orbital floor route through the lower eyelid (trans-septal) or via a transconjunctival route inferotemporally or superotemporally. Triamcinolone (Kenalog) 40 mg/1 cc or methylprednisolone (Depo-Medrol) 40 mg are common formulations. The authors prefer Kenalog, as it is readily accessible and is nontoxic if there is inadvertent injection into the eye. Duration of effect is 1 to 3 months, but the authors do not recommend using it more frequently than every 2 to 3 months due to concern for ocular hypertension with highly frequent use. Although IOP elevations are lower than with intravitreal corticosteroids, so, too, is efficacy—a common theme. There is a small risk of globe perforation with the procedure, but this is rare in skilled hands.

INTRAVITREAL CORTICOSTEROIDS

Corticosteroids can be delivered into the vitreous either as a bolus injection in the form of triamcin-olone or as implantable devices, which include the dexamethasone implant (Ozurdex), the injectable fluocinolone acetonide implant (Yutiq), and the surgically implanted fluocinolone aceto-nide device (Retisert). Much like periocular therapy, these can be used for treatment of uveitic mac-ular edema, for control of inflammation involving the posterior segment, or for both.

Intravitreal triamcinolone (IVT) is injected as a single bolus of 2 mg/0.05 cc to 4 mg/0.1 cc (Table 3.2). Patients need to be alerted to the fact that their vision will instantly be clouded by large floaters, as the drug is insoluble, and these will clear rapidly within a few days. Once injected, drug levels in the vitreous decay with approximately first-order kinetics. Duration of effect is variable but is in the range of 1 to 3 months, less so in vitrectomized eyes. In addition to the usual risks of any intravitreal injection, numerous reports of sterile inflammatory reactions to IVT have been reported, which appear to be more common with the preserved form (Kenalog) than with the preservative-free form (Triesence).

An alternative to triamcinolone is the dexamethasone 0.7 mg injectable device. The implant floats in the vitreous, is biodegradable, and elutes the drug with approximately zero-order kinetics after an initial burst. Although intended to last 6 months, its duration of action may be considerably less than that. In a comparative effectiveness trial of periocular triamcinolone 40 mg, IVT 4 mg, and the dexamethasone implant for uveitic macular edema, IVT and the dexamethasone implant were equally effective and appeared to last about 8 weeks. If the implant migrates into the anterior

TABLE 3.2 ■ Local Therapies

	Dose	Frequency of Use	Kinetics	Setting of Use	Rate of Incisional Glaucoma Surgery at 3 Years
Periocular triamcinolone	40 mg	2–3 months	Bolus	Clinic	-
Intravitreal triamcinolone	2–4 mg	2–3 months	Bolus	Clinic	-
Dexamethasone intravitreal implant (Ozurdex)	0.7 mg	2–3 months	Zero-order	Clinic	-
Fluocinolone injectable implant (Yutiq)	0.18 mg	3 years	Zero-order	Clinic	6%
Fluocinolone surgical implant (Retisert)	0.59 mg	3 years	Zero-order	Operating room	40%

chamber, it will rapidly cause corneal decompensation. Wound leak is a rare but possible complication as well, with vitrectomized patients being at higher risk. In theory, its zero-order kinetics should mean that its duration of effect is less affected by vitrectomy and that its IOP profile is better than IVT. In the POINT Trial, the only trial directly comparing the two for uveitis, increase in IOP was no different between the two.

A second injectable implant that can be delivered in the clinic is the fluocinolone acetonide 0.18 mg device (Yutiq), which is about one-third the dose of the surgically implanted fluocinolone acetonide device (Retisert). It elutes a steady dose of drug for 3 years, which is its main advantage. Its IOP profile is somewhat favorable, with only 6% of treated patients requiring surgical glaucoma therapy in the two phase III trials performed thus far. Its drawbacks are similar to that of the dexamethasone implant, namely the rare potential for wound leak and for anterior chamber migration.

Retisert is surgically implanted in the operating room, releases an initial burst of fluocinolone, and then steadily elutes drug at more than three times the dose of the injectable implant. This higher dose provides superior inflammatory control but at the cost of much more aggressive glaucoma: about 30% of patients at 2 years required incisional glaucoma surgery and almost 40% at 3 years in the MUST Trial. Its implantation in the operating room is both a disadvantage and an advantage. Because the implant is sutured to the sclera, it remains fixed and cannot migrate into the anterior chamber, thus making it suitable for people with aphakia and with pseudophakia with zonular loss or ruptured posterior capsules (e.g., sulcus intraocular lenses [IOLs], anterior chamber intraocular lens [ACIOLs], sutured IOLs).

OTHER INJECTABLE THERAPIES

Intravitreal methotrexate 400 µg/0.1 cc is an old drug that is safe in the eye and has been used for decades to treat primary vitreoretinal lymphoma. Retrospective data have been promising that it provides good control of inflammation involving the posterior segment. Its main drawback is keratopathy. Intravitreal sirolimus 440 µg/0.02 cc and suprachoroidal triamcinolone 4 mg/0.1 cc are other local therapies that, as of this writing, are under investigation and are not commercially available.

TOPICAL THERAPY

Topical therapies are the single most common route of corticosteroid administration for the eye. They are generally effective for treating anterior chamber inflammation in all but the most severe cases. For anterior uveitis, moderate-strength corticosteroids such as prednisolone acetate 1% (Pred Forte) or dexamethasone sodium phosphate 0.1% QID to q1h are appropriate for acute flares and

TABLE 3.3 ■ Topical Therapies

	Potency	Cost	Risk of IOP Increase
Difluprednate 0.05% (Durezol)	High	High	High
Prednisolone acetate 1% (Pred Forte)	Medium	Low	Moderate
Dexamethasone sodium phosphate 0.1%	Medium	Low	Moderate
Prednisolone acetate 0.1% (Pred Mild)	Low	Variable	Low
Fluorometholone 0.1%	Low	Variable	Low
Rimexolone 1% (Vexol)	Low	High	Low

IOP, Intraocular pressure.

then can be tapered slowly (Table 3.3). The strongest topical therapy available is difluprednate 0.05% (Durezol). It has approximately double the potency of prednisolone acetate 1% but similarly carries a greater risk of increased IOP, particularly in children, to such an extent that the authors avoid its use in the pediatric population. It is also very expensive to the point of being unaffordable to some patients. Although high-quality data are lacking, it furthermore appears to have better efficacy for uveitic macular edema than the weaker topical corticosteroids.

Milder topical corticosteroids, such as prednisolone acetate 0.1% (Pred Mild), fluorometholone 0.1%, and rimexolone 1% (Vexol), are generally too weak to be of benefit in uveitis. However, there are some exceptions to this general rule. For instance, low doses of rimexolone may be effective in chronically suppressing the herpetic iritis that can follow some cases of herpetic keratitis. Rimexolone causes little corticosteroid response, which makes it a superior choice to stronger topical corticosteroids to avoid adverse side effects, provided it sufficiently suppresses inflammation. Topical nonsteroidal antiinflammatory drops have little to no role in treating uveitis or uveitic macular edema.

THERAPEUTIC SURGERY FOR UVEITIS

Clearly, surgery can have a critical role in diagnosing challenging cases and treating uveitic complications like cataract and glaucoma. However, surgery to control intraocular inflammation itself is another matter. In anterior uveitis, surgery has no such role. In stark contrast, in idiopathic intermediate uveitis (pars planitis), vitrectomy with cryoablation or photocoagulation of the peripheral retina can be highly effective, even curative, in some cases. This is reserved for cases that do not respond to local therapy, do respond but require frequent local therapy, or do not respond to local and initial systemic therapy and thus require significant escalation of IMT.

Surgery as therapy for noninfectious panuveitis has had more mixed results. This diagnosis is a different entity from pars planitis, and, quite frankly, noninfectious panuveitis is a highly heterogeneous disease, replete with a wide range of severities and systemic associations. There are retrospective studies showing that vitrectomy reduces inflammation and allows for dose reduction of systemic medications or frequency of local treatments. Vitrectomy causes the vitreous cavity to be filled with aqueous humor, which bathes the posterior segment in its immunosuppressive factors, such as calcitonin gene-related peptide, vasointestinal protein, TGF-β2, melanocyte-stimulating hormone, and soluble fas ligand, among others. This is one mechanism by which vitrectomy has an immunomodulatory effect. Another is the removal of proinflammatory factors sequestered within the vitreous, although this effect can be temporary. Regardless of the biologic mechanisms, these studies suffer from the same drawbacks as other retrospective, uncontrolled studies. Because modern, small-gauge vitrectomy is fairly safe, pars plana vitrectomy is a reasonable therapeutic option in unilateral panuveitis requiring escalation of IMT. Ideally, the eye would be at least temporarily quieted with high-dose local or systemic corticosteroids in the preoperative period, as operating on inflamed eyes, although sometimes necessary for diagnostic and/or therapeutic purposes, carries the risk of provoking severe flares.

CHAPTER 4

First Episode of Acute Iritis

Harpal S. Sandhu

History of Present Illness (HPI)

A 32-year-old man with no past ocular or medical history complains of 3 days of light sensitivity and redness in his left eye. He woke up with the symptoms and thought that maybe he had gotten something into his eye while sleeping. The symptoms have not improved and, he reports, have probably gotten worse.

Exam

	OD	OS
Vision	20/20	20/25 −
IOP	14	9
Lids and lashes:	Normal	Normal
Sclera/conjunctiva:	White and quiet	See Fig. 4.1
Cornea:	Clear	Clear
Anterior chamber (AC):	Deep and quiet	3+ cells, 2+ flare
Iris:	Flat	Flat
Lens:	Clear	Clear
Anterior vitreous:	Clear	Clear

Dilated Fundus Examination (DFE)

Nerve:	Cup-to-disc (c/d) 0.3, pink, sharp	c/d 0.3, pink, sharp
Macula:	Good foveal reflex	Good foveal reflex
Vessels:	Normal caliber and course	Normal caliber and course
Periphery:	Unremarkable	Unremarkable

Further Questions to Ask

- Have you had any trauma to the left eye (OS) or the fellow eye?
- Any recent illnesses or hospitalizations?
- Have you used any new medications recently?
- Have you gone camping or had any tick bites recently?

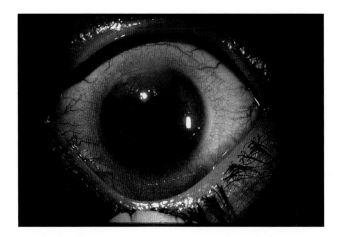

Fig. 4.1 Color external photograph of the left eye shows severe ciliary flush.

- Perform a review of systems with particular focus on joints, skin, lungs, and the gastrointestinal tract.

The patient answers no to all questions.

Assessment

- Acute anterior uveitis, OS

Differential Diagnosis

- Idiopathic noninfectious anterior uveitis
- HLA-B27-associated anterior uveitis
- Sarcoidosis
- Syphilis
- Less likely: Lyme disease, tuberculosis

Working Diagnosis

- Idiopathic noninfectious anterior uveitis OS

Management

- Prednisolone acetate 1% every 2 hours (q2h) OS
- Cyclopentolate 1% three times a day (TID) OS
- Follow up in 1 week

Follow-up

HPI

The patient returns the following week. He says all his symptoms have improved, although he has had difficulty seeing up close ever since he started "the dilating drop."

Exam

	OD	OS
Vision	20/20	20/20
IOP	16	12
Lids and lashes:		Normal
Sclera/conjunctiva:		White and quiet
Cornea:		Clear
AC:		Trace cells, 1+ flare
Iris:		Flat
Lens:		Clear
Anterior vitreous:		Clear
DFE		Unchanged

Management

- Stop cycloplegia
- Taper topical corticosteroid to four times a day (QID) OS × 1 week, then TID OS × 1 week, then twice a day (BID) OS × 1 week, then daily OS × 1 week
- Follow up in 4 weeks

Key Points

- Unilateral first episodes of isolated, nongranulomatous anterior uveitis do not necessitate a laboratory evaluation for the underlying cause.
- This presentation typically responds well to intensive topical therapy with cycloplegia to prevent synechiae.
- Bilateral involvement, granulomatous features (e.g., "mutton-fat keratic precipitates (KP)"), and repeat episodes are generally indications for initiating a systemic evaluation.
- Intraocular pressure (IOP) can be high, low, or normal in acute anterior uveitis. Low is not uncommon and implies a cyclitis in addition to iritis. Viral causes of anterior uveitis classically cause ocular hypertension due to trabeculitis, although this can also be seen in noninfectious anterior uveitis on occasion.
- Flare alone is not an indication for treatment. Anterior chamber cells are a much superior indicator of inflammatory activity.

CHAPTER 5

Keratouveitis Secondary to Retained Lens Fragments

Harpal S. Sandhu

History of Present Illness (HPI)

A 67-year-old man presents 3 months after uncomplicated cataract extraction/intraocular lens implant (CE/IOL) right eye (OD) complaining of decreased vision and mild photophobia in the right eye. It has been progressive over the last 5 days. On postoperative day 1 after cataract surgery, he was 20/25− with 1+ white cells in the anterior chamber (AC) and trace corneal stromal edema, improving to 20/20 and a normal exam by week 1.

Exam

	OD	OS
Vision	20/60	20/20
Intraocular pressure (IOP)	25	15
Lids and lashes:	Normal	Normal
Sclera/conjunctiva:	White and quiet	White and quiet
Cornea:	See Fig. 5.1	Clear
AC:	2+ white cell	Deep and quiet
Iris:	Flat	Flat
Lens:	Posterior chamber intraocular lens (PCIOL)	PCIOL
Anterior vitreous:	2+ anterior vitreous cells	Clear

Dilated Fundus Examination (DFE)

Nerve:	Cup-to-disc (c/d) 0.4	c/d 0.4
Macula:	Flat, no edema	Unremarkable
Vessels:	Normal caliber and course	Normal caliber and course
Periphery:	Unremarkable	Unremarkable

Further Questions to Ask

- Do you have any history of cold sores or genital ulcers?

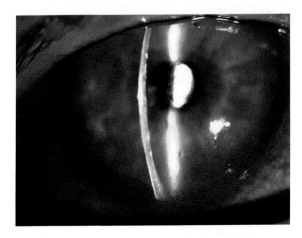

Fig. 5.1 Color slit lamp photograph of the right eye shows mild corneal stromal edema centrally and inferiorly. (From Pandit RT, Coburn AG. Sudden corneal edema due to retained lens nuclear fragment presenting 8.5 years after cataract surgery. *J Cataract Refract Surg.* 2011;37[6]:1165–1167.)

- Have you ever had zoster on your face or head?

He answers no to all questions.

Assessment

Unilateral keratouveitis with ocular hypertension OD after cataract surgery

Differential Diagnosis

- Herpetic keratouveitis
- Retained lens fragment

Testing

- The patient needs gonioscopy (See Fig. 5.2) and a scleral depressed examination to rule out retained lens fragments.

Diagnosis

- Retained lens fragment in the AC OD

Management

- Start pilocarpine 1% four times a day (QID) OD and prednisolone acetate 1% QID
- Urgent anterior segment surgery to remove the lens fragment

Follow-up

HPI: Surgery was uneventful, and postoperative day 1 showed some persistent edema and iritis, as expected. Prednisolone acetate 1% QID and moxifloxacin QID OD were prescribed. The patient follows up 1 week postoperatively and reports his vision is much improved.

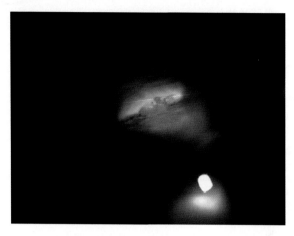

Fig. 5.2 Gonioscopic color photograph of the inferior angle of the right eye. There is a small, white lens fragment in the inferior angle. (From Pandit RT, Coburn AG. Sudden corneal edema due to retained lens nuclear fragment presenting 8.5 years after cataract surgery. *J Cataract Refract Surg.* 2011;37[6]:1165–1167.)

Exam

	OD
Vision	20/20
IOP	21
Lids and lashes:	Normal
Sclera/conjunctiva:	White and quiet
Cornea:	Clear
AC:	Deep and quiet
Iris:	Flat
Lens:	PCIOL

Key Points

- Corneal edema and iritis that occur after resolution of initial postoperative inflammation is unusual and mandates a high level of suspicion for retained lens fragments
- Most of these cases present within the first 1 or 2 months after surgery. Delayed presentations of many months and even years have been described but are quite rare.
- Small fragments can remain hidden in the vitreous base and only become symptomatic when they migrate into the anterior chamber, causing corneal edema, iritis, and ocular hypertension.
- Classically, the corneal edema is configured in a sectoral "wedge shape" but can also be predominantly central in location.
- The presence of a lens fragment in the anterior chamber is a time-sensitive situation that requires prompt surgical evacuation due to the risk of corneal decompensation. After diagnosis, it is advisable to begin topical miotic therapy, like pilocarpine. Constriction of the pupil sequesters the fragment in the anterior chamber, allowing for easy removal through a clear corneal wound.
- Herpetic disease can present in an almost identical fashion with endotheliitis causing corneal edema, iritis, and ocular hypertension. A thorough scleral depressed examination of the fundus and gonioscopic examination of the angle can distinguish the two.

CHAPTER 6

Cytomegalovirus (CMV) Anterior Uveitis

Harpal S. Sandhu

History of Present Illness (HPI)

A 58-year-old man with no significant past medical history presents for follow-up of anterior uveitis in the left eye (OS). He has been seen multiple times by outside ophthalmologists and has been on topical steroids for 2 months. He reports he has never been able to get off the steroids completely. He has had testing for an underlying cause of uveitis, all of which have been negative, including human immunodeficiency virus (HIV), syphilis, purified protein derivative (PPD), Lyme serologies, HLA-B27, angiotensin-converting enzyme (ACE), lysozyme, and a chest computed tomography (CT) scan to assess for pulmonary sarcoidosis. He notes some blurred vision OS, which has waxed and waned since the onset of the uveitis but has never been normal.

Ocular medications:
- Prednisolone acetate 1% three times a day (TID) OS
- Timolol twice a day (BID) OS

Exam

	OD	OS
Vision	20/20	20/25 −
IOP	14	24
Lids and lashes:	Normal	Normal
Sclera/conjunctiva:	White and quiet	Trace injection
Cornea:	Clear	Clear, a few fine keratic precipitates (KP)
Anterior chamber (AC):	Deep and quiet	1+ cells
Iris:	Flat	See Fig. 6.1
Lens:	Clear	Clear
Anterior vitreous:	Clear	Clear

Dilated Fundus Examination (DFE)

Nerve:	Normal, cup-to-disc (c/d) 0.4	Normal, c/d 0.5
Macula:	Good foveal reflex	Good foveal reflex
Vessels:	Normal caliber and course	Normal caliber and course
Periphery:	Unremarkable	Unremarkable

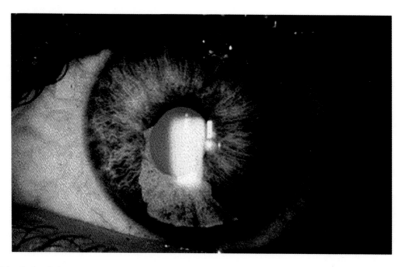

Fig. 6.1   Color slit lamp photograph of the left eye shows sectoral atrophy of the inferior iris. (From Van der Lelij A, Ooijman FM, Kiljstra A, Rothova A. Anterior uveitis with sectoral iris atrophy in the absence of keratitis: A distinct clinical entity among herpetic eye diseases. *Ophthalmology.* 2000;107[6]:1164−1170.)

Further Questions to Ask

- Have you ever had trauma to the eye? Have you ever had a hyphema/bleeding inside the eye?
- Have you ever had shingles on your face or head?

He answers no to all questions.

Assessment

Chronic hypertensive anterior uveitis OS

Differential Diagnosis

- Herpes simplex virus (HSV) 1/2−associated anterior uveitis
- Varicella zoster virus (VZV)−associated anterior uveitis
- Cytomegalovirus (CMV)−associated anterior uveitis
- Rubella-associated anterior uveitis
- Idiopathic
- Fuchs heterochromic iridocyclitis
- Less likely: Posner−Schlossman

Working Diagnosis

- Herpesviridae-associated anterior uveitis
- Hypertensive iritis with sectoral iris atrophy is highly suggestive of a herpetic etiology. The hypertensive uveitis syndrome Posner−Schlossman is generally episodic, and Fuchs is a diagnosis of exclusion. Polymerase chain reaction (PCR) of the aqueous humor would confirm the diagnosis.

Testing

- Anterior chamber tap for PCR

Management

- Acyclovir 400 mg by mouth (PO) five times a day while awaiting PCR results
- Continue prednisolone acetate 1% TID OS and timolol BID OS
- Follow up in 1 week

Follow-up

The patient returns 1 week later. There have been no changes in his symptoms. PCR was positive for CMV. The patient was switched to valganciclovir 900 mg PO BID. Six weeks later, the patient's vision improves to 20/20 OS, intraocular pressure (IOP) is 20, and the anterior chamber is quiet off all topical therapy.

Key Points

- CMV is an underappreciated cause of hypertensive anterior uveitis in immunocompetent patients.
- Sectoral iris atrophy, ocular hypertension, and inability to wean off topical steroids are all suggestive of Herpesviridae, and PCR allows further differentiation between HSV, VZV, CMV, and rubella. This is important for management, as acyclovir and valacyclovir are generally ineffective against CMV.
- Alternatives to systemic valganciclovir include topical ganciclovir 0.15% ophthalmic ointment four to six times a day to the affected eye.
- Similar to cases of HSV and VZV, lower doses of these drugs can be used for chronic prophylaxis if necessary.
- Rubella is another cause of hypertensive anterior uveitis and is thought to be the etiology of some cases of Fuchs heterochromic iridocyclitis.

CHAPTER 7

Chronic Anterior Uveitis

Harpal S. Sandhu

History of Present Illness (HPI)

A 46-year-old woman with a history of anterior uveitis in the left eye (OS) associated with HLA-B27 presents to you from an outside ophthalmologist for a second opinion. She had her first episode of iritis 7 years ago. She responded well to drops and did not recur for almost a year. In the last 1 to 2 years, her flares have become more frequent and difficult to control. She is currently being treated for her third flare this year and has grown tired of the recurrences and frequent trips to the ophthalmologist's office. She has had extensive testing for an underlying cause and only HLA-B27 was positive.

She is 3 weeks into this current flare. Her symptoms have subsided, and she has just started tapering her drops as per the usual routine.

Ocular medications:

- Prednisolone acetate 1% three times a day (TID) OS

Exam

	OD	OS
Vision	20/20	20/20
IOP	14	21
Lids and lashes:	Normal	Normal
Sclera/conjunctiva:	White and quiet	White and quiet
Cornea:	Clear	Clear
Anterior chamber (AC):	Deep and quiet	Trace cells, 1+ flare
Iris:	Flat	Flat
Lens:	Clear	Trace posterior subcapsular cataract (PSC), off contor
Anterior vitreous:	Clear	1+ cells

Dilated Fundus Examination (DFE)

Nerve:	Cup-to-disc (c/d) 0.3, pink, sharp	c/d 0.3, pink, sharp
Macula:	Good foveal reflex	Good foveal reflex
Vessels:	Normal caliber and course	Normal caliber and course
Periphery:	Unremarkable	Unremarkable

Questions to Ask

- Do you have any other manifestations of HLA-B27-associated disease, like low back pain?
- What is the longest period you have gone without drops in the last year?
- Have you ever had high eye pressure from using steroid drops?

The patient denies any low back pain or other joint problems. She has not gone any longer than 5 weeks without topical therapy this year. She recalls once having eye pressures in the 20s when she was using the corticosteroid drop every hour for a while, but it came down once she was using the drop less frequently.

Assessment

- Chronic HLA-B27-associated anterior uveitis OS
- By definition (Standardization of Uveitis Nomenclature), any uveitis that consistently recurs within 3 months of discontinuing therapy is defined as chronic disease

Management

- Extend the length of time over which the topical steroids are tapered (i.e., reduce by one drop per day every 2 weeks)
- Hold at prednisolone acetate 1% daily OS indefinitely

Follow-up

HPI

You have seen the patient once since the initial consultation. She follows up over 3 months later. She is pleased that her symptoms have been well controlled since then.

Exam

	OD	OS
Vision	20/20	20/20
IOP	14	17
Lids and lashes:	Normal	Normal
Sclera/conjunctiva:	White and quiet	White and quiet
Cornea:	Clear	Clear
AC:	Deep and quiet	Deep and quiet
Iris:	Flat	Flat
Lens:	Clear	Trace PSC, off center
Anterior vitreous:	Clear	1+ cells

Management

- Continue chronic prednisolone acetate 1% daily OS
- Consider tapering to every other day (QOD) OS at next visit
- Follow up in 3 months

Key Points

- Chronic disease calls for chronic therapy. In the case of anterior uveitis, this can take the form of chronic topical corticosteroids.
- It can be helpful in these cases to take an extensive history, where one attempts to ascertain what doses of topical corticosteroid have provided sufficient suppression of inflammation in the past. This allows the clinician to determine a "minimum suppressive dose" for the individual patient. If the history is inconclusive, then clinical experience with the patient is the only means of determining the minimum suppressive dose.
- The author is comfortable treating patients with one to two drops per day of topical corticosteroid in those whose intraocular pressure (IOP) responds only minimally to such doses.
- Patients who require significantly more topical corticosteroid than that should be considered for chronic systemic therapy in the form of low-dose prednisone or systemic immunomodulatory therapy.
- Patients must of course be made aware of the risks of chronic topical corticosteroid use, namely increased IOP, acceleration of cataract development, and increased susceptibility to ocular surface infections. Patients should not regularly wear contact lenses if they are on chronic topical corticosteroids.

CHAPTER 8

Hypopyon Uveitis

Harpal S. Sandhu

History of Present Illness (HPI)

A 52-year-old woman with no past ocular history is referred to you for anterior uveitis in the left eye (OS). She presented to an outside ophthalmologist 1 week ago with decreased vision and photophobia. Outside records note 4+ white cells in the anterior chamber. She was started on difluprednate six times a day OS and cyclopentolate three times a day (TID) OS. Follow-up 5 days later noted still "3 to 4+ cells" OS. Difluprednate was increased to once every hour (q1h). She was seen the following day and still had not significantly improved, and was sent to you the following day.

The patient complains of profound vision loss and light sensitivity. She claims she had normal vision before this episode.

Past Medical History (PMH)

Coronary artery disease status post (s/p) stent

Exam

	OD	OS
Vision	20/20	Count fingers (CF) 3′
IOP	20	8
Lids and lashes:	Normal	Normal
Sclera/conjunctiva:	White and quiet	2+ injection
Cornea:	Clear	Clear
AC:	Deep and quiet	See Fig. 8.1
Iris:	Flat	Poor view, flat
Lens:	Clear	Poor view

Dilated Fundus Examination (DFE)

Nerve:	Cup-to-disc (c/d) 0.3, pink, sharp	No view
Macula:	Good foveal reflex	
Vessels:	Normal caliber and course	
Periphery:	Unremarkable	

Further Questions to Ask

- Have you had any trauma to this eye or the fellow eye?
- Have you ever had surgery on this eye or the other eye?
- Have you been sick recently? Any recent hospitalizations, fevers, chills, or infections?
- Do you use injection drugs?
- Have you had any other new symptoms in the rest of your body, like new rashes, joint pains, tick bites, oral or genital ulcers, or bloody stools?

She responds that she cannot recall ever having any trauma to either eye, and she has definitely never had surgery on either eye. She denied any recent infections or hospitalizations. She does note that she has had a rash on both lower extremities for over a month, which her cardiologist told her was "low-grade cellulitis." She has a few aches and pains but nothing that she considers out of the ordinary and nothing that has changed of late. She denies injection drug use (Figs. 8.1 and 8.2).

B scan OS: retina attached, no significant vitreous opacities

Assessment

- Explosive anterior chamber inflammation OS resistant to topical corticosteroids

Differential Diagnosis

- Noninfectious anterior uveitis, specifically:
  - HLA-B27-associated anterior uveitis
  - Behçet's disease
- Endogenous endophthalmitis
- Less likely: syphilis, sarcoidosis

Working Diagnosis

- Noninfectious anterior uveitis associated with psoriasis, with or without psoriatic arthritis

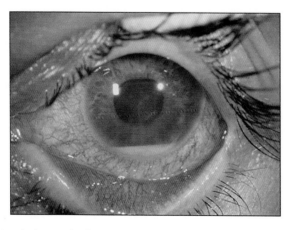

Fig. 8.1 Color external photograph of the left eye shows significant ciliary flush, conjunctival injection, significant flare, and a 1-mm hypopyon. (From Forrester J, Dick A, McMenamin P, et al. *The Eye*. 4th ed. Saunders; Philadelphia, PA 2015: p. 14, Figure 1−10.)

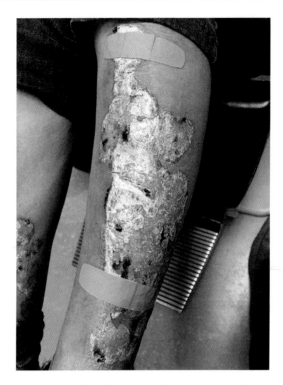

Fig. 8.2 Color external photograph of the left lower extremity shows a large, silver-gray, scaly plaque on the extensor surface. She has similar lesions on the right lower extremity (not centered).

Testing

- The presence of a hypopyon should always alert one to the distinct possibility of infectious endophthalmitis, particularly one that has not responded to topical steroids. In this case, because there were no routes of exogenous entry, only endogenous endophthalmitis is possible. Assuming one can trust the patient's responses, she has no risk factors for endogenous endophthalmitis either. This leaves noninfectious uveitis as the diagnosis by default. However, given the resistance to intensive topical steroids and the fact that some patients are not always entirely truthful about risks factors for endogenous endophthalmitis (intravenous [IV] drug use, for instance), an anterior chamber paracentesis for bacterial polymerase chain reaction (PCR) and Gram stain is advisable. The patient should be seen the next day to ensure stability.
- Check HLA-B27, fluorescent treponemal antibody absorption (FTA-ABS), rapid plasma reagin (RPR), angiotensin-converting enzyme (ACE), lysozyme, chest x-ray

Management

- Close observation. Continue present management, await results of testing, and see back in 1 day.

Follow-up

HPI

The patient returns the following day. Her complaints are the same. PCR was negative, and Gram stain was negative for organisms.

Exam

	OD	OS
Vision	20/20	CF 3′
IOP	21	8
Lids and lashes:	Normal	Normal
Sclera/conjunctiva:	White and quiet	White and quiet
Cornea:	Clear	Clear
AC:	Deep and quiet	1-mm hypopyon
		4+ white cells
		3+ flare
Iris:	Flat	Flat
Lens:	Clear	Poor view

Working Diagnosis

- Noninfectious anterior uveitis OS associated with psoriasis

Management

- Add prednisone 60 mg by mouth (PO) daily.
- Follow-up in 1 week.

Further Follow-up

HPI

The patient returns 1 week later. She notes that her vision is still very blurry but starting to improve and that her light sensitivity has resolved. HLA-B27 returned positive.

Exam

	OD	OS
Vision	20/20	20/200
IOP	20	12
Lids and lashes:	Normal	Normal
Sclera/conjunctiva:	White and quiet	White and quiet
Cornea:	Clear	Clear
AC:	Deep and quiet	1/2+ white cells
		3+ flare
Iris:	Flat	Flat
Lens:	Clear	Better view, trace PSC

Diagnosis

- Same: Severe anterior uveitis associated with HLA-B27 and psoriasis

Management

- Taper prednisone by 10 mg a week
- Taper topical difluprednate
- Follow-up in 3 to 4 weeks

Extended Follow-up

The patient was eventually tapered to prednisone 5 mg and off topical drops over the course of 2 to 3 months. Vision returned to 20/30, limited by early posterior subcapsular cataract (PSC) cataract.

Key Points

- HLA-B27 is the most common cause of noninfectious hypopyon uveitis in the developed world. Behçet's disease is a distant second cause.
- As noted earlier, suspicion should be high for infectious endophthalmitis and only allayed by a lack of risk factors for infection, other supporting evidence of systemic autoimmune disease associated with uveitis, and/or negative testing of intraocular samples, as seen in this case. If risk factors for endogenous endophthalmitis are present (none was present in this case), then a tap of the anterior chamber (AC) or vitreous followed by injection of broad-spectrum antimicrobials is indicated.
- Once one is confident that the uveitis is noninfectious in origin, escalating therapy is indicated. Although most cases of anterior uveitis can be quieted with topical therapy, a minority of cases will require systemic corticosteroids for acute flares, and a subset of those will require steroid-sparing immunomodulatory therapy for chronic suppression.
- Psoriasis is weakly associated with uveitis, whereas psoriatic uveitis that is HLA-B27 positive is much more strongly associated with it.
- In cases associated with systemic disease that evolves into chronic uveitis, multispecialty collaboration is critical to determine the appropriate steroid-sparing immunomodulatory agent. An appropriate agent in this case would have efficacy for both uveitis and psoriasis. Methotrexate and anti–tumor necrosis factor-α (TNF-α) agents would both be appropriate. The efficacy of anti-interleukin (IL)-12/23 agents (e.g., ustekinumab, tildrakizumab), which treat the cutaneous manifestations of psoriasis well, is still being defined for uveitis.

CHAPTER 9

Herpetic Keratitis and Iritis

Harpal S. Sandhu ◼ Danielle Trief

History of Present Illness (HPI)

A 39-year-old man with no significant past medical history complains of 2 days of tearing, light sensitivity, and blurry vision in his left eye (OS). It started first with some foreign body sensation and has progressed since then. His other eye is fine. He denies getting anything in the eye or being hit in the eye and denies contact lens use.

Exam

	OD	OS
Vision	20/20	20/40+
IOP	12	25
Lids and lashes:	Normal	Normal
Sclera/conjunctiva:	White and quiet	Trace injection
Cornea:	Clear	See Fig. 9.1
AC:	Deep and quiet	1+ white cell
Iris:	Flat	Flat
Lens:	Clear	Clear
Anterior vitreous:	Clear	Clear

Dilated Fundus Examination (DFE)

Nerve:	Normal, cup-to-disc (c/d) 0.3	Normal, c/d 0.3
Macula:	Good foveal reflex	Good foveal reflex
Vessels:	Normal caliber and course	Normal caliber and course
Periphery:	Unremarkable	Unremarkable

Questions to Ask

- Do you have any history of cold sores?
- Have you had previous episodes like this one?
- Do you have any vesicular rashes on your head or elsewhere on your body?

He responds that he has had cold sores from time to time. He has no rashes. He has never had an episode like this.

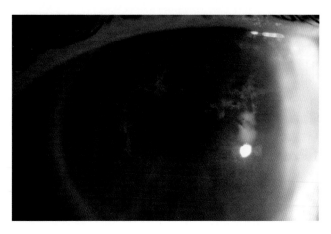

Fig. 9.1 Color slit lamp photograph of the left eye under normal illumination shows a particularly long dendriform lesion on the corneal epithelium nasal and superior to the visual axis. A few stellate keratic precipitates (KPs) were noted, which are less well visualized in this image.

Assessment

- Herpetic epithelial keratitis with iritis OS
- Ocular hypertension OS secondary to herpes

Differential Diagnosis

- Herpes simplex virus (HSV) 1 (more likely) or 2
- Varicella zoster virus (VZV)

Working Diagnosis

- HSV 1/2

Testing

- None

Management

- Acyclovir 400 mg by mouth (PO) five times a day or valacyclovir 1000 mg PO twice a day (BID) for 10 days
- Polysporin ointment to prevent bacterial superinfection
- Observe borderline intraocular pressure (IOP)
- Follow up in 1 week

Follow-up

HPI

The patient follows up a little over a week later. He states that his vision is still a bit blurry, but the eye is more comfortable.

Exam

	OD	OS
Vision	20/20	20/30+
IOP	12	19
Lids and lashes:	Normal	Normal
Sclera/conjunctiva:	White and quiet	White and quiet
Cornea:	Clear	Dendrite resolved, a few stellate KP
AC:	Deep and quiet	1+ cell
Iris:	Flat	Flat
Lens:	Clear	Clear
Anterior vitreous:	Clear	Clear
DFE:	Unchanged	Unchanged

TESTING

Check corneal sensation. Sensation was only mildly reduced by Cochet–Bonnet.

Management

- Finish out 10-day course of acyclovir
- Continue Polysporin ointment
- Add prednisolone acetate 1% four times a day (QID) left eye (OS)

Further Follow-up

The patient returns about a week later. He states that his symptoms are much improved. Vision has improved to 20/25, IOP is 18, and the anterior chamber (AC) is quiet. He was tapered off topical corticosteroids over the next 3 weeks without recurrence of inflammation or keratitis.

Key Points

- Herpesviridae are a family of ubiquitous viruses. HSV 1 and 2 and VZV can lie dormant in the nerve ganglia and reactivate throughout a patient's lifetime.
- Simultaneous epithelial keratitis and iritis as a primary presentation, as in this case, are uncommon but can occur. Iritis is more commonly seen either in isolation during episodes of reactivation or in association with stromal keratitis.
- Corticosteroids are relatively contraindicated in herpetic epithelial keratitis, as they can potentiate viral replication. Even with the simultaneous presence of iritis, it is advisable to treat with antivirals first until the epithelial keratitis has healed and then add corticosteroids if inflammation persists. Of note, some clinicians do treat this type of case with simultaneous antivirals and topical corticosteroids.
- Alternatively, trifluridine eight times a day can be used, but it can cause corneal epithelial toxicity and punctal occlusion, so the authors prefer systemic treatment. Ganciclovir 0.15% gel is another alternative therapy.

- For VZV, the antiviral dose is greater (i.e., acyclovir 800 mg PO five times a day or valacyclovir 1000 mg PO three times a day [TID]).
- Ocular hypertension is caused by herpetic trabeculitis and will often resolve with treatment of the underlying disease. For highly elevated IOPs that warrant treatment, prostaglandin analogues should be avoided, as they may contribute to reactivation.

CHAPTER 10

Juvenile Idiopathic Arthritis (JIA)

Henry J. Kaplan

History of Present Illness

"My rheumatologist asked me to have an eye examination." A 6-year-old girl with a recent diagnosis of juvenile idiopathic arthritis (JIA) is referred to an ophthalmologist for a routine eye examination. The child has no complaints, and the parents have not noticed any problem with her vision or eyes. She was diagnosed with JIA at 4 years of age, and previous eye examinations every 3 months have been normal. Her joint symptoms have been controlled with oral methotrexate (15 mg/m^2) weekly (Fig. 10.1).

Exam

	OD	OS
Visual acuity	20/20	20/40
Intraocular pressure (IOP) (mm Hg)	12	10
Sclera/conjunctiva	Clear, no injection	Clear, no injection
Cornea	Clear with nongranulomatous (NG) keratic precipitates (KPs) in Arlt triangle	Clear with NG KPs in Arlt triangle
Anterior chamber (AC)	1+ flare, 1+ cell	1+ flare, 3+ cell
Iris	Round pupil	Intermittent posterior synechiae (see Fig. 10.1)
Lens	Clear	Clear
Vitreous cavity	Clear	2+ vitreous cells
Retina/optic nerve	Normal	Swollen optic nerve head with normal retina

Questions to Ask

- Has her vision changed in either eye since seeing her ophthalmologist?
- What diagnostic tests has she had to confirm her diagnosis of JIA?
- Has anyone in her family had a viral infection like herpesvirus, measles, or mumps?
- Does she have a skin rash?
- Has she been hospitalized for any serious infections, or has she been exposed to anyone with a serious infection like tuberculosis (TB)?

Her vision has not changed before seeing her eye doctor until recently. She had several blood tests to establish a diagnosis of JIA, but the family does not know the exact results. No one in the family has had a recent viral infection, and the patient does not have a skin rash and has not been hospitalized for a serious infection.

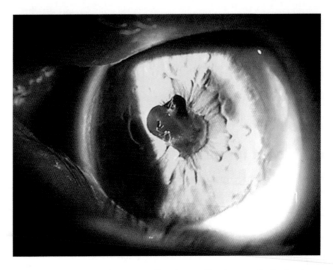

Fig. 10.1   Posterior synechiae and focal capsular fibrosis resulting from metaplastic changes in iris epithelium, OS.

Assessment

- Anterior uveitis both eyes (OU), with optic disc edema and cystoid macular edema (CME) left eye (OS)

Differential Diagnosis

- JIA-associated anterior uveitis
- Infectious anterior uveitis (herpes simplex virus, varicella zoster virus, cytomegalovirus, TB, borreliosis, syphilis)
- Intermediate uveitis (pars planitis)

Working Diagnosis

- JIA-associated anterior uveitis OU, OS > OD (right eye)

Testing

- Antibody testing:
  - Antinuclear antibodies (ANA) positive, antineutrophil cytoplasmic antibodies (ANCA) negative
  - Rheumatoid factor (immunoglobulin M [IgM]-RF): negative
- HLA-B27: negative

In patients with an established diagnosis of JIA, no further workup is necessary. The presence of optic disc edema OS is secondary to the intraocular inflammation in that eye. If inflammation in the OS resolves and optic disc edema persists for several months, then further evaluation is required. For atypical cases of anterior uveitis, the potential infectious causes, noted earlier, should be further investigated by detailed history and laboratory testing as indicated. Coordination with a pediatric rheumatologist is strongly encouraged.

Management

- Topical corticosteroid (e.g., prednisolone acetate suspension 1%), OU, every 4 to 6 hours (q4–6h) while awake
- Topical cyclopentolate hydrochloride 0.5%, 1 qtt, OU twice a day to three times a day (BID to TID)
- Follow up in 2 weeks

Follow-up Care

- The patient returned after 2 weeks without a noticeable improvement. She was continued on topical corticosteroid and cycloplegic therapy OU and changed from oral to subcutaneous methotrexate (15 mg/m^2) to increase bioavailability.
- Follow up in 1 month.

Follow-up

The patient returns with improved visual acuity (VA) OS to 20/25, no anterior chamber (AC) inflammation OU, and resolving optic disc edema OS. Topical corticosteroids were slowly tapered OU, and cycloplegia was stopped.

Key Points

- Uveitis screening by an ophthalmologist has to start immediately after a diagnosis of JIA, and screening should be continued throughout childhood at appropriate intervals. A recent study of JIA concluded that almost all children developed uveitis within 4 years of diagnosis after arthritis onset and that the most important predictor for the development of uveitis was ANA positivity.
- Many patients with JIA will present with asymmetric disease, including the presence of optic disc edema. The latter does not require further evaluation unless it persists after the resolution of intraocular inflammation.

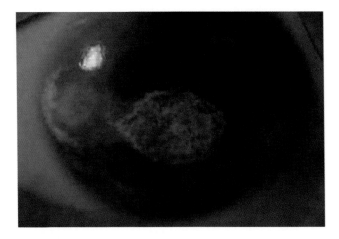

Fig. 10.2   Band keratopathy in JIA-associated uveitis.

- As much as 80% of anterior uveitis cases in pediatrics are associated with JIA. The cumulative incidence of JIA-associated uveitis is 12.4% in the oligoarticular group, 4.3% in the polyarticular group, and 1.8% in the systemic group.
- Three major complications of JIA-associated anterior uveitis are band keratopathy (Fig. 10.2), cataract, CME, and glaucoma. Cataract surgery is technically demanding, but "small incision surgery" and control of perioperative inflammation can result in satisfactory surgical outcomes. Persistent CME without active inflammation can be treated with periocular or intravitreal corticosteroids or intravitreal anti–vascular endothelial growth factor (VEGF) agents.
- The leading cause of permanent vision loss in JIA-associated anterior uveitis is glaucoma, which is frequently not responsive to medical therapy. Thus filtering procedures to decrease intraocular pressure is often required.
- Early identification of JIA-associated uveitis with prompt and aggressive therapy should be started to prevent complications and visual loss. Disease-modifying antirheumatic drugs (DMARDs), such as methotrexate, infliximab, or adalimumab, will often have to be administered to achieve the therapeutic goal of complete absence of intraocular inflammation. If there is no response to topical therapy at 1 month, DMARDs should be added or increased with the support of a rheumatologist.

CHAPTER 11

Tubulointerstitial Nephritis and Uveitis Syndrome (TINU)

Manfred Zierhut ■ Aleksandra Radosavljevic ■ Jelena Karadzic

History of Present Illness

A 42-year-old female with past medical history of biopsy-proven interstitial nephritis since 2008 presented for the first time 2 years after the onset of nephritis to the eye clinic with anterior uveitis that started 5 months ago. She was treated with systemic corticosteroids (CS). The treatment was stopped a month ago, and 3 days later she noticed worsening of vision (Figs. 11.1 and 11.2).

Exam

	OD	OS
Visual acuity	20/40	20/25
IOP	15	15
Sclera/conjunctiva	Minimal ciliary injection	Minimal ciliary injection
Cornea	Small granulomatous KP in lower half (see Fig. 11.1)	Larger granulomatous KP in lower half (see Fig. 11.2)
Anterior chamber (AC)	Deep, 1–2+ cells	Deep, 2+ cells
Iris	Unremarkable	Unremarkable
Lens	Clear	Clear
Anterior vitreous	+2 cells	+2 cells
Retina	See Fig. 11.3	See Fig. 11.3

Questions to Ask

- Have you ever had any numbness, tingling, weakness on one side of the body, or bowel or bladder problems? Is there any history of neurologic disorders in the family?
- Have you noticed any recent ticks or tick bites on your body?
- Have you had any cough, lung problems, or episodes of fever?

She answers no to all of these questions.

Assessment

- Intermediate uveitis left eye greater than right eye (OS > OD)

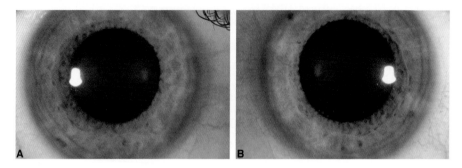

Fig. 11.1 (A, B) Anterior segment photograph of both eyes with granulomatous keratic precipitate (KP).

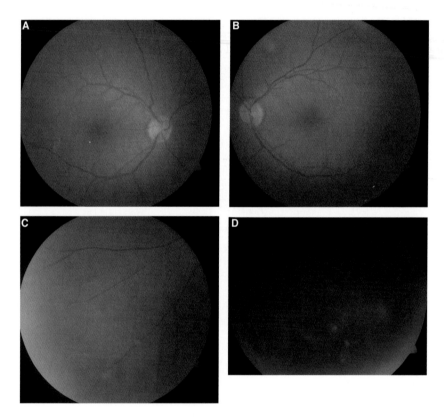

Fig. 11.2 Fundus photograph showing moderately hazy media (A, B) and snow balls in the periphery (C, D). Optic nerve and posterior pole had normal findings. There were no signs of vascular sheathing.

Differential Diagnosis

- Tubulointerstitial nephritis and uveitis (TINU) syndrome
- Sarcoid-associated intermediate uveitis
- Multiple sclerosis (MS)–associated intermediate uveitis

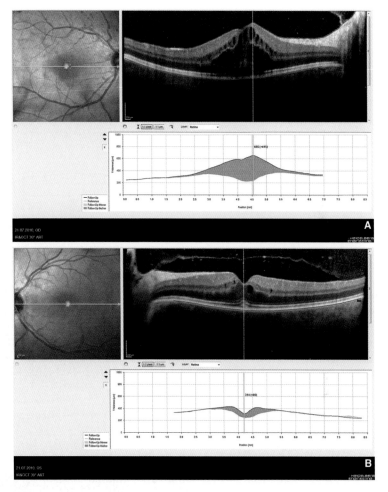

Fig. 11.3 Optical coherence tomography of both eyes showing cystoid macular edema OU, OD > OS, and trace posterior vitreous cell.

- Pars planitis
- Less likely: Lyme-associated, tuberculous, or syphilitic intermediate uveitis; granulomatosis with polyangiitis; vitreoretinal lymphoma

Working Diagnosis

- Intermediate uveitis both eyes (OU), OS > OD

Testing

- Under the suspicion of TINU a urinalysis was done and disclosed an increased β2-microglobulin (> 1.2, normal ≤ 0.3) with proteinuria. All other laboratory data were within normal limits.
- For atypical cases, check:

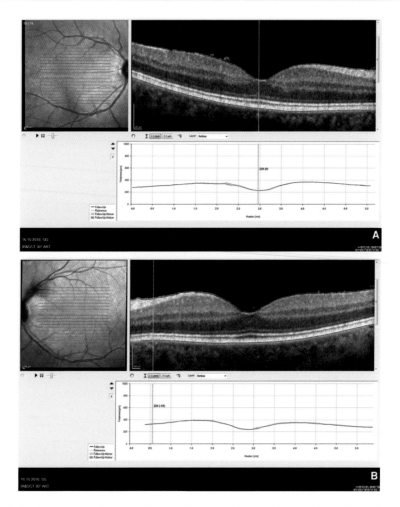

Fig. 11.4 Optical coherence tomography of both eyes at last follow-up showing normal macular structure (after 7 years of follow-up).

- Fluorescent treponemal antibody absorption (FTA-ABS), rapid plasma reagin (RPR) (negative)
- Lyme antibody with Western blot (negative)
- QuantiFERON or purified protein derivative (PPD) (negative)

Management

- Systemic prednisone 1 mg/kg for 1 week than slowly tapered by 10 mg every 1 week until 20 mg, then by 2.5 mg every week until 10 mg, then very slow tapering, depending on the activity of uveitis
- Local treatment included topical prednisolone 1% five times per day and tropicamide three times per day
- Follow up in 2 weeks

Follow-up

The patient reported nearly complete resolution of her symptoms after 2 months of treatment. Vision was 20/20 OU.

However, the patient had a relapse of intraocular inflammation and acute renal failure after 9 months of treatment while on prednisone 5 mg every day. The CS dose was raised to 20 mg of prednisone per day for 7 days with slow reduction by 2.5 mg every week over the next 3 months until discontinued, and she remained stable.

Two years and 5 months after the first examination, the patient had a relapse of intermediate uveitis with decreased vision due to cystoid macular edema (CME) in both eyes (visual acuity [VA] OD 20/25, OS 20/40). A treatment regimen with systemic CS and local nonsteroidal anti-inflammatory drug (NSAID) was initiated, and after 1 month of treatment CME resolved (VA OU 20/20). The patient was followed for the next 7 years and had two mild relapses of intraocular inflammation and minimal macular edema that responded well to systemic CS treatment.

On the last visit, VA OU: 20/20, intraocular pressure (IOP) OD: 15 mm Hg, and OS: 19 mm Hg. She had +1/2 cells in the anterior chamber, +1 vitreous cells, and occasional snow balls. She was treated with local therapy of nepafenac two times per day and prednisolone 1% once per day (Figs. 11.3 and 11.4).

Management Algorithm

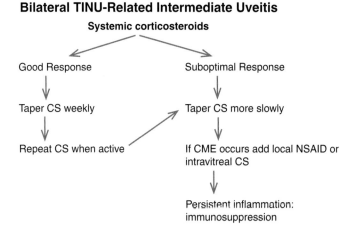

Key Points

- TINU can present as anterior, intermediate, or posterior uveitis.
- In most cases, the interstitial nephritis is self-limited, and the renal prognosis is good.
- Many patients with TINU-related pars planitis can have asymmetric disease and mild presentations and can frequently be monitored without therapy.
- More severe cases of vitreal inflammation require systemic CS treatment.
- CME is the most common cause of vision loss in these patients.

CHAPTER 12

Blau-Jabs Syndrome (Granulomatous Arthritis, Dermatitis and Uveitis)

Henry J. Kaplan

History of Present Illness

A 7-year-old Caucasian boy complains of blurred visual acuity (VA), photophobia, and intermittent pain in both eyes (OU) over the past 12 months. Since age 3 he has had exacerbations of a papulonodular, tender, reddish-brown rash on his face (Fig. 12.1) and trunk (Fig. 12.2), as well as multiple firm subcutaneous nodules. The skin manifestations usually resolve with systemic corticosteroids.

Exam

	OD	OS
Visual acuity	20/80	20/40
IOP (mm Hg)	22	21
Sclera/ conjunctiva	Clear. No injection.	Clear. No injection.
Cornea	Band keratopathy (BK) with subepithelial corneal opacities inferiorly	No BK but subepithelial corneal opacities (see Fig. 12.2A)
AC	2+ flare and 2+ cells	2+ flare and 2+ cells
Iris	Pinpoint pupil with intermittent posterior synechiae for 360 degrees	Intermittent posterior synechiae for 360 degrees
Lens	3+ Posterior subcapsular cataract (PSC)	1+ PSC
Vitreous cavity	2+ vitreous cells	2+ vitreous cells
Retina/optic nerve	Fundus view blocked by pinpoint pupil and PSC	Disseminated chorioretinal lesions obscured by PSC and vitritis (see Fig. 12.2B)

Questions to Ask

- Have you had a biopsy of your skin lesions, and what did it show?
- Do you have any joint symptoms?
- Are you having shortness of breath, and have you had a recent chest x-ray?
- Have you had genetic testing to rule out sarcoidosis?

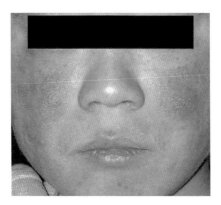

Fig. 12.1 Butterfly-shaped skin rash on the cheeks. (Picture credit: *Ophthalmology*. 2003;110(10): 2040–2044, by Elsevier.)

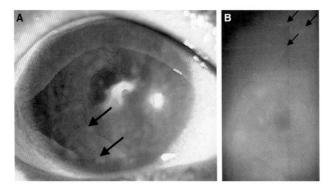

Fig. 12.2 (A) Subepithelial corneal deposits (*arrows*), posterior synechiae, left eye (OS). (B) Disseminated chorioretinal lesions (*arrows*) obscured by PSC and vitritis, OS. (Picture credit: *Ophthalmology*. 2003;110 (10):2040–2044, by Elsevier.)

His skin biopsy revealed a granulomatous dermatitis with noncaseating granulomas. His joints swell symmetrically with moderate redness, warmth, and tenderness involving the interphalangeal joints of the hands and feet (Fig. 12.3). He has no shortness of breath, and a recent chest x-ray was normal. Genetic testing revealed a *CARD15/NOD2* mutation that excludes early-onset sarcoidosis as the cause of symptoms.

Assessment

- Granulomatous panuveitis OU with secondary cataract and chorioretinal lesions, associated with cutaneous eruptions and symmetrical polyarthritis

Differential Diagnosis

- Jabs/Blau syndrome
- Sarcoidosis

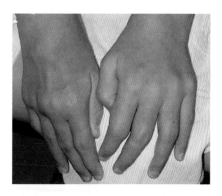

Fig. 12.3 Deformed hands secondary to chronic interphalangeal joint inflammation. (Picture credit: *Ophthalmology*. 2003;110(10):2040–2044, by Elsevier.)

- Multifocal choroiditis with panuveitis
- Lymphoma or other bone marrow disorder
- Infectious retinitis (tuberculosis [TB], herpesviruses, Lyme disease)
- Inflammatory bowel disease

Working Diagnosis

- Jabs/Blau syndrome, with panuveitis OU (secondary cataract, chorioretinitis, and ocular hypertension) and granulomatous dermatitis and polyarthritis

Testing

- The triad of panuveitis, granulomatous dermatitis, and polyarthritis with a *CARD15/NOD2* mutation establishes the diagnosis of Jabs/Blau syndrome and excludes early-onset sarcoidosis.

Management

- Topical corticosteroids, cycloplegia, and antiglaucoma medications were used to control the anterior uveitis. Systemic glucocorticoids (0.75 mg/kg/day) were used to control bilateral chorioretinitis. Low-dose systemic glucocorticoids are generally sufficient to control intraocular inflammation in the quiescent stage of the disease.
- Patient scheduled to return at 2 weeks.

Follow-up

Two weeks later, anterior chamber (AC) inflammation is starting to resolve but VA remains the same. Intraocular pressure (IOP) is 18 mm Hg OU. The patient will be followed monthly until intraocular inflammation and IOP are well controlled, with resolution of retinal lesions.

Key Points

- The triad of panuveitis, granulomatous dermatitis, and polyarthritis suggests Jabs/Blau syndrome in a young person.

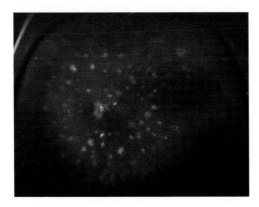

Fig. 12.4 Disseminated chorioretinal lesions, some with fibrotic scar formation. Peripapillary nodular lesions are present as well. (Picture credit: *Am J Ophthalmol.* 2018;187:158–166, by Elsevier.)

- Pulmonary involvement in this disease is rare compared with sarcoidosis.
- Cataract surgery will be necessary to improve VA right eye (OD), and if IOP is not controlled on medical therapy, a surgical filtering procedure will need to be considered.
- If the therapeutic response to corticosteroids is unsatisfactory or a maintenance dose of prednisone >7.5 mg/day is needed for prolonged periods, treatment with biologics such as anti–tumor necrosis factor (TNF) agents should be considered.
- Lesion size in disseminated chorioretinitis secondary to Jabs/Blau syndrome can vary and can be larger than 1 disc diameter (Fig. 12.4).

CHAPTER 13

Postoperative Uveitis

Harpal S. Sandhu

History of Present Illness (HPI)

A 63-year-old woman underwent cataract surgery in the left eye (OS) about 3 months ago. The case was reportedly uncomplicated, and a one-piece intraocular lens (IOL) was placed in the capsular bag. Since then, she has had multiple episodes of what her cataract surgeon called "rebound iritis." She was tapered off prednisolone acetate four times a day (QID) from postoperative week 1 to 4, promptly experienced a slight decrease in vision, and was noted to have white cells in the anterior chamber. Another week of prednisolone acetate QID was initiated, resulting in near resolution of the inflammation according to the surgeon's notes, followed by another taper over 3 weeks. She presented postoperative week 8 with a similar presentation to week 4. Another 4 weeks of identical management with recurrent iritis again at week 12 then followed. At that point, she was referred to you on prednisolone acetate 1% twice a day (BID).

Past Ocular History

- Keratoconjunctivitis sicca both eyes (OU), controlled with preservative-free artificial tears and topical cyclosporine 0.05% BID OU

Past Medical History

- Gastroesophageal reflux disease
- Osteoarthritis
- Sjogren syndrome

Exam

	OD	OS
Visual acuity	20/25	20/30+
Intraocular pressure (IOP)	15	14
Sclera/conjunctiva	White and quiet	White and quiet
Cornea	Clear	A few large keratic precipitates (KPs)
Anterior chamber (AC)	Deep and quiet	2+ white cells
		1+ flare
Iris	Unremarkable	Unremarkable, no transillumination defect (TIDs)
Lens	2+ nuclear sclerosis (NS)	See Fig. 13.1
Anterior vitreous	clear	2+ white cells, 0 haze

Dilated Fundus Examination (DFE)

Nerve:	Cup-to-disc (c/d) 0.2, pink, sharp	c/d 0.2, pink, sharp
Macula:	Flat	Flat
Vessels:	Normal caliber and course	Normal caliber and course
Periphery:	Unremarkable	Unremarkable

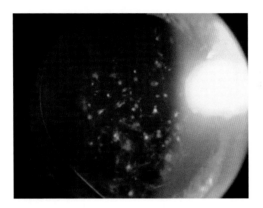

Fig. 13.1 Slit lamp photograph of the left eye demonstrates a one-piece posterior chamber intraocular lens (PCIOL) with inflammatory cells/deposits on the IOL, or "lens precipitates." The haptics are clearly within the capsular bag. (From Murthy SI, Pappuru RR, Latha KM, et al. Surgical management in patient with uveitis. *Indian J Ophthalmol* 2013;61:284–290.)

Questions to Ask

- Acquire a copy of the operative report. Was there manipulation of uveal tissue? Was there iris prolapse out of the wound? Were hooks or a Malyugin ring used?
- Do you have any other history of rheumatic or autoimmune disease beyond what you have told us?
- Have you ever had any other eye problems, like inflammation in the eye or blepharitis?

There was no report of iris prolapse out of the wound. Iris hooks were used during the case. The patient was diagnosed with Sjogren syndrome two decades ago but no other autoimmune diseases. Upon prompting, she does recall that she had an episode of "iritis" in one of her eyes years ago, which resolved quickly "with just a few drops."

Assessment

- Anterior uveitis and intermediate uveitis OS (predominantly anterior) beginning after cataract surgery

Differential Diagnosis

- Retained lens fragments
- Indolent (subacute/chronic) endophthalmitis

- Exuberant inflammation from intraoperative manipulation of uveal tissue
- Unmasking of uveitis associated with systemic autoimmune disease
- De novo noninfectious uveitis beginning after surgery (i.e., postsurgical uveitis)

Working Diagnosis

- Indolent endophthalmitis OS

Testing

- Gonioscopy and scleral depressed examination to assess for retained lens fragments. Both tests were performed and were negative.
- Anterior chamber tap for polymerase chain reaction (PCR)

Management

- Increase topical steroids to 6 to 8 times a day OS
- Follow up in 1 to 2 weeks

Follow-up

HPI

The patient returns 1 week later. She notes no changes. PCR was negative for organisms.

Exam

	OD	OS
Visual acuity	20/25	20/25−
IOP	15	17
Sclera/conjunctiva	White and quiet	White and quiet
Cornea	Clear	A few large KP
AC	Deep and quiet	1/2+ white cells
		1+ flare
Iris	Unremarkable	Unremarkable, no TIDs
Lens	2+ NS	PCIOL with lens precipitates
Anterior vitreous	Clear	2+ white cells

Working Diagnosis

- Postsurgical uveitis vs. unmasking of a uveitic syndrome associated with systemic disease

Testing

- Although there can be false-negative results with PCR, it is generally a highly sensitive test, and thus an infectious cause is now quite unlikely. Retained lens fragments have also been ruled out with a thorough examination, including gonioscopy and scleral depressed examination of the fundus. The patient is now in postoperative week 14, and thus continued inflammation from surgical manipulation of the uvea, although possible, is increasingly unlikely. Although the patient has a history of Sjogren syndrome, this disease is only rarely associated with intraocular inflammation. Thus testing for an underlying systemic disease associated with anterior uveitis is indicated.

- Check HLA-B27, angiotensin-converting enzyme (ACE), lysozyme, rapid plasma reagin (RPR), fluorescent treponemal antibody absorption (FTA-ABS), QuantiFERON or purified protein derivative (PPD), and a chest x-ray.

Further Follow-up

All testing was negative. The patient was gradually tapered down to a maintenance dose of prednisolone acetate 1% every other day (QOD) OS. At postoperative month 6, her disease remained quiescent and vision 20/25 + OS.

Diagnosis

- Postsurgical chronic anterior and intermediate uveitis OS, associated with Sjogren syndrome

Key Points

- Uveitis after cataract surgery that persists after several months and multiple courses of high-dose topical corticosteroids requires one to entertain a broad differential diagnosis. One should have a high suspicion for infectious causes of indolent endophthalmitis (e.g., *Propionibacterium acnes*, fungi).
- Other common causes, such as retained lens fragments and dislocated haptics chafing against the iris, can usually be determined by a thorough examination. Ultrasound biomicroscopy can be helpful if the latter diagnosis is still in question after a good examination. Iris transillumination defects and a predominance of pigmented cells over white cells in the anterior chamber are other signs of this diagnosis.
- Once infection has been ruled out, the clinician should consider the typical causes of noninfectious anterior uveitis. Occasionally, endogenous uveitis associated with systemic autoimmune disease will be unmasked by intraocular surgery.
- A history of uveitis is a risk factor for severe and/or prolonged postoperative inflammation. Knowledge of this history before surgery would have allowed for aggressive pre- and perioperative antiinflammatory therapy to decrease the risk of precisely this complication (see chapter 75).
- Albeit rare, surgery in and of itself can cause chronic uveitis. However, this diagnosis is one of exclusion. Although some advocate IOL explantation in these cases, the author generally treats them in the same fashion as any idiopathic uveitis and reserves IOL explantation for refractory disease.
- The definitive treatment of *P. acnes*–associated uveitis (i.e., indolent endophthalmitis) involves vitrectomy, IOL explantation, capsulectomy, and injection of intravitreal antibiotics, typically clindamycin.

CHAPTER 14

Bilateral Pigment Dispersion

Harpal S. Sandhu

History of Present Illness (HPI)

A 35-year-old healthy woman with no significant past medical or ocular history is referred to the uveitis clinic by an outside ophthalmologist for "bilateral acute anterior uveitis." She reports that her symptoms started a little over a month ago. Her eyes started to become red and very light sensitive. The referral note mentions that she was started on prednisolone acetate 1% four times a day (QID) both eyes (OU) for "4+ cells" in both anterior chambers and timolol 0.5% twice a day (BID) OU for an intraocular pressure (IOP) of 32 OU upon presentation. Since then, the photophobia and redness have decreased somewhat, she says, but not completely. The referral note goes on to add that despite some symptomatic relief, the cellularity has remained unchanged.

Exam

	OD	OS
Visual acuity	20/25 pinhole (PH) 20/20	20/40 PH 20/20
IOP	28	27
Sclera/conjunctiva	Trace injection	Trace injection
Cornea	Clear stroma, pigment on inferior endothelium	Clear, pigment on inferior endothelium
Anterior chamber (AC)	4+ pigmented cells, 2+ flare	4+ pigmented cells, 2+ flare
Iris	See Figs. 14.1 and 14.2	See Figs. 14.1 and 14.2
Lens	Clear	Clear
Anterior vitreous	1+ pigmented cells	1+ pigmented cells

Questions to Ask

- Have you been hit in the head or the eyes recently?
- Have you been told that you have glaucoma, or has anyone in your family had glaucoma?
- Have you ever suffered from cold sores? Have you ever had shingles?
- Have you been ill recently? If so, how was your illness treated?
- Are you on any medications now or have you recently been on any medications that you have not told us about?

She denies any trauma to the head or eyes or any eye problems, and she has never heard anyone in her family mention any eye problems besides cataracts in her grandparents. She has no history of cold sores. She had a bad case of what her doctor told her was bronchitis, and she was treated with a 7-day course of oral moxifloxacin.

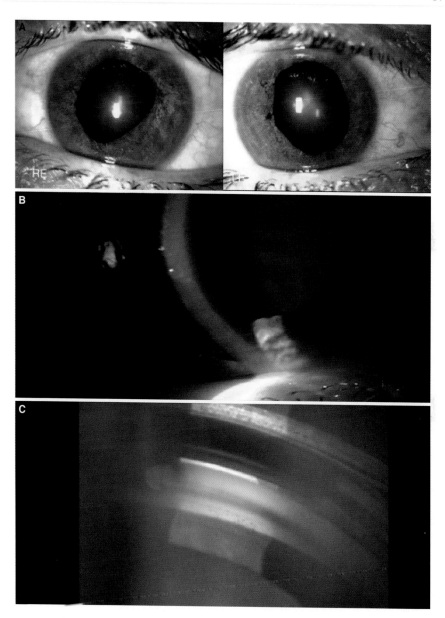

Fig. 14.1 (A) Color external photographs of both eyes. The pupils are mid-dilated, and both irises have multiple areas of depigmentation. (B) Slit lamp photograph shows deposition of pigment on the corneal endothelium. (C) Gonioscopy reveals abnormal pigmentation of the angle. (Reproduced from Rueda-Rueda T, Sánchez-Vicente LJ, Moruno-Rodríguez A, Monge-Esquivel J, Muñoz-Morales A, López-Herrero F. Bilateral acute iris depigmentation and bilateral acute iris transillumination syndrome. *Arch Spanish Society Opthalmol [English Edition]*. 2019;94:355–358.)

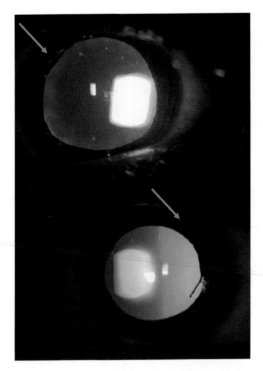

Fig. 14.2 Color slit lamp photograph of both eyes under retroillumination shows iris transillumination defects *(blue arrows)*. (Reproduced from Rueda-Rueda T, Sánchez-Vicente LJ, Moruno-Rodríguez A, Monge-Esquivel J, Muñoz-Morales A, López-Herrero F. Bilateral acute iris depigmentation and bilateral acute iris transillumination syndrome. *Arch Spanish Society Opthalmol [English Edition]*. 2019;94:355–358.)

Assessment

- Acute, symptomatic pigment dispersion OU

Differential Diagnosis

- Bilateral acute iris transillumination syndrome (BAIT)
- Bilateral acute depigmentation of the iris (BADI)
- Pigment dispersion syndrome OU
- Less likely: traumatic pigment dispersion, herpetic anterior uveitis

Working Diagnosis

- BAIT/BADI
- There are no leukocytes (white cells) on examination, only pigmented cells. The lack of true inflammatory cells and the bilateral nature make herpetic uveitis less likely, and the acute symptomatology is inconsistent with pigment dispersion syndrome. This leaves BAIT or BADI, which is essentially a milder form of BAIT (see Key Points), as the diagnosis.

Testing

- Baseline glaucoma evaluation should be performed, but can be deferred to a later time when the patient is more comfortable. This involves corneal pachymetry, visual field testing, and optic nerve optical coherence tomography (OCT) to measure retinal nerve fiber layer thickness in addition to gonioscopy, which has already been performed.

Management

- Increase prednisolone acetate 1% to every 2 hours (q2h) OU
- Add dorzolamide 2% BID OU to timolol 0.5% BID OU

Follow-up

HPI

After 2 weeks, the patient reports her symptoms are a quite a bit better, though not completely resolved. She wears sunglasses all the time outdoors now. She has no new issues to report.

Exam

	OD	OS
Visual acuity	20/25 PH 20/20	20/30 PH 20/20
IOP	24	24
Sclera/conjunctiva	White and quiet	White and quiet
Cornea	Clear stroma, pigment on inferior endothelium	Clear, pigment on inferior endothelium
AC	3+ pigmented cells, 2+ flare	3+ pigmented cells, 2+ flare
Iris	Areas of depigmentation, same as prior Mid-dilated pupil	Areas of depigmentation, same prior Mid-dilated pupil
Lens	Clear	Clear
Anterior vitreous	1+ pigmented cells	1+ pigmented cells

Management

- Taper prednisolone acetate 1% slowly: QID × 2 weeks, three times a day (TID) × 2 weeks, BID × 2 weeks, daily × 2 weeks, every other day (QOD) × 2 weeks, then stop
- Continue timolol–dorzolamide BID OU

Further Follow-up

After another 3 months, pigment in the anterior chamber finally resolved to trace levels. The patient has some photophobia only in highly illuminated environments that is tolerable with tinted lenses. IOP never fell below 23 while on therapy, so timolol–dorzolamide was continued indefinitely in both eyes.

Key Points

- BAIT syndrome is a rare cause of acute pigment dispersion in the eye associated with iris transillumination defects and elevated IOP, both of which can vary from mild to profound. Mydriasis, poor pupillary reaction to light, and female predilection are features of the syndrome.
- Patients are typically symptomatic with photophobia, which is sometimes intense, and complain of redness (conjunctival injection and/or hyperemia). In cases of profound iris atrophy, photophobia can persist even after resolution of pigmented cells in the anterior chamber.
- Although symptoms are generally responsive to intensive topical corticosteroids and tend to resolve, IOP elevations are more difficult to treat and can require indefinite medical therapy and occasionally even surgical intervention.
- The etiology of this condition is unknown. There is a strong association with antecedent flulike illnesses, which implicates an infectious etiology or postinfectious immune response. A large fraction of cases has been linked to systemic moxifloxacin. However, cases have developed in the absence of systemic moxifloxacin, and there have been no reported cases with topical moxifloxacin, a commonly used agent, thus weakening this association. Counseling against further use of systemic moxifloxacin is a reasonable precaution, but the benefit is unclear.
- BADI is thought to be a milder presentation of the same syndrome as BAIT, but with more prominent iris depigmentation and less severe symptoms. This case interestingly shows features of both, which adds credence to the idea that they exist along a spectrum of the same disease.
- Other rare but serious causes of pigment dispersion, such as intraocular foreign bodies or uveal melanoma, tend to be unilateral and are associated with other examination features, and thus are readily distinguished from this bilateral entity.

CHAPTER 15

Episcleritis

Harpal S. Sandhu

History of Present Illness

A 39-year-old woman with no past medical history presents for the first time to the eye clinic complaining of redness and irritation in the left eye (OS) for 3 days. It is just in the left-hand corner of the left eye and has not improved at all since it started.

Exam

	OD	OS
Visual acuity	20/20	20/20
Intraocular pressure (IOP)	12	13
Sclera/conjunctiva	White and quiet	See Fig. 15.1
Cornea	Clear	Clear
Anterior chamber (AC)	Deep and quiet	Deep and quiet
Iris	Unremarkable	Unremarkable
Lens	Clear	Clear
Anterior vitreous	Clear	Clear

Questions to Ask

- How bad is your pain? How would you rate it out of 10?
- Have you had any change in your vision?
- Have you had any discharge from the eye?
- Do you wear contact lenses?
- Do you think you could have gotten anything in your eyes?
- Has anything like this ever happened before?
- Have you started any new medications recently?

She rates her pain as mild ("2 out of 10") but a nuisance. She answers no to the remaining questions.

Assessment

Sectoral inflammation of episclera and/or conjunctiva OS

Differential Diagnosis

- Episcleritis
- Scleritis
- Less likely: conjunctivitis, allergic or viral

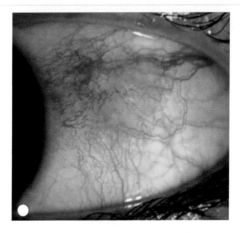

Fig. 15.1 Color external photograph of the left eye shows a sectoral area of moderate injection temporally. The external examination of both eyes is otherwise normal, and there are no follicles or papillae on the palpebral conjunctiva. (From *Kanski's Clinical Ophthalmology*. 9th ed. Fig 9.2A, by Elsevier.)

Working Diagnosis

- Episcleritis OS
- The lack of a blue or violaceous hue in the inflamed area and relatively mild pain are much more consistent with episcleritis than scleritis.

Testing

- Place 1 drop of phenylephrine 2.5% on the OS—the redness largely blanches in response. This further supports a diagnosis of episcleritis.
- No laboratory testing is indicated for a first episode. If there are frequent or worsening episodes, consider testing similar to that for scleritis:
  - Antinuclear antibodies (ANA), angiotensin-converting enzyme (ACE), lysozyme, chest x-ray, antineutrophil cytoplasmic antibodies (ANCA), rheumatoid factor, HLA-B27, uric acid, baseline metabolic profile (BMP), rapid plasma reagin (RPR), fluorescent treponemal antibody absorption (FTA-ABS), QuantiFERON, or plasma protein derivative (PPD)

Management

- Ibuprofen 800 mg by mouth (PO) three times a day (TID). (Inquire about kidney function before beginning high-dose nonsteroidal antiinflammatory drugs [NSAIDs]. Check blood urea nitrogen [BUN] and creatinine if there is any uncertainty.)
- Artificial tears as needed (PRN)
- Ranitidine 150 mg PO twice a day (BID) for gastrointestinal (GI) prophylaxis (alternative: omeprazole 20 mg PO daily)
- Follow up in 2 to 3 weeks

Follow-up

The patient returns as scheduled and reports nearly complete resolution of her symptoms. Ibuprofen was discontinued without recurrence.

Key Points

- Episcleritis represents inflammation of the vascularized, fibroelastic layer of tissue superficial to the sclera. The degree of injection and pain are significantly less than those of scleritis. Scleral edema, which is sometimes visible at the slit lamp in scleritis, is absent in episcleritis.
- Episcleritis can present as either simple episcleritis, as in this case, or as a more nodular form.
- Unlike scleritis, it carries very little risk of vision-threatening complications and is much less likely to be associated with a systemic disease.
- Most episcleritis is thus idiopathic and noninfectious in etiology. Many cases are self-limited and require no treatment. In more symptomatic or prolonged cases, systemic, high-dose NSAIDs are the author's treatment of choice.
- If there are contraindications to systemic NSAIDs (e.g., renal disease, peptic ulcer disease), low- or medium-potency topical corticosteroids are a reasonable alternative, as are topical NSAIDs like ketorolac 0.5% TID to four times a day (QID). Rebound inflammation can sometimes be an issue with the former treatment, although the author has found mixed efficacy with the latter. A randomized controlled trial of topical ketorolac versus artificial tears found no significant difference between the two (Williams et al., *Eye* 2005).

CHAPTER 16

Refractory Scleritis in an Older Woman

Harpal S. Sandhu

History of Present Illness (HPI)

A 68-year-old woman with a history of non—insulin-dependent diabetes mellitus type 2, rheumatoid arthritis, and scleritis left eye (OS) complains of increasing pain and redness in her OS. Her scleritis has been difficult to control in the past, and last year the dosing of adalimumab was increased from 40 mg subcutaneous (SC) every 2 weeks to every week. She had to discontinue adalimumab 3 weeks ago because of an ulcer in her foot, as per the recommendations of her rheumatologist and primary care physician. Shortly after that, she reports the OS became very painful and red. She rates the pain as 8 to 9 out of 10. Her vision is a bit blurry, but she denies any major change.

Eye-Related Medications

- Ibuprofen 800 mg by mouth (PO) three times a day (TID)
- Adalimumab 40 mg SC every week (held as of 3 weeks ago)

Exam

	OD	OS
Vision	20/25	20/40
Intraocular pressure (IOP)	14	14
Lids and lashes:	Normal	Normal
Sclera/conjunctiva:	White and quiet	See Fig. 16.1
Cornea:	Clear	Clear
Anterior chamber (AC):	Deep and quiet	Deep and quiet
Iris:	Flat	Flat
Lens:	1+ nuclear sclerosis (NS)	2+ NS 1+ posterior subcapsular cataract (PSC)
Anterior vitreous:	Clear	Clear
Dilated fundus examination (DFE):		Deferred

Further Questions to Ask

- What is the status of your foot ulcer? Are you on antibiotics and getting wound care? Is it almost healed?

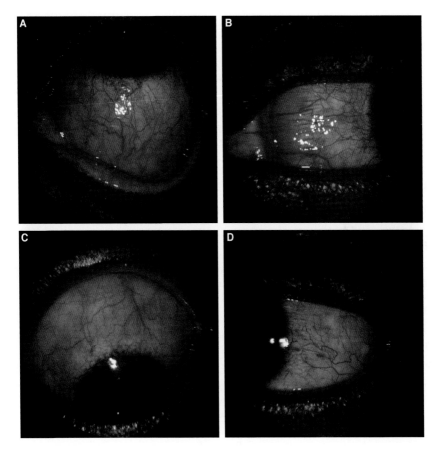

Fig. 16.1   (A) Color external photograph shows deep red injection of the inferior conjunctiva and sclera, which did not blanche with topical phenylephrine 5%. (B) Nasal view. (C) Superior view. (D) Temporal view.

Assessment

Diffuse anterior scleritis flare OS

Differential Diagnosis

- Rheumatoid arthritis is the leading cause of noninfectious scleritis, and in this case has already been established as the underlying systemic disease.

Management

- Prednisolone acetate 1% six times a day OS as a temporizing measure until immunomodulatory therapy (IMT) is resumed
- Continue ibuprofen 800 mg PO TID
- Follow up in 2 weeks

Follow-up

HPI

The patient follows up 2 weeks later. She reports only mild improvement in pain and redness. She still rates her pain as 7 to 8 out of 10. Unfortunately, her ulcer has not yet healed, and she is unsure when she will be able to resume adalimumab.

Examination	Unchanged in both eyes from last examination

Assessment

Diffuse anterior scleritis flare OS unresponsive to topical steroids

Management

- In a patient with severe pain from a scleritis flare and in whom systemic antiinflammatory and/or IMTs are contraindicated, local therapy is the only remaining option.
- Inject subconjunctival triamcinolone 2 to 4 mg (0.05 to 0.1 cc) per quadrant
- Taper off topical prednisolone acetate

Follow-up

HPI

The patient returns 3 weeks later. She happily reports that she has been at times pain-free since the last visit and only occasionally feels some pain, which she easily tolerates. She has no pain at the moment. She is still using the prednisolone acetate 1% once a day.

Exam

	OD	OS
Vision	20/25	20/30−
IOP	14	14
Lids and lashes:	Normal	Normal
Sclera/conjunctiva:	White and quiet	See Fig. 16.2
Cornea:	Clear	Clear
AC:	Deep and quiet	Deep and quiet
Iris:	Flat	Flat
Lens:	1+ NS	2+ NS 1+ PSC
Anterior vitreous:	Clear	Clear

Key Points

- The single most common association with scleritis is rheumatoid arthritis. Presentations can range from mild to severe, necessitating IMT.

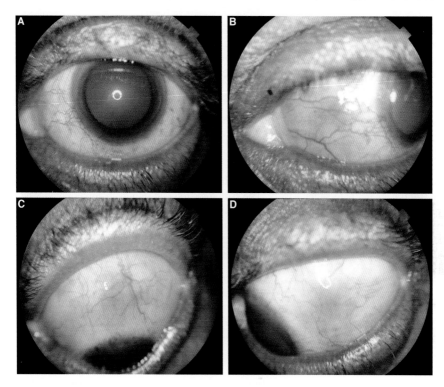

Fig. 16.2 (A) Color external photograph of the left conjunctiva and sclera showing vastly improved anterior scleral inflammation. (B) Nasal view. (C) Superior view. (D) Temporal view.

- Forms include diffuse anterior scleritis, nodular anterior scleritis, necrotizing scleritis, scleromalacia perforans, and posterior scleritis.
- Local therapies include sub-Tenon's or subconjunctival steroids. These carry the risk of scleral thinning and thus should be used with caution, reserved for difficult cases such as this one. They are contraindicated in necrotizing scleritis.
- Other noninfectious associations include the systemic vasculitides, HLA-B27 antigen, inflammatory bowel disease, sarcoidosis, lupus, relapsing polychondritis, and rarely gout.
- Infectious causes include syphilis, tuberculosis, Lyme disease, herpes viruses, and rarely fungi.
- Drug-induced causes include immune checkpoint inhibitors, erlotinib (an epidermal growth factor receptor [EGFR] inhibitor for lung cancer), bisphosphonates, and procainamide .
- There is evidence that antineutrophil cytoplasmic antibodies (ANCA)—associated scleritis responds better to rituximab than to other IMT agents.
- Cases where no underlying systemic disease has been identified and that do not respond to empiric trials of antiinflammatory therapy should be considered for scleral biopsy. Sometimes this is the only means of making a diagnosis of infectious scleritis or ocular surface squamous neoplasia masquerading as scleritis.

CHAPTER 17

Necrotizing Scleritis

Peter Yuwei Chang ■ C. Stephen Foster

History of Present Illness

A 54-year-old Caucasian female with long-standing rheumatoid arthritis complains of severe right eye (OD) pain and redness for 1 week. The symptoms respond minimally to ibuprofen. She has had similar pain in both of her eyes in the past couple of years and was treated with topical corticosteroid drops and oral nonsteroidal antiinflammatory drugs (NSAIDs) by her ophthalmologist.

Her current medications include methotrexate 15 mg by mouth (PO) weekly, prednisone 7.5 mg PO daily, and ibuprofen 400 mg every 4 to 6 hours as needed (Fig. 17.1).

Exam

	OD	OS
Visual acuity	20/100	20/20
Intraocular pressure (IOP)	14	14
Sclera/conjunctiva	3+ superior conjunctival injection with necrotic and avascular sclera	Diffuse scleral thinning nasally
Cornea	Moderate temporal haze without thinning	Clear
Anterior chamber (AC)	Trace cells	Deep and quiet
Iris	Unremarkable	Unremarkable
Lens	1+ nuclear sclerosis (NS) and trace posterior subcapsular cataract (PSC)	1+ NS
Anterior vitreous	Clear	Clear

Questions to Ask

- How are your joint symptoms?
- Have you had any upper or lower respiratory tract problems, including nosebleed, sinus pain, or bloody sputum?
- Any pain in your earlobes?
- Any known kidney problem?
- Have you had ocular rosacea or severe blepharitis in the past?

She states that her rheumatoid arthritis has gradually worsened despite systemic therapy, the dose of which has remained the same for the past year. She denies upper respiratory tract or pulmonary symptoms. There is no known nephropathy.

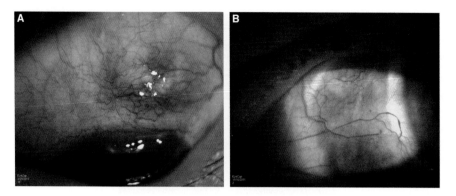

Fig. 17.1 Slit lamp photograph demonstrating actively inflamed and necrotic sclera of the right eye (A) and diffuse scleral thinning of the left eye (B).

Assessment

- Necrotizing scleritis OD with evidence of past scleritis left eye (OS)

Differential Diagnosis

- Rheumatoid arthritis
- Granulomatosis with polyangiitis (GPA, or formerly Wegener granulomatosis)
- Polyarteritis nodosa
- Systemic lupus erythematosus
- Relapsing polychondritis
- Ocular rosacea
- Atopy
- Herpesviruses
- Tuberculosis
- Syphilis

Working Diagnosis

- Necrotizing scleritis secondary to rheumatoid arthritis

Testing

- In this case, the patient had a known diagnosis of rheumatoid arthritis, so the scleritis is presumed to be related to this. However, when encountering a patient with necrotizing scleritis without known systemic disease, the following laboratory and radiographic testing should be conducted:
  - Rheumatoid factor, anti-citrulline peptide antibodies
  - Antinuclear antibodies (ANA)
  - Antineutrophil cytoplasmic antibodies (ANCA)
  - Circulating immune complexes
  - Complement levels
  - QuantiFERON, purified protein derivative (PPD)

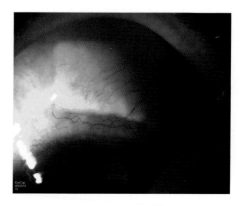

Fig. 17.2 Slit lamp photograph of the right eye after inflammatory control with aggressive immunosuppressive therapy and scleral patch surgery.

- Fluorescent treponemal antibody absorption (FTA-ABS), rapid plasma reagin (RPR)
- Herpes simplex virus (HSV) and varicella zoster virus (VZV) immunoglobulin G (IgG) and immunoglobulin M (IgM)
- Sinus and chest radiographs
- Blood urea nitrogen (BUN)/creatinine, urinalysis
- For cases resistant to antiinflammatory therapy, scleral biopsy should be considered to look for immunofluorescent staining for anti-HSV or VZV antibodies

Management

- Prednisone was increased immediately to 60 mg every day (QD)
- Methotrexate was discontinued, and intravenous cyclophosphamide commenced immediately
- Careful monitoring for scleral or corneal perforation

Follow-up

The patient's scleritis became quiescent after alkylating therapy and slow prednisone taper. Her cyclophosphamide was discontinued after 9 months, and she eventually resumed methotrexate, but at a higher dose given subcutaneously. She subsequently underwent scleral patch surgery for reinforcement (Fig. 17.2).

Key Points

- Necrotizing scleritis is a poor prognosticator for systemic disease. Its presence in rheumatoid arthritis is associated with increased cardiovascular mortalities. Therefore rheumatology should be alerted immediately so that systemic therapy can be aggressively modified.
- If necrotizing scleritis is not severe and not rapidly progressing, the first choice of therapy is antimetabolites, including methotrexate, azathioprine, and mycophenolate. Cyclosporine can be used as an adjunct therapy to the antimetabolites, but is often not effective as a monotherapy. In more recalcitrant cases, tumor necrosis factor-alpha (TNF-α) inhibitors

such as adalimumab and infliximab have both shown efficacy. In rapidly progressive cases, alkylators (cyclophosphamide, chlorambucil) or rituximab is preferred.

■ Extreme corneal thinning or perforation requires reinforcement. Donor sclera, fascia lata, periosteum, or artificial materials can be used. To maintain its integrity, the material must be covered by conjunctiva. Extreme corneal marginal ulceration or keratolysis may require corneal grafting, usually as a lamellar patch graft.

CHAPTER 18

Ebola Uveitis

Aaron Lindeke-Myers ▦ Steven Yeh ▦ Jessica G. Shantha

History of Present Illness

A 28-year-old female in Monrovia, Liberia, presents with blurry vision in both eyes (OU). She has a past medical history of Ebola virus disease (EVD) diagnosed 6 months before her initial presentation. Vision loss in the right eye (OD) occurred 3 days after discharge from an Ebola treatment unit with subsequent loss of vision in the left eye (OS). Other associated symptoms include pain, light sensitivity, and tearing OU (Fig. 18.1).

Exam

	OD	OS
Visual acuity	Hand motion	Hand motion
Intraocular pressure (IOP)	20	19
Sclera/conjunctiva	Trace injection	Trace injection
Cornea	Corneal edema, keratic precipitates	Corneal edema, keratic precipitates
Anterior chamber (AC)	1+ cell	2+ cell with hyphema
Iris	Engorged Vessels	Engorged vessels
Lens	Posterior synechiae 360 degrees	Posterior synechiae 360 degrees
Anterior vitreous	2–3+ vitritis	2–3+ vitritis

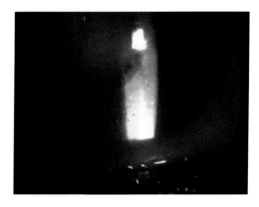

Fig. 18.1 Slit lamp photograph of the right eye shows a uveitic white cataract with corneal edema. There are keratic precipitates on the corneal endothelium. No chorioretinal lesions were noted in either eye.

Questions to Ask

- Have you had recent fever, myalgia, weight loss, headache, vomiting, diarrhea, or unexplained bleeding?
- Any recent rashes or history of sexually transmitted diseases?
- Do you have a previous history of other infections?
- Do you have a past medical history of any other illnesses?
- Did you have vision problems before you developed Ebola?

The patient answers no to all these questions. She had significant constitutional symptoms 6 months ago at the time of EVD, but those have long since resolved.

Assessment

- Panuveitis OU

Differential Diagnosis for Panuveitis

- Infectious: Ebola, syphilis, tuberculosis, toxoplasmosis
- Inflammatory
- Idiopathic
- Less likely: metastatic malignancy, primary vitreoretinal lymphoma, Chikungunya virus

Working Diagnosis

- Ebolavirus-associated panuveitis OU
- The patient had a history of EVD and presented previously with fever, headache, vomiting, and diarrhea and was positive for Ebola ribonucleic acid (RNA) by reverse transcription polymerase chain reaction (RT-PCR). There was no history of systemic herpetic disease or other infectious diseases endemic to West Africa.

Further Testing

- RT-PCR of Ebola virus via anterior chamber (AC) fluid paracentesis
- Blood for Ebola virus immunoglobulin G (IgG) antibody
- Purified protein derivative (PPD) to rule out tuberculosis and rapid plasma reagin (RPR) to rule out syphilis
- Based on review of symptoms, consider other inflammatory laboratory tests and imaging such as a chest x-ray or computed tomography (CT) chest (deferred in this case).

Management

- Difluprednate 0.05% four times a day (QID) OU to treat the anterior segment inflammation
- Prednisolone 40 mg by mouth (PO) daily with a tapering regiment for posterior segment disease

Follow-up

After acute EVD had resolved, serologies were positive for Ebola IgG and negative for human immunodeficiency virus (HIV), syphilis, and tuberculosis, leading to the diagnosis of EVD-associated panuveitis. Serologic testing may be limited in a resource-limited setting like West

Africa. The patient's symptoms improved after treatment with topical corticosteroids, although the visual acuity remained limited due to dense vitreous opacity, posterior synechiae, and cataract. Follow-up is ongoing with ophthalmologists in Monrovia.

Key Points

- Ten to thirty-four percent of EVD survivors develop uveitis at a median time of 2 to 3 months after EVD diagnosis; however, this can occur anywhere from during the acute viral infection to several months after systemic illness.
- Uveitis may be anterior, intermediate, posterior, or panuveitis.
- Relapses of uveitis may occur up to 12 months after first occurrence of Ebola-associated uveitis in up to 9% of patients with Ebola uveitis.
- Ebola-associated uveitis may cause severe vision loss and permanent blindness if untreated. However, if the uveitis is recognized early, interventions can prevent long-term vision-threatening complications from sequelae of uveitis.
- Less commonly reported Ebola-related ocular manifestations include scleritis, keratitis, and optic neuropathy.
- It is important for survivors of EVD and Marburg virus disease, a related filovirus, to receive regular eye care for up to a year after resolution of the initial infection. Individuals who develop uveitis should receive prompt treatment with corticosteroids and/or antivirals to reduce the risk of vision loss due to uveitis.
- Experimental antiviral medications (e.g., favipiravir, remdesivir) can be considered, if available with appropriate regulatory approvals. Oral favipiravir has been reported as an adjunctive therapy in the successful management of EVD uveitis.

CHAPTER 19

Iris Mass and Panuveitis in a Child

Frederick R. Blodi ▓ Aparna Ramasubramanian

History of Present Illness

A 4-year-old healthy male with no past medical history presents to the eye clinic complaining of redness of the right eye (OD) for 2 weeks. He had been placed on topical prednisolone four times a day (QID) OD without improvement.

Exam

	OD	OS
Visual Acuity	Fix and follow	Fix and follow
Intraocular pressure (IOP)	16	14
Sclera/conjunctiva	Conjunctival congestion inferiorly	White and quiet
Cornea	Clear	Clear
Anterior chamber (AC)	2+ cells 1+ flare	Deep and quiet
Iris	Posterior synechiae, iris mass at 6 o'clock (see Fig. 19.1A and B)	Unremarkable
Lens	Pigment on anterior lens surface	Clear
Anterior vitreous	2+ vitreous cell	Clear
Dilated fundus examination (DFE)	See Fig. 19.2A	See Fig. 19.2B

Anterior segment fluorescein angiography (FA), fundus FA, and optical coherence tomography (OCT) were all pursued.

Questions to Ask

- Has the patient had fevers, chills, cough, shortness of breath, joint pain/swelling/stiffness, diarrhea, blood in urine/stool, skin rashes, or oral/genital ulcers?
- Any history of weight loss?
- Any recent history of travel or contact with sick people?

The patient had a history of diarrhea several months before presentation, which resolved after 3 weeks without treatment. He and his parents replied no to all other questions.

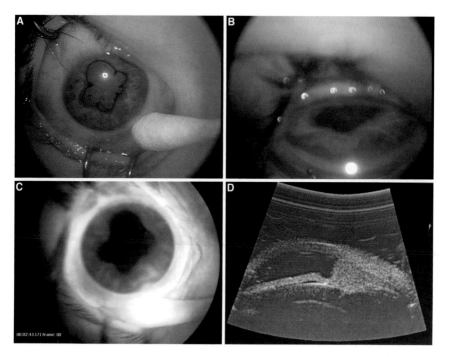

Fig. 19.1 (A) External photograph of the right eye shows multiple posterior synechiae, pigment on the anterior lens capsule, an irregular pupil, and an angle mass inferonasally. (B) A magnified view of the mass. (C) Anterior segment fluorescein angiography showed leakage from the iris mass without neovascularization of the iris. (D) Ultrasound biomicroscopy demonstrates a solid iris mass.

Assessment

- Panuveitis OD
- Angle mass OD
- Chorioretinal lesions and papillitis left eye (OS)

Differential Diagnosis

- Infectious: toxoplasmosis, toxocariasis, Lyme disease, Herpesviridae, syphilis
- Lymphoma
- Inflammatory nodule or granuloma (i.e., sarcoidosis, tuberculosis, leprosy, or other granulomatous disease)

Working Diagnosis

- Sarcoidosis or idiopathic inflammatory iris mass

Testing

- In patients with a presentation of an angle mass, such as this one, the following workup should be performed:

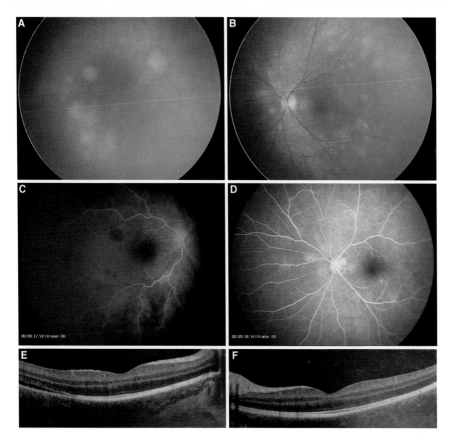

Fig. 19.2 (A) Color fundus photograph of the right eye. There are multiple chorioretinal lesions, mild vitreous hemorrhage inferiorly, and mild disc edema. (B) Color fundus photograph of left eye demonstrates multiple yellow chorioretinal lesions. (C and D) Fundus fluorescein angiography of both eyes shows early hypofluorescence and late hyperfluorescence of the chorioretinal lesions. (E) Spectral-domain OCT of the right eye shows shallow subretinal fluid temporally. (F) Spectral-domain OCT of the left eye shows no subretinal fluid.

- Complete blood count (CBC), complete metabolic panel (CMP), toxoplasmosis serologies, toxocariasis serologies, Epstein-Barri virus (EBV) serologies, antinuclear antibodies (ANA), C-reactive protein (CRP), erythrocyte sedimentation rate (ESR), angiotensin-converting enzyme (ACE), lysozyme, Lyme serology with reflex Western blot, rapid plasma reagin (RPR), fluorescent treponemal antibody absorption (FTA-ABS), antineutrophil cytoplasmic antibodies (ANCA), purified protein derivative (PPD), or QuantiFERON
- Chest x-ray
- Fine needle aspiration biopsy can be performed after retinoblastoma is ruled out, and viral polymerase chain reaction (PCR) and cytology can be performed.

Management

- Laboratory workup (see Testing) was all negative.

- Fine needle aspiration biopsy of the iris mass was undertaken. Cytology showed benign mature lymphocytes with few macrophages. Immunohistochemistry was not suggestive of lymphoma. Giemsa and acid-fast bacillus (AFB) stain was also negative on the aspirate.
- Patient was started on oral prednisone 1 mg/kg with a valacyclovir cover. PCR was not available, and hence the antiviral was started.

Follow-up

One month later, the lesions were flat at the level of the retinal pigment epithelium. Subretinal fluid had resolved. Disc edema was improving. The angle mass had resolved. The oral steroid was slowly tapered over 3 months with no recurrence of symptoms.

Final Diagnosis

- Idiopathic inflammatory mass

Key Points

- Although it is an uncommon presentation, an iris mass in children warrants a broad differential diagnosis (see Diagnostic Algorithm).
- Fine needle aspiration biopsy can be useful to rule out metastatic lesions and lesions associated with leukemia or lymphoma.
- Inflammatory granulomas are the most common and resolve with systemic immunosuppressive agents.

Diagnostic Algorithm

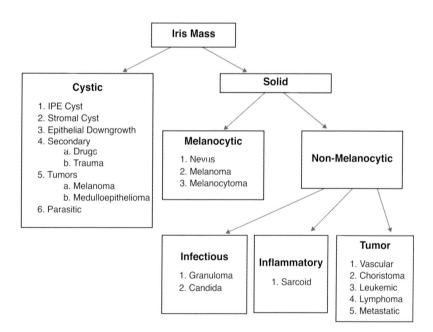

CHAPTER *20*

Toxic Anterior Segment Syndrome

Harpal S. Sandhu

History of Present Illness (HPI)

A 70-year-old woman presents for her postoperative day 1 appointment after cataract surgery right eye (OD). She underwent an uncomplicated phacoemulsification with implantation of a one-piece intraocular lens into the capsular bag. She complains of some foreign body sensation and mild discomfort but otherwise no significant pain. After taking off her shield, she immediately complains that her vision is significantly worse than before the surgery.

- Questions to ask the patient:
  - Were you told before surgery that your cataract was particularly bad or complex?
  - Were there any complications during the surgery?
- Questions for the cataract surgeon:
  - How dense was the cataract? What total phacoemulsification energy was used?
  - Were any surgical adjuvants used?
  - What prophylactic medications, if any, were used perioperatively?

Based on preoperative notes and the operative report, the cataract was described as 2 to 3+ nuclear sclerosis (NS), and the total phacoemulsification energy was not unusual. No surgical adjuvants were used during the case other than standard viscoelastics. Subconjunctival cefazolin and dexamethasone were used at the end of the case as prophylaxis. The patient reports that she was told the surgery went smoothly and that her cataract was fairly standard (Fig. 20.1).

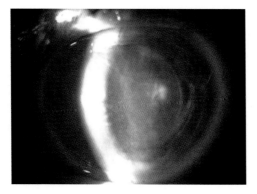

Fig. 20.1 Color slit lamp photograph of the cornea and anterior segment showing severe corneal edema from limbus to limbus and an intraocular lens in the capsular bag. (From Unal M, Yücel I, Akar Y, et al. Outbreak of toxic anterior segment syndrome associated with glutaraldehyde after cataract surgery. *J Cataract Refact Surg* 2006;32[10]:1696–1701.)

Exam

	OD	OS
Vision	20/400	20/25
IOP	29	13
Lids and lashes:	Normal	Normal
Sclera/conjunctiva:	1+ injection	White and quiet
Cornea:	See Fig. 20.1	Clear
AC:	3+ cells	Deep and quiet
Iris:	Slightly irregular pupil	Flat
Lens:	Posterior chamber intraocular lens (PCIOL)	Clear
Dilated fundus examination (DFE):	Poor view	Not performed

Assessment

Severe anterior segment inflammatory reaction immediately after cataract surgery.

Differential Diagnosis

- Toxic anterior segment syndrome (TASS) OD
- Infectious endophthalmitis OD

Testing

- B scan OD should be performed to evaluate the posterior segment, given that the fundus cannot be visualized through such severe corneal edema. B scan shows that the retina is attached and the vitreous is relatively clear.

Working Diagnosis

- TASS OD

Management

- Start intensive topical corticosteroid (e.g., prednisolone acetate 1% or difluprednate 0.05% every hour [q1h] OD, cycloplegia three times a day (TID), and intraocular pressure (IOP) control with timolol twice a day (BID) OD)
- Follow up in 1 day

Follow-up

HPI

You see the patient the following day. She notes that her vision is a bit better but still blurry. She has no pain.

Exam

	OD	**OS**
Vision	20/200	20/20
IOP	19	15
Lids and lashes:	Normal	Normal
Sclera/conjunctiva:	White and quiet	White and quiet
Cornea:	Similar corneal edema	Clear
AC:	2+ cells	Deep and quiet
Iris:	Irregular	Flat
Lens:	PCIOL	Clear

Diagnosis

- TASS
- The fact that the patient's condition has not worsened and in fact actually improved somewhat on intensive topical corticosteroid therapy alone rules out infectious endophthalmitis.

Management

- Continue present management
- Follow-up can be spaced out somewhat now that infectious endophthalmitis has been excluded

Further Follow-up

HPI

One month postoperatively, the patient follows up again after having been seen multiple times since the surgery. She notes that her vision is much improved.

Exam

	OD	**OS**
Vision	20/25	20/20
IOP	19	15
Lids and lashes:	Normal	Normal
Sclera/conjunctiva:	White and quiet	White and quiet
Cornea:	Clear	Clear
AC:	Deep and quiet	Deep and quiet
Iris:	Irregular	Flat
Lens:	PCIOL	Clear

Key Points

- TASS is a rare complication of anterior segment surgery. Prognosis is generally good, but there can be severe cases that do not resolve with medical therapy.
- Management involves intensive topical corticosteroid therapy and management of IOP. Long-term complications of refractory glaucoma and corneal decompensation are unfortunately possible.
- Unlike infectious endophthalmitis, TASS usually presents on postoperative day 1 or 2, pain is usually a minor feature or entirely absent, and there is generally little to no vitreal involvement, which can be confirmed by ultrasound.
- Patients typically present with severe "limbus-to-limbus" corneal edema, a fairly specific and dramatic finding. Anterior chamber (AC) reaction is severe and can involve fibrin in the AC and/or hypopyon. Iris ischemia results in irregular, poorly dilating pupils in some cases.
- Outside of direct patient care, investigation into possible causes in the operating room should be undertaken. Contaminated equipment, surgical adjuvants, preservatives, and heavy metals have all been implicated in TASS.
- Delayed presentations of TASS have been described, and these can be difficult to distinguish from postoperative endophthalmitis. AC tap for microbial testing is advisable in such cases.

CHAPTER 21

Pars Planitis

Harpal S. Sandhu

History of Present Illness

A 15-year-old healthy boy with no past medical history presents for the first time to the eye clinic complaining of blurred vision in his left eye (OS). He noticed some change about a month ago and now notices a significant difference between the two eyes, especially when he plays football. He also complains of floating spots in the OS (Figs. 21.1 and 21.2).

Exam

	OD	OS
Visual acuity	20/20	20/40 −
Intraocular pressure (IOP)	15	14
Sclera/conjunctiva	White and quiet	White and quiet
Cornea	Clear	Clear
AC	Deep and quiet	{1/2}+ white cells, 1+ flare
Iris	Unremarkable	Unremarkable
Lens	Clear	Clear
Anterior vitreous	Clear	1+ cells

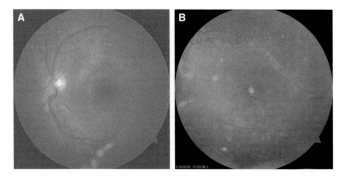

Fig. 21.1 (A) Color fundus photograph of the left eye shows hazy media consistent with vitritis and multiple snowballs. (B) Color fundus photograph of the left eye temporal to the macula shows vascular sheathing.

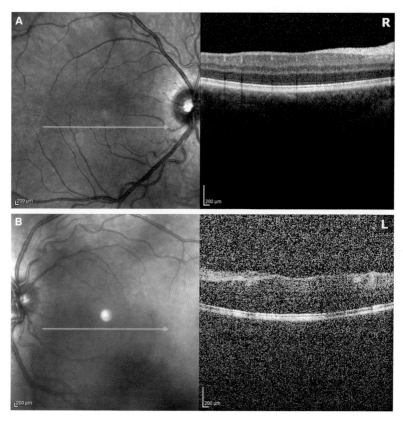

Fig. 21.2 (A) Optical coherence tomography (OCT) of the right eye shows normal macular structure and trace posterior vitreous cell. (B) OCT of the left eye shows normal macular structure without cystoid macular edema but with degraded image quality, increased hyperreflectivity of the vitreous, and posterior vitreous cells consistent with vitreal inflammation.

Questions to Ask

- Do you notice anything in the right eye (OD)?
- Have you ever had any numbness, tingling, weakness on one side of the body, or bowel or bladder problems? Is there any history of neurologic disorders in the family?
- Have you noticed any recent ticks or tick bites on your body? Do you go camping at all or spend much time outdoors?

He answers no to all of the questions.

Assessment

- Intermediate uveitis OS > OD with mild periphlebitis both eyes (OU)

Differential Diagnosis

- Pars planitis
- Sarcoid-associated intermediate uveitis

- Syphilitic intermediate uveitis
- Less likely: Lyme-associated, tuberculous-, or multiple sclerosis (MS)—associated intermediate uveitis

Working Diagnosis

- Pars planitis OU, OS > OD

Testing

- In patients with a classic presentation of pars planitis, such as this one, no further workup is necessary. This includes children and young adults presenting with predominantly vitreal inflammation out of proportion to the anterior chamber (AC) cell with or without mild periphlebitis.
- For atypical cases, check:
  - Fluorescent treponemal antibody absorption (FTA-ABS), rapid plasma reagin (RPR)
  - Lyme antibody with reflex Western blot
  - QuantiFERON or purified protein derivative (PPD)
  - Angiotensin-converting enzyme (ACE), lysozyme, and chest x-ray (CXR)
- Patients should be asked periodically on follow-up about neurologic symptoms because of the association with MS. If neurologic review of systems (ROS) is positive, perform magnetic resonance imaging (MRI) brain and orbits. Tumor necrosis factor-alpha (TNF-α) inhibitors, which can be used to treat chronic, bilateral pars planitis, are contraindicated in demyelinating disease. This patient's ROS was negative.

Management

- Sub-Tenon's triamcinolone 40 mg OS
- Follow up in 1 month

Follow-up

The patient reports nearly complete resolution of his symptoms. Vision is 20/20 OU (Figs. 21.3 and 21.4).

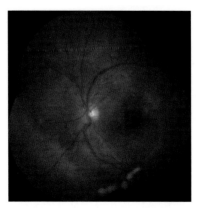

Fig. 21.3 Color fundus photograph of the left eye shows clear media and some residual snowballs.

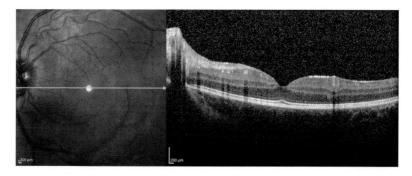

Fig. 21.4 OCT of the left eye shows normal macular structure in addition to greatly improved image quality and normal reflectivity of the vitreous, consistent with resolved vitritis.

Management Algorithm

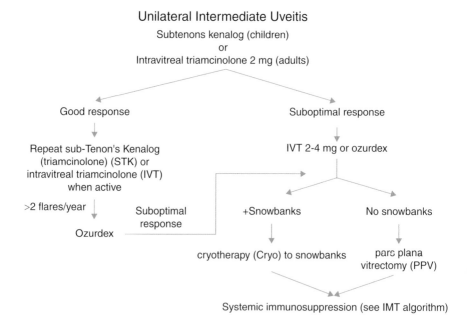

Key Points

- Pars planitis is an idiopathic inflammatory disease that localizes primarily to the vitreous and pars plana. There may be mild, associated AC inflammation, as well as retinal vascular inflammation in this entity. The disease typically starts in childhood or adolescence.

- Many patients with pars planitis can have asymmetric disease, and mild presentations, such as the OD, can frequently be monitored without therapy.
- More severe periphlebitis out of proportion to vitreal inflammation should heighten one's concern for MS. Peripheral nonperfusion can lead to neovascularization in the retinal periphery and consequent vitreous hemorrhage.
- Cystoid macular edema (CME) is the most common cause of vision loss in these patients and warrants treatment, usually with local therapy for unilateral presentations.
- Retinal tears and rhegmatogenous retinal detachment are infrequent but possible complications of pars planitis. As such, complaints of new floaters must be evaluated promptly.
- Vitrectomy with ablation of the peripheral retina is a reasonable approach to more severe cases of unilateral pars planitis, but it is unclear if bilateral vitrectomy is superior to systemic immunomodulatory therapy for bilateral disease.

CHAPTER 22

Lyme Disease

Peter Yuwei Chang ■ C. Stephen Foster

History of Present Illness

A 28-year-old male presents with gradually worsening vision and floaters in both eyes (OU) for several weeks. There is mild redness, pain, and sensitivity to light. Past medical history is unremarkable except that he recently developed joint and muscle aches after returning from a camping trip in Delaware.

Exam

	OD	OS
Visual acuity	20/50	20/40
Intraocular pressure (IOP)	12	14
Sclera/conjunctiva	Trace injection	Trace injection
Cornea	Clear	Clear
Anterior chamber (AC)	Trace cells	Trace cells
Iris	Unremarkable	Unremarkable
Lens	Clear	Clear
Anterior vitreous	2+ cells, 2+ haze	2+ cells, 2+ haze
Optic nerve	Hyperemic	Hyperemic
Macula	Flat	Flat
Vessels	Scattered sheathing (Fig. 22A)	Scattered sheathing (Fig. 22B)
Periphery	Inferior snowballs (Fig. 22.1)	Inferior snowballs

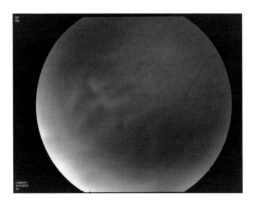

Fig. 22.1 Photograph showing snowballs in the inferior periphery of the right eye.

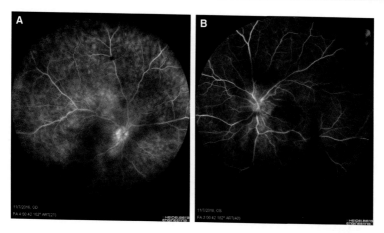

Fig. 22.2 Wide-field fluorescein angiography demonstrating optic nerve and retinal vascular leakage of the right eye (A) and the left eye (B), as well as diffuse multifocal choroidal hyperfluorescence OU.

Questions to Ask

- Do you recall any tick bite or unusual rash?
- Besides joint and muscle pain, did you have fever, malaise, or fatigue?
- Have you noticed any facial weakness? How about tingling, numbness, or weakness elsewhere in the body?
- Any cough, shortness of breath, or chest pain?

He does not recall a tick bite, but he indeed had mild fever and malaise for a week after his camping trip.

Assessment

- Intermediate uveitis with optic nerve inflammation and retinal vasculitis, OU

Differential Diagnosis

Diseases commonly associated with intermediate uveitis:
- Lyme disease
- Sarcoidosis
- Multiple sclerosis
- Syphilis
- Tuberculosis
- Whipple disease
- Pars planitis (idiopathic)

Working Diagnosis

- Lyme-associated intermediate uveitis, OU

Testing

- Enzyme-linked immunosorbent assay (ELISA) serum Lyme antibody screening, with reflex confirmatory Western blot
  - Both may be negative in the initial 2 to 4 weeks after infection, as it takes time for antibodies to develop
- For atypical cases or those that fail to improve with oral or intravenous (IV) antibiotics, consider:
  - Fluorescent treponemal antibody absorption (FTA-ABS), rapid plasma reagin (RPR)
  - QuantiFERON or purified protein derivative (PPD)
  - Angiotensin-converting enzyme (ACE), lysozyme
  - Chest x-ray or computed tomography (CT) scan
  - Magnetic resonance imaging (MRI) brain

Management

- Doxycycline 100 mg twice a day (BID) for 10 to 21 days
  - Alternatives: amoxicillin 500 mg three times a day (TID) or cefuroxime 500 mg BID for 14 to 21 days
- Neurologic involvement (including ocular disease involving the posterior segment): may need IV therapy; in Europe, oral antibiotics appear to be as effective as IV therapy for meningitis. In the United States, IV therapy is used more commonly. Antibiotic treatment for neurologic involvement is controversial and the type of antibiotic and dosages should be confirmed by a neurologic infectious disease specialist.
  - Ceftriaxone 2 g once daily
  - Cefotaxime 2 g every 8 hours (q8h)
  - Penicillin G 18 to 24 MU/day divided every 4 hours (q4h)
- Topical corticosteroids for nummular keratitis and anterior uveitis, and oral corticosteroids for posterior segment inflammation, once proper antibiotic therapy has been started

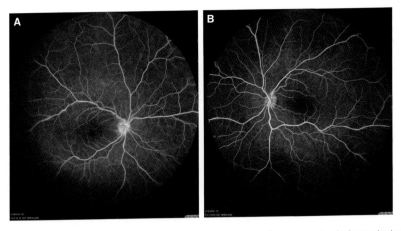

Fig. 22.3 Fluorescein angiography demonstrating resolution of the optic nerve and retinal vascular leakage, as well as vitreous opacities, of the right eye (A) and the left eye (B).

Follow-up

Because of optic nerve inflammation and affected visual acuity, the patient was started on oral doxy-cycline and prednisone concurrently. After 3 weeks, his eyes were completely quiet, with resolved optic nerve and retinal vascular leakage on fluorescein angiography. Ocular inflammation remained quiescent after corticosteroid taper.

Key Points

- Lyme disease is caused by *Borrelia burgdorferi sensu lato,* a group of spirochetes transmitted by *Ixodes* ticks. It is characterized by skin, musculoskeletal, neurologic, and cardiac manifestations.
- Endemic areas in the United States include states in the Northeast, Mid-Atlantic, and upper Midwest; Austria and Slovenia have the highest prevalence in Europe.
- Many patients do not recall tick bite.
- Lyme disease is divided into three stages:
  - Early localized stage
    - Self-limited over 3 to 4 weeks
    - Systemic: Erythema migrans (70% to 80%); fever, malaise, fatigue, myalgia, arthralgia
    - Ocular: Follicular conjunctivitis and episcleritis
  - Early disseminated stage
    - Days to weeks after tick bite
    - Systemic: Erythema migrans away from tick bite site, cranial neuropathy (with bilateral Bell palsy very characteristic of Lyme disease), peripheral neuropathy, and heart block of varying degrees
    - Ocular: Bilateral intermediate uveitis with significant vitreous inflammation is by far most common, but virtually all parts of the eye can be inflamed, ranging from keratitis to orbital inflammation
  - Late disseminated stage
    - Months to years after tick bite
    - Systemic: Chronic monoarthritis or oligoarthritis (80%), cranial neuropathies, radiculoneuritis, meningitis, encephalomyelitis, benign intracranial hypertension, encephalopathy
    - Ocular: Same as early disseminated stage
- Judicious use of topical, local, and systemic corticosteroids is appropriate as long as proper antibiotic therapy has been commenced

CHAPTER 23

Amyloidosis

Sivakumar R. Rathinam

History of Present Illness

A 27-year-old woman complained of decreased vision in both eyes (OU) for the past 30 days, which was gradual in onset and painless. She has also had numbness and a tingling sensation in both feet for about 6 months. She then developed a trophic ulcer in her right foot after painless swelling.

Exam

	OD	OS
Visual acuity	20/80	20/80
Intraocular pressure (IOP)	38	14
Sclera/conjunctiva	White and quiet	White and quiet
Cornea	Clear	Clear
Anterior chamber (AC)	Deep and quiet	Deep and quiet
Iris	Normal	Normal
Lens	Whitish deposits on posterior lens capsule (see Fig. 23.1)	Whitish deposits on posterior lens capsule (similar to Fig. 23.1)
Anterior vitreous	Vitreous opacities attached to the posterior lens capsule as pseudopodial attachments	Vitreous opacities attached to the posterior lens capsule as pseudopodial attachments

Dilated fundus examination (DFE) See Fig. 23.2

Vitreous	Vitreous membranes	
Optic disc	Cup-to-disc ration (CDR) 0.7, sharp	
Vessels	Normal	
Macula	Normal	
Periphery	Hazy, attached	Hazy, attached

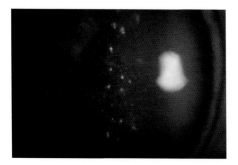

Fig. 23.1 Anterior segment photograph of the right eye showing vitreous opacities attached to the posterior lens capsule in "pseudopodial" morphology.

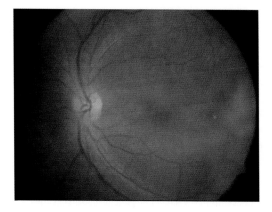

Fig. 23.2 Color fundus photograph of the left eye with dense vitreous opacities.

Questions to Ask

- Have you had floaters in either eye? Have they changed over time?
- Has anyone in your family had similar complaints?
- Any history of neurologic disorders in your family?
- Has anyone in your family had leprosy?

She responds that she has had floaters for the last 3 months that have been steadily increasing. Her brother has had a similar problem with vision and also has a foot drop. At one point, he underwent a biopsy, which was positive for amyloidosis. She has no contacts with leprosy.

Assessment

- Intermediate uveitis OU

Differential Diagnosis

- Pars planitis
- Sarcoid-associated intermediate uveitis
- Syphilitic intermediate uveitis
- Lyme disease–associated uveitis
- Multiple sclerosis with intermediate uveitis
- Vitreous amyloidosis

Working Diagnosis

- Vitreous amyloidosis due to the presence of pseudopodia lentis and close family history

Testing

- Complete blood count (CBC), rapid plasma reagin (RPR), fluorescent treponemal antibody absorption (FTA-ABS), purified protein derivative (PPD), Lyme serology, angiotensin-converting enzyme (ACE), lysozyme, and chest x-ray
- To confirm vitreous amyloidosis, a vitreous biopsy is necessary

Management

- Pars plana vitrectomy (PPV) OU with vitreous biopsy
- Topical timolol and dorzolamide three times a day (TID) right eye (OD) for secondary open angle glaucoma
- Glaucoma filtering surgery OD can be considered in the future if intraocular pressure (IOP) is not controlled

Follow-up

The patient underwent uneventful PPV OU. The patient reported nearly complete resolution of her symptoms. Vision improved to 20/40 OU. IOP declined to 19 OD. Vitreous biopsy was positive for amorphous acellular material that stained with Congo red consistent with amyloidosis (Fig. 23.3). She later underwent superficial peroneal nerve biopsy, which showed severe axonal loss and amyloid deposits stained by Congo red. All other testing was negative.

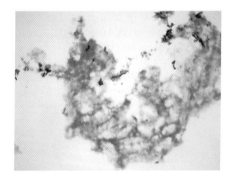

Fig. 23.3 Histopathology slide of the vitreous biopsy specimen shows amyloid deposits stained by Congo red.

Management Algorithm

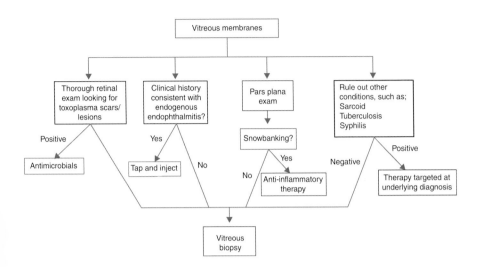

Key Points

- The well-described clinical signs of vitreous amyloidosis are pseudopodia lentis, glass wool vitreous, and retinal perivascular amyloid deposits.
- Pseudopodia lentis are distinct white opacities (foot plates) on the posterior lens capsule that can be traced further through clear vitreous into the gray-white meshwork of opacified vitreous.
- Vitreous amyloidosis is almost always related to mutant transthyretin (TTR), which is a plasma protein carrier of thyroxine and vitamin A.
- Glaucoma can occur in cases of ocular amyloidosis resulting from conjunctival and episcleral perivascular amyloid deposits, elevated episcleral venous pressure, and intratrabecular meshwork deposition.
- Mutations in the transthyretin gene have been found in familial amyloid polyneuropathy (FAP). Val130Met substitution is found to be associated most commonly with FAP.
- Vitreous amyloidosis can be the initial manifestation of FAP.
- FAP is a type of amyloidosis with autosomal dominant inheritance pattern, with incomplete penetrance and variable expressivity.
- In FAP, vitreous involvement varies between 5.4% and 35%.
- Trabecular punch biopsy can also be sent for testing amyloid deposits.
- During vitrectomy, the vitreous usually cuts like waxy paper.
- The main intraoperative challenge is to thoroughly remove the amyloidotic vitreous without causing an iatrogenic retinal break because of abnormally strong vitreoretinal adhesions in these cases.

CHAPTER 24

Retinoblastoma

Mohammad Ali Sadiq ■ Swathi Kaliki ■ Aparna Ramasubramanian

History of Present Illness

A 13-year-old boy presented with a history of decreased vision and pain in the right eye (OD) for the past 2 months. He reported a history of blunt trauma to this eye around the time his symptoms began. He had been treated for a presumed traumatic uveitis for the past 2 months.

Exam

	OD	OS
Visual acuity	20/30	20/20
Intraocular pressure (IOP)	30	18
Sclera/conjunctiva	White and quiet	White and quiet
Cornea	Deposits on the corneal endothelium mimicking keratic precipitates (see Fig. 24.1B)	Clear
Anterior chamber (AC)	Hypopyon-like layering of white material inferiorly (see Fig. 24.1A)	Deep and quiet
Iris	Unremarkable	Unremarkable
Lens	White deposits on the anterior lens capsule.	Clear
Anterior vitreous	Vitreous seeding (see Fig. 24.1D)	Clear

Dilated Fundus Examination (DFE) (See Fig. 24.1D)

Nerve:	cup-to-disc (c/d) 0.2, pink, sharp
Macula:	Normal
Vessels:	Normal caliber and course
Periphery:	Unremarkable

Questions to Ask

- Do you have any symptoms in the left eye?
- Is there any family history of cancer?
- Any previous history of medical treatment other than for traumatic uveitis?

The patient and his family respond no to all of these questions.

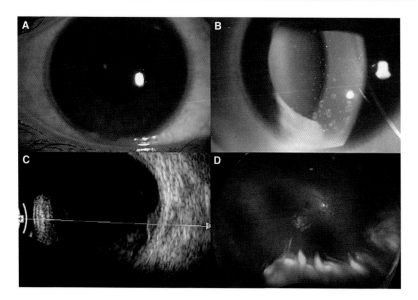

Fig. 24.1 (A) Color external photograph of the right eye shows a subtle pseudohypopyon in the anterior chamber. (B) Slit lamp photograph of the right eye reveals large white deposits on the corneal endothelium mimicking keratic precipitates. Deposits were also noted on the anterior lens capsule. These deposits are consistent with dispersed tumor cells. (C) B scan ultrasonography demonstrates an intraocular mass with calcification, with echoes in the vitreous suggestive of vitreous seeds. (D) Color fundus photograph of the right eye reveals a solid tumor mass in the inferior and inferonasal mid-periphery with diffuse vitreous seeding.

Testing

- B scan ultrasonography is essential to better characterize the mass lesion and narrow the differential (see Fig. 24.1C).

Assessment

- Anterior segment seeding OD with intraocular calcified mass and vitreous seeding

Differential Diagnosis

- Retinoblastoma
- Medulloepithelioma
- Leukemia or lymphoma
- Fungal or *Toxocara* endophthalmitis

Working Diagnosis

- Retinoblastoma with anterior segment seeding OD

Further Testing

- In patients with a typical presentation of retinoblastoma (with posterior segment findings) and anterior segment seeding, further workup for inflammatory etiologies is unnecessary.

However, in patients in whom the source of anterior segment findings is not obvious, further testing needs to be performed to evaluate for possible inflammatory etiologies. These include:

- Fluorescent treponemal antibody absorption (FTA-ABS) and rapid plasma reagin (RPR) to assess for syphilis
- Lyme antibody with reflex Western blot
- QuantiFERON or purified protein derivative (PPD) to assess for tuberculosis
- Angiotensin-converting enzyme (ACE), lysozyme, and chest x-ray to assess for sarcoidosis
- Complete blood count (CBC) to assess for leukemia
- Anterior segment and posterior segment ultrasonography to assess the presence of calcification (already performed)
- Optical coherence tomography (OCT) to assess anterior segment structures
- Magnetic resonance imaging (MRI) to assess for tumor extension outside the orbit, optic nerve invasion, or presence of a pinealoblastoma

Management

- Chemotherapy alone or in combination with intravenous, intraarterial, or intravitreal chemotherapy
- Metastatic workup (when high-risk retinoblastoma is suspected), which includes lumbar puncture, bone marrow aspiration, and bone and liver radionucleotide scans
- Genetic testing and counseling of the family regarding expectations and future management

Follow-up

The patient's inflammatory and infectious testing, CBC, and MRI were normal. The patient received six cycles of intravenous chemotherapy and eight monthly injections of intravitreal melphalan. He showed partial response to treatment with complete regression of the solid tumor, minimal decrease in vitreous seeds, and an increase in anterior chamber seeds. Right eye enucleation followed by implant placement was performed. Histopathology showed persistent retinoblastoma at the root of ciliary body, iris, and anterior chamber.

Key Points

- In any child presenting with atypical uveitis, a detailed fundus examination should be performed to look for mass lesion.
- Anterior chamber seeding in patients with retinoblastoma may present with pseudouveitis, pseudohypopyon, and increased intraocular pressure. Therefore these findings may initially be mistaken for anterior uveitis.
- Fluorescein angiography will show leakage and staining of active retinoblastoma lesions.
- A computed tomography (CT) scan can show the presence of calcifications, although this is typically avoided due to the risk of radiation exposure.
- Fine needle aspiration biopsy is avoided due to the risk of seeding; however, if all testing is inconclusive, it can be carefully performed.
- Prompt management is recommended in patients with retinoblastoma and anterior segment seeding, as it presents a high risk for metastasis.

- Treatment includes intravitreal, intraarterial, and/or systemic chemotherapy.
- Radiation treatment either with plaque brachytherapy or external beam radiation is reserved for patients who fail chemotherapy.
- Enucleation followed by histopathologic evaluation and a metastatic workup is indicated if unresponsive to conservative treatment.

CHAPTER 25

Intraocular Foreign Body and Uveitis

Henry J. Kaplan

History of Present Illness

"**CC:** I think something is in my left eye!" A backyard gate was closed with a chain and lock. The combination to the lock was lost, and so a 54-year-old man used a hammer and chisel in an attempt to break a link in the chain. After hitting the steel chisel with a hammer, he felt a sharp pain in the left eye (OS). His vision was still fairly good, and the sharp pain subsided, so he decided to wait until the next day before seeing a doctor. On awakening, he had mild discomfort OS and noticed sensitivity to light.

Exam

	OD	OS
Visual acuity	20/25	20/40
Intraocular pressure (IOP)	14	12
Sclera/conjunctiva	Clear. No injection.	Focal conjunctival injection and a small (2 mm) laceration at 9:00 near the corneal limbus.
Cornea	WNL	Clear without laceration. Few fine nongranulomatous keratic precipitate (KP) inferiorly.
Anterior chamber (AC)	No flare or cell.	1+ flare and 1+ cells
Iris	WNL	Pupil small but reactive to light and without an APD.
Lens	1+ NS	1+ NS
Vitreous cavity	Clear without vitreous cells	1+ vitreous cells
Retina/optic nerve	WNL	IOFB, ≈2 mm in diameter, lying on retinal surface just below optic disc with adjacent hemorrhage (see Fig. 25.1)

Questions to Ask

- Were you wearing glasses or protective lenses at the time of the injury?
- What was your vision like in both eyes (OU) before the accident?
- Have you had any previous eye surgery?
- Did you put any drops or ointment in your eye before visiting us?
- When was the last time you had something to eat and/or drink?
- Are you allergic to any antibiotics? Do you have other allergies?

He only wears glasses to read small print and was not wearing any protective lenses at the time of the accident. His visual acuity (VA) before the injury was 20/25 OU, and he had no history of

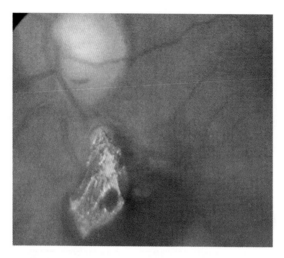

Fig. 25.1 IOFB lying on retinal surface, inferior to optic disc, OS. (From *Kanski's Clinical Ophthalmology*. Elsevier; 2016: Fig 22.28B.)

previous eye surgery. No drops or ointment were placed in his OS before the visit. He had breakfast at 8:00 AM, 8 hours ago. He is allergic to latex, but has no allergies to antibiotics.

Assessment

- Penetrating ocular injury, OS, with mild anterior uveitis

Differential Diagnosis

- Metallic intraocular foreign body (IOFB)
- Nonmetallic IOFB
- Traumatic anterior uveitis
- Idiopathic anterior uveitis

Working Diagnosis

- Metallic IOFB, OS, with traumatic anterior uveitis

Testing

- B-scan ultrasound (Fig. 25.2)
- Orbital computed tomography (CT) scan (Fig. 25.3)

Management

- A protective rigid shield, without a patch, should be placed over the OS and the patient brought to the operating room (OR) as soon as possible for surgery under general anesthesia. Simultaneous closure of the scleral laceration, pars plana vitrectomy, and removal of the metallic IOFB by either an IOFB forceps or rare earth magnet. Topical cycloplegic, corticosteroid, and antibiotic drops are instilled at the conclusion of the

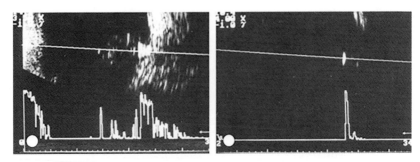

Fig. 25.2 (*Left panel*) B-scan of intraocular metallic foreign body demonstrating typical initial high spike with repetitive spikes or reverberations posteriorly. (*Right panel*) Decreasing the amplification on the B-scan eliminates all lower echo spikes, and the foreign body echo remains the sole high spike. (From Guthoff RF, Labriola LT, Stachs O. Diagnostic ophthalmic ultrasound. In S Srini Vas, ed. *Ryan's Retinal Imaging and Diagnostics*. 2013: Figure 9.32, e246.)

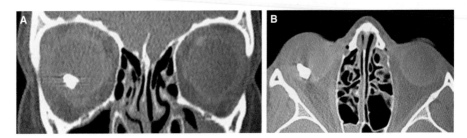

Fig. 25.3 (A) Axial and (B) coronal CT scan cuts of a different patient with intraocular metallic foreign body OD. (From *Kanski's Clinical Ophthalmology*. Elsevier; 2016: Fig 22.30B.)

procedure, as well periocular injection of an antibiotic. No need for intraocular or systemic antibiotic therapy because metal-on-metal contact produces a red hot iron foreign body with rare complication of intraocular infection.

- Patient scheduled to be seen next day.

Follow-up

- On return VA is still 20/40 OS with mild anterior uveitis. Posterior segment examination confirms removal of IOFB without operative complication. Topical cycloplegia, corticosteroid, and antibiotic therapy were continued.
- On postoperative day (POD) #7, the patient returns with improved VA of 20/25 and resolved anterior uveitis. Topical cycloplegia and antibiotics were discontinued. Topical corticosteroids were tapered over the next 2 weeks.

Key Points

- IOFB can produce a penetrating or perforating injury of the globe. A penetrating injury enters the globe and remains within the eye; a perforating injury enters and exits the globe, usually posterior to the equator.
- Intraocular surgical approach can either be simultaneous repair of laceration and removal of IOFB or initial closure of the entrance site and delayed repair, 7 to 14 days later, if there is a perforating injury or massive choroidal hemorrhage.
- When a metallic IOFB, principally iron or copper, is left in the eye, metallosis may occur, the result of oxidative damage to the tissues of the eye. A retained iron IOFB may cause

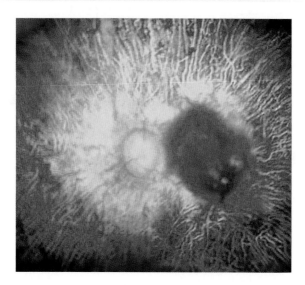

Fig. 25.4 Peripheral RPE degeneration resulting from long-standing retained iron metallic foreign body (From *Kanski's Clinical Ophthalmology*. Elsevier; 2016: Fig 22.11C and Fig 22.11D.)

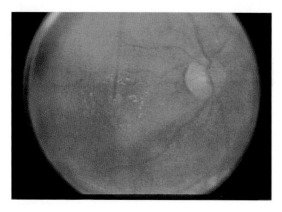

Fig. 25.5 Golden refractile spots in the macula in chronic chalcosis. (This image was originally published in the Retina Image Bank® website. Author: David Callanan. Title: Chalcosis. Retina Image Bank. Year 2014; Image Number 15750. © The American Society of Retina Specialists.)

siderosis, but only if left within the eye for months or years, causing heterochromia, peripheral retinal pigment epithelium (RPE) degeneration (Fig. 25.4) and gradual loss of vision with retinal vascular narrowing.

- In contrast, a retained copper IOFB may cause chalcosis if not removed shortly after penetration into the eye. A sterile endophthalmitis may occur acutely, or if not removed, chronic chalcosis can result in a Kayser–Fleischer ring, greenish heterochromia, sunflower cataract, and refractile deposits in the macula (Fig. 25.5).
- Prognosis is usually related to the severity of the injury and complications that may develop as a result—for example, infectious endophthalmitis, retinal detachment, hemorrhagic choroidal detachment, or proliferative vitreoretinopathy.

CHAPTER 26

Eales Disease

Marion Ronit Munk ■ Kim Anne Strässle

History of Present Illness

A 33-year-old male, born in Sri Lanka, who has lived in Switzerland since 2013, presents himself at the eye clinic complaining of vision loss for 4 months in his left eye (OS). He just returned from a holiday in Sri Lanka. When the symptoms started, he noticed blurred vision, followed by floaters and a feeling of pressure in his OS. At the time he was using a steroid cream due to psoriasis-like lesions on his extremities. He denied other health issues and had no systemic medications. In the past few weeks he was seen by two other ophthalmologists—the first prescribed a new pair of glasses, which did not help; the second diagnosed a vitreous hemorrhage in the OS.

Exam

	OD	OS
Visual acuity	20/20	20/30
Intraocular pressure (IOP)	14	15
Sclera/conjunctiva	White and quiet	White and quiet
Cornea	Arcus superior	Arcus superior
Anterior chamber (AC)	Deep, cells 0.5+	Deep, cells 0.5+
Iris	Unremarkable	Unremarkable
Lens	Clear	Clear

The vitreous showed 1+ vitreous cells right eye (OD) and vitreous hemorrhage OS. Funduscopy OD revealed intraretinal dot hemorrhages and pronounced neovascularization elsewhere (NVE). OS showed vitreous hemorrhage, intraretinal hemorrhage, and NVE (Fig. 26.1A and B, Fig. 26.2A and B, and Fig. 26.3A and B).

Questions to Ask

- Have you ever had aphthous ulcers, joint pain, or thrombosis?
- Is there any history of eye illnesses in the family?
- Were you born preterm?
- Have you had radiation in the past?
- Do you have diabetes?
- Were you ever diagnosed with sickle cell disease or anemia?

The patient denies all of these questions.

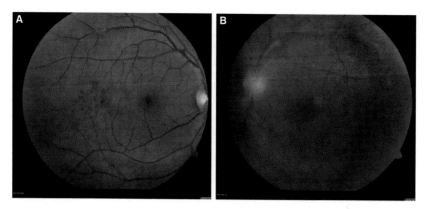

Fig. 26.1 (A and B) The vitreous showed 1 + vitreous cells OD and vitreous hemorrhage OS. Funduscopy OD revealed intraretinal dot hemorrhages and pronounced neovascularization elsewhere (NVE). OS showed vitreous hemorrhage, intraretinal hemorrhage, and NVE.

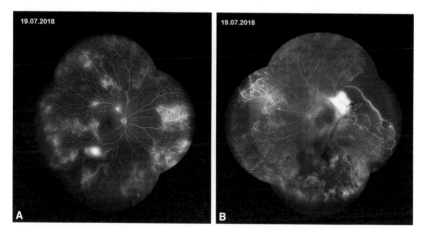

Fig. 26.2 (A and B) Wide field fluorescein angiography OU confirms NVE and depicts peripheral retinal vascular leakage and nonperfusion. There is phlebitis OS > OD and blockage due to vitreous hemorrhage OS.

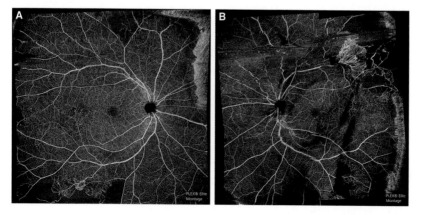

Fig. 26.3 (A and B) The montage wide field swept source/optical coherence tomography (OCT)/angiography color-coded retina slabs highlight the vascular abnormalities, including intraretinal microvascular anomalies (IRMAS), areas of flow voids, and retinal neovascularization. Image artifacts OS are due to vitreous hemorrhage.

Assessment

- Occlusive vasculitis with neovascularization and vitreous hemorrhage OS > OD of unknown origin

Differential Diagnosis

- Proliferative diabetic retinopathy both eyes (OU) with vitreous hemorrhage OS
- Retinal vascular occlusion
- Hyperviscosity sydrome
- Sarcoidosis
- Syphilis
- Tuberculosis-associated retinal vasculitis
- Eales disease
- Retinopathy of prematurity
- Familial exudative retinopathy
- Behçet disease

Working Diagnosis

- Occlusive vasculitis with neovascularization and vitreous hemorrhage OS > OD of unknown origin

Testing

Occlusive vasculitis, neovascularization, and extensive retinal ischemia need further diagnostic workup. Diabetes, sickle cell disease, hyperviscosity syndrome, and autoimmune diseases such as sarcoidosis and Behçet must be ruled out. Furthermore, infectious diseases as an underlying cause, such as tuberculosis and syphilis, must be excluded.

Laboratory and Imaging Workup

- Blood test:
  - Fluorescent treponemal antibody absorption (FTA-ABS), rapid plasma reagin (RPR): Negative
  - HbA1c: 5.6%
  - Angiotensin-converting enzyme (ACE), lysozyme, interleukin-2 (IL-2) receptor: within normal limits (WNL)
  - HLA B51: Negative
  - QuantiFERON: Positive
  - Coagulation tests: WNL
  - Differential blood count: WNL
  - Blood smear: Unremarkable
- Chest x-ray: Unremarkable
- Sputum: Negative for *Mycobacteria*

Management

Due to lack of evidence of any other underlying disease and a positive QuantiFERON test, the patient was diagnosed with Eales disease.

- OD: Panretinal laser photocoagulation (PRP)

- OS: Vitreoretinal surgery, endolaser photocoagulation, and intravitreal bevacizumab and triamcinolone
- Antituberculostatic drugs

Follow-up

During follow-up the patient developed high intraocular pressure (IOP) OS due to corticosteroid responsiveness; however, IOP was well controlled with medical treatment.

Four months after the first consultation, neovascularization OS fully regressed, symptoms resolved, and visual acuity was 20/20 OU. Due to persistent active NVE OD, the patient will receive additional PRP. Figs. 26.4 (A and B), 26.5 (A and B), and 26.6 (A and B).

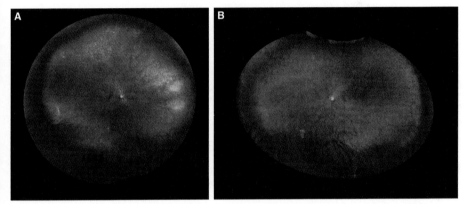

Fig. 26.4 (A) The montage wide field Optomap OD shows clear media, regressing NVE, and laser spots throughout the periphery. (B) The montage wide field Optomap OS reveals clear media, regressed NVE, laser spots throughout the periphery, and ghost vessels at the superior arcade.

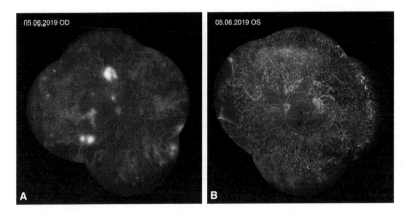

Fig. 26.5 (A and B) Wide field fluorescein angiography OD shows persistent NVE despite PRP; OS shows sufficient PRP throughout the fundus. No NVE is visible.

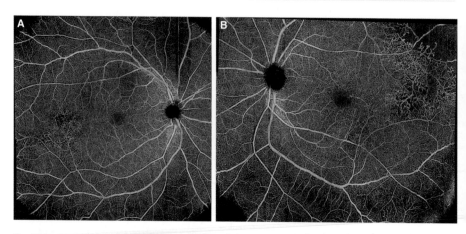

Fig. 26.6 (A and B) The montage wide field swept source/optical coherence tomography (SS/OCT)/angiography color-coded retina slabs highlight the vascular abnormalities, including IRMAS, and areas of flow voids. No retinal neovascularization is visible OD due to the smaller field of view compared with initial presentation.

Management Algorithm

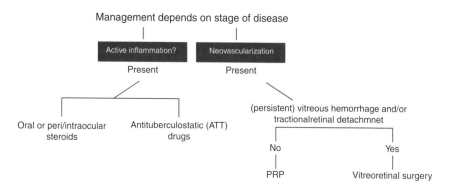

Key Points

- Eales disease is a diagnosis of exclusion, is more frequently observed in the Indian continent, and occurs mainly in young healthy males.
- It is characterized by venous inflammation, vascular occlusion, retinal neovascularization, and recurrent vitreous hemorrhages.
- The cause is unknown, the underlying etiology seems multifactorial, and it seems associated with *Mycobacterium tuberculosis,* as respective deoxyribonucleic acid (DNA) was detected in a significant number of patients using polymerase chain reaction (PCR).

- All other possible underlying conditions must be ruled out, and the patient should test positive for tuberculosis for the diagnosis to be made.
- Management depends on the stage of the disease and includes corticosteroids in the active inflammatory stage, PRP in cases of retinal neovascularization, and vitreoretinal surgery in cases of (persistent) vitreous hemorrhage and tractional retinal detachment.
- The role of antituberculosis therapy (ATT) is controversial.

CHAPTER 27

Posterior Scleritis

Christopher Conrady ■ Albert Vitale

History of Present Illness

A 75-year-old female with past medical history significant for hypertension, chronic kidney disease, and a prior carotid endarterectomy of the left internal carotid presented with acute-onset blurry vision, tearing, eye pain, and redness of the right eye (OD).

Exam

	OD	OS
Visual acuity	20/25 – 2	20/20 – 2
Intraocular pressure (IOP)	14	14
Sclera/conjunctiva	White and quiet	White and quiet
Cornea	Clear	Clear
Anterior chamber (AC)	Deep and quiet	Deep and quiet
Iris	Unremarkable	Unremarkable
Lens	Clear	Clear
Anterior vitreous	Clear	Clear
Posterior segment	Choroidal folds	Within normal limits

Because of the finding of choroidal folds, optical coherence tomography (OCT) and ultrasound were performed (Figs. 27.1 and 27.2).

Questions to Ask

- Do you have ocular pain, with or without eye movement?
- Do you have an associated systemic rheumatic disease, autoimmune disease, or systemic vasculitis or is there any family history of such diseases?
- Do you have any sinus issues, including epistaxis?
- Do you have a history of a sexually transmitted disease or exposure to other infectious diseases?
- Do you have a history of ocular or systemic neoplastic disease?

She answers yes to ocular pain with and without eye movement. Otherwise, she answers no.

Assessment

- Unilateral posterior scleritis OD

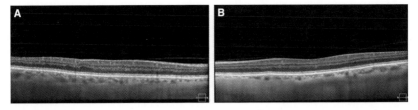

Fig. 27.1 Optical coherence tomography (OCT). (A) Enhanced-depth OCT of the right eye shows normal macular structure but significant choroidal thickening. (B) Enhanced-depth OCT of the left eye shows normal macular structure and normal choroid.

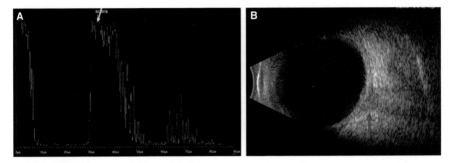

Fig. 27.2 Ultrasonography. (A) A-scan identified scleral thickening (*yellow arrow*), whereas (B) B-scan ultrasonography identified sub-Tenon's fluid consistent with a "T-sign" (*red arrow*) of the right eye. Left eye was unremarkable (images not shown).

Systemic Disease Associations

- Rheumatoid arthritis
- Granulomatous polyangiitis
- Polyarteritis nodosa
- Ankylosing spondylitis
- Psoriasis
- Systemic lupus erythematous
- Sarcoidosis
- Tuberculosis
- Syphilis

Differential Diagnosis

- Choroidal tumor (melanoma, hemangioma, metastasis)
- Orbital neoplasia (immunoglobulin G [IgG] 4—related disease)
- Annular ciliochoroidal detachment
- Exudative retinal detachment
  - Choroidal neovascularization (CNVM)
  - Central serous chorioretinopathy (CSCR)
  - Vogt-Koyanagi-Harada disease (VKH) (bilateral posterior scleritis)
- Uveal effusion syndrome

Working Diagnosis

- Idiopathic posterior scleritis OD

Testing

- In patients with classic presentations, such as the woman described here, testing for systemic rheumatologic, autoimmune, and noninfectious diseases should be undertaken to identify potentially treatable conditions that might affect systemic health, morbidity, and mortality, as well as to exclude infectious diseases before the introduction of systemic treatment with steroids or immunomodulatory therapy (IMT).
- For most cases check:
  - Fluorescent treponemal antibody absorption (FTA-ABS), rapid plasma reagin (RPR)
  - Purified protein derivative (PPD) or QuantiFERON gold
  - Rheumatoid factor, anti-cyclic citrullinated peptide antibody (CCP)
  - Cytoplasmic antineutrophil cytoplasmic antibodies (cANCA) and perinuclear antineutrophil cytoplasmic antibodies (pANCA) with myeloperoxidase (MPO)/proteinase 3 (PR-3) antibodies
  - Antinuclear antibodies (ANA)
  - Angiotensin-converting enzyme (ACE), lysozyme, and chest x-ray
  - HLA-B27
  - Complete blood count (CBC), complete metabolic panel (CMP)
- Patients should be periodically asked about the development of associated symptoms, such as joint pain, sinus issues/epistaxis, shortness of breath, and skin rashes.

Management

- Oral prednisone taper once the results of infectious laboratory tests have returned (60 mg for 2 weeks then 50 mg, 40 mg, 35 mg, 30 mg, 25 mg, 20 mg, 15 mg, 10 mg, and 5 mg for 1 week each)
- Follow up in 1 month with repeat ultrasonography
- Refer to rheumatology if associated systemic autoimmune disease is identified during workup

Follow-up

The patient follows up 1 month later. She reports nearly complete resolution of her symptoms. Vision is 20/25 both eyes (OU) (Fig. 27.3).

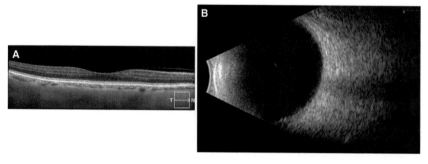

Fig. 27.3 (A) OCT identified resolution of choroidal thickening and (B) B-scan ultrasonography showed complete resolution of sub-Tenon fluid of the right eye. Left eye was unremarkable (images not shown).

Management Algorithm

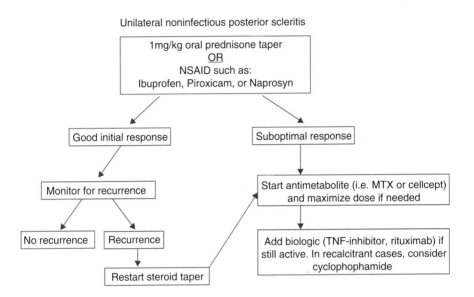

Unilateral noninfectious posterior scleritis

1mg/kg oral prednisone taper
OR
NSAID such as:
Ibuprofen, Piroxicam, or Naprosyn

Good initial response

Suboptimal response

Monitor for recurrence

Start antimetabolite (i.e. MTX or cellcept) and maximize dose if needed

No recurrence

Recurrence

Add biologic (TNF-inhibitor, rituximab) if still active. In recalcitrant cases, consider cyclophophamide

Restart steroid taper

Key Points

- Posterior scleritis represents 10% of all cases of scleritis and is twice as common in women as in men.
- Although idiopathic posterior scleritis is more common overall, systemic disease associations are much more likely in patients over the age of 50.
- Moderate to severe pain is the hallmark of presentation and may be associated with orbital signs, including extraocular motility disturbances and proptosis.
- Early diagnosis and treatment control posterior scleral inflammation and limit vision loss.
- If disease relapses or is difficult to control with oral steroids, corticosteroid-sparing IMT should be instituted beginning with an antimetabolite such as methotrexate or mycophenolate mofetil (CellCept) and then advancing to a biologic such as infliximab, adalimumab, or rituximab as needed. In recalcitrant cases, a cytotoxic agent such as cyclophosphamide should be considered.
- Posterior scleritis may occur in isolation but is not infrequently associated with anterior scleritis. Anterior uveitis, optic disc swelling/hyperemia, and subretinal fluid may also be observed.
- Underlying systemic rheumatologic conditions, autoimmune conditions, and infectious conditions should always be excluded and treated, given their potential to significantly affect patient morbidity and mortality.

KEY IMAGING MODALITIES FOR DIAGNOSIS

- **B-scan ultrasonography**: Scleral thickening, nodularity, pathognomonic T-sign due to fluid collection within sub-Tenon's/posterior episcleral space with extension around optic nerve.
- **Enhanced-depth OCT**: Increased choroidal thickness, subretinal fluid.
- **Fluorescein and indocyanine green angiography**: Useful in distinguishing posterior scleritis from entities presenting with subretinal fluid or neurosensory detachments (CSCR, CNVM, VKH)

CHAPTER 28

Multifocal Choroiditis with Panuveitis

Harpal S. Sandhu

History of Present Illness

A 25-year-old woman with no past medical history and a long-standing history of myopia presents for the first time to the eye clinic complaining of distorted vision in her right eye (OD). She first noticed that her vision was a little blurry about a month ago, which also coincided with more floaters than she is used to. She had assumed that these symptoms were insignificant and would resolve, but then 2 weeks later she noticed a grayed-out area of vision paracentrally OD, so she decided to present to the eye clinic.

Exam

	OD	OS
Visual acuity	20/40	20/20
Intraocular pressure (IOP)	18	19
Sclera/conjunctiva	White and quiet	White and quiet
Cornea	Clear	Clear
Anterior chamber (AC)	2+ white cells 1+ flare	Deep and quiet
Iris	Unremarkable	Unremarkable
Lens	Clear	Clear
Anterior vitreous	2+ white cells	Clear

Dilated Fundus Examination (DFE) (See Fig. 28.1)

Nerve	Cup-to-disc (c/d) 0.1, peripapillary
atrophy	
Macula	Lacquer cracks
Vessels	Normal caliber and course
Periphery	Unremarkable

Questions to Ask

- Have you noticed anything in the left eye (OS)?
- Have you had any recent illnesses or hospitalizations?

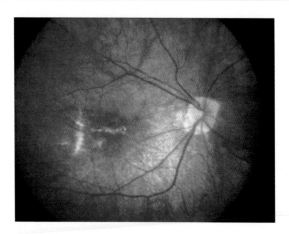

Fig. 28.1 Color fundus photograph of the right eye shows lacquer cracks and a small submacular hemorrhage. There were no peripheral lesions. (Modified from Schroeder K, Meyer-ter-Vehn T, Fassnacht-Riederle H, Guthoff R. Course of disease in multifocal choroiditis lacking sufficient immunosuppression: A case report. *J Med Case Rep* 2016;10:298.)

- Are you having or have you recently had any other symptoms in the rest of your body, such as joint pains, new rashes, breathing problems, problems with bowel movements, or oral or genital ulcers?
- Have you had any tick bites recently?
- Have you ever traveled outside the country?
- Have you had any trauma or surgery to the eye?
- Do you use injection drugs?
- Do you practice safe sex?
- What is your glasses prescription?

The patient answers no to the first seven questions. She has always used barrier protection during sex. She hands over her glasses, and the Rx is $-9.00 +0.75 \times 180$ OD, $-8.50 +0.50 \times 145$ OS.

Fluorescein angiography (FA) and optical coherence tomography (OCT) were pursued to further investigate the cause of metamorphopsia and subretinal hemorrhage (Fig. 28.2).

Assessment

- Panuveitis with occult multifocal choroiditis (MFCPU) by angiography OD
- Choroidal neovascularization OD
- High myopia OU with secondary lacquer cracks

Differential Diagnosis

- Idiopathic
- Sarcoidosis
- Syphilis
- Less likely: tuberculosis, atypical *Mycobacteria*, subacute fungal infection

Working Diagnosis

- Noninfectious MFCPU, but rule out infectious causes before starting therapy.

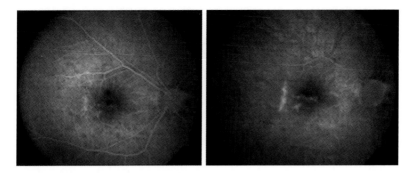

Fig. 28.2 Fluorescein angiogram of the right eye shows early hyperfluorescence in the area of the lacquer crack, as well as multiple hypofluorescent spots in areas where there were no funduscopically visible lesions (*left panel, early frame*), suggestive of occult choroiditis. In the late frame (*right panel*), the area of early, discrete hyperfluorescence has increased in size and intensity, suggestive of choroidal neovascularization. OCT OD (*not shown*) confirmed the presence of shallow subretinal fluid. (Modified from Schroeder K, Meyer-ter-Vehn T, Fassnacht-Riederle H, Guthoff R. Course of disease in multifocal choroiditis lacking sufficient immunosuppression: A case report. *J Med Case Rep* 2016;10:298.)

- The patient has no risk factors for common infectious causes of multifocal choroiditis, nor is she immunosuppressed. Her young age, female gender, and myopic refraction are classic for idiopathic MFCPU.

Testing

- FA and OCT already performed, as noted earlier
- Indocyanine green (ICG) (not performed) is a superior test for identifying areas of choroiditis
- Check fluorescent treponemal antibody absorption (FTA-ABS), rapid plasma reagin (RPR), QuantiFERON or purified protein derivative (PPD), angiotensin-converting enzyme (ACE), lysozyme, and chest x-ray (CXR)

Management

- Start prednisone 60 mg by mouth (PO) daily once infectious laboratory tests are negative
- Prednisolone acetate 1% four times a day (QID) OD, cyclopentolate 1% twice a day (BID) OD
- Defer anti–vascular endothelial growth factor (VEGF) treatment for now, as new inflammatory choroidal neovascularization (CNV) will often respond to antiinflammatory therapy
- Follow up in 2 weeks

Follow-up

The patient has the appropriate diagnostic tests performed, all of which are negative. However, she does not return to the clinic as scheduled in 2 weeks, nor does she reschedule.

She returns 8 months later complaining of severe loss of vision OD. She admits that she never started the prednisone, as prescribed, and only used the eye drops intermittently. However, she is now very concerned about her vision (Figs. 28.3 and 28.4).

Exam

	OD	OS
Visual acuity	20/200	20/29
IOP	14	18
Sclera/conjunctiva	White and quiet	White and quiet
Cornea	Clear	Clear
AC	2+ white cells 1+ flare	1+ white cells 1+ flare
Iris	Posterior synechiae	Unremarkable
Lens	1+ Posterior subcapsular cataract (PSC)	Clear
Anterior vitreous	2+ white cells	1+ white cells

DFE See Fig. 28.5

Nerve	c/d 0.1, peripapillary
atrophy	
Macula	Lacquer cracks, multiple
atrophic spots	
Vessels	Normal caliber and course
Periphery	Multiple punched-out spots
	Throughout the fundus

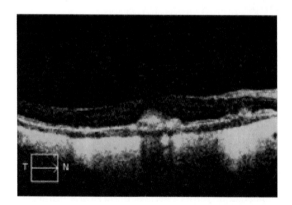

Fig. 28.3 OCT of the right eye shows hyperreflective subfoveal material, which can represent either an active inflammatory lesion or choroidal neovascularization. (Modified from Schroeder K, Meyer-ter-Vehn T, Fassnacht-Riederle H, Guthoff R. Course of disease in multifocal choroiditis lacking sufficient immunosuppression: A case report. *J Med Case Rep* 2016;10:298.)

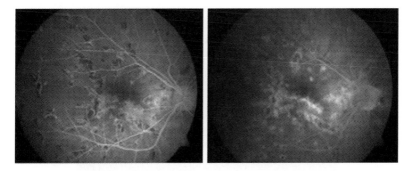

Fig. 28.4   Early (*right panel*) and late (*left panel*) phase FA shows many more lesions, most of which block early, but some of which are hyperfluorescent early due to retinal pigment epithelium (RPE) window defects. There is late staining of several of the lesions in the nasal macula. (Modified from Schroeder K, Meyer-ter-Vehn T, Fassnacht-Riederle H, Guthoff R. Course of disease in multifocal choroiditis lacking sufficient immunosuppression: A case report. *J Med Case Rep* 2016;10:298.)

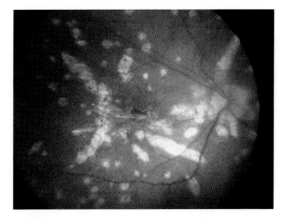

Fig. 28.5   Color fundus photograph of the right eye shows multiple atrophic spots of varying sizes, morphology, and degrees of pigmentation throughout the macula. (Modified from Schroeder K, Meyer-ter-Vehn T, Fassnacht-Riederle H, Guthoff R. Course of disease in multifocal choroiditis lacking sufficient immunosuppression: A case report. *J Med Case Rep* 2016;10:298.)

Assessment

- MFCPU OU, worsening
- High myopia OU

Management

- Start prednisone 60 mg PO daily and topical prednisolone acetate 1% BID both eyes (OU) and Cyclogyl 1% OU every day

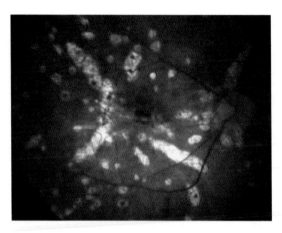

Fig. 28.6 Color fundus photograph of the right eye shows no new lesions in the posterior pole. The only change was variable degrees of pigmentation. (Modified from Schroeder K, Meyer-ter-Vehn T, Fassnacht-Riederle H, Guthoff R. Course of disease in multifocal choroiditis lacking sufficient immunosuppression: A case report. *J Med Case Rep* 2016;10:298.)

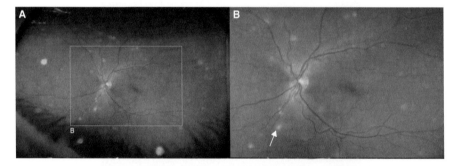

Fig. 28.7 An example of infectious multifocal choroiditis secondary to disseminated *Mycobacterium chimaera* in a cardiothoracic surgery patient. Note the deep, active, multifocal, inflammatory lesions throughout the fundus in the left-hand panel (A). The right-hand panel (B) is a magnified image of the posterior pole. (From Zweifel SA, Mihic-Probst D, Curcio CA et al. Clinical and histopathologic ocular findings in disseminated Mycobacterium chimaera infection after cardiothoracic surgery. *Ophthalmology* 2017;124[2]:178–188.)

Follow-up

The patient's anterior chamber and vitreal inflammation resolved, and vision improved to 20/100 OD and 20/25 OS. As prednisone was slowly tapered to zero over 7 months, mycophenolate mofetil 1000 mg PO BID and adalimumab 40 mg subcutaneous (SC) q2 weeks were added, and the disease remained quiescent (Fig. 28.6). Reactivated CNV necessitated multiple treatments with intravitreal bevacizumab 1.25 mg/0.05 cc, but these became inactive about 6 months after initiating therapy.

Key Points

- MFCPU is an inflammatory disease of unknown cause characterized by multiple chorioretinal lesions throughout the fundus of varying size that can eventually number in the hundreds.

- Active chorioretinal lesions appear gray-yellow and become more "punched-out" with varying degrees of pigmentation as they become inactive. Sometimes subretinal fibrosis will develop at the site of a lesion or will bridge two lesions.

- The chorioretinal scars of punctate inner choroidopathy (PIC), pathologic myopia, and presumed ocular histoplasmosis syndrome (POHS) can sometimes appear similar to MFCPU. However, the latter is readily distinguished from these three by active anterior chamber or vitreal inflammation, or their sequelae.

- PIC, MFCPU, and the subretinal fibrosis with uveitis syndrome share multiple overlapping features and may represent a single disease with varying degrees of severity.

- Multiple infectious diseases can present as MFCPU, including atypical *Mycobacteria* (Fig. 28.7) and endogenous bacterial and fungal endophthalmitis. A careful history aimed at identifying risk factors for infection (see "Questions to Ask" earlier) is essential.

- CNV is a common structural complication of the disease, arising in about 40% of cases, and is the main cause of vision loss.

- Treatment is aimed at controlling inflammation and treating CNV. Local and systemic corticosteroids are the mainstays of treatment, and systemic immunomodulatory therapy (IMT) is frequently needed. Whereas photodynamic therapy was used in the past for this complication, anti-VEGF therapy is now the treatment of choice for CNV secondary to MFCPU.

CHAPTER 29

Common Variable Immunodeficiency with Granulomatous Panuveitis

Henry J. Kaplan

Cutaneous nodules, granulomatous uveitis and oligoarthritis in child

History of Present Illness

A 5-year-old girl presented with a complaint of red eye and blurred vision left eye (OS) for the past 4 months. She had a history of pneumonia at 4 years of age, which required hospitalization. Shortly afterward she developed a swollen, painful right knee and left interphalangeal joint. For the past 6 months, erythematous, plaquelike, and scaly lesions were observed on her right hand (Fig. 29.1), buttocks, and feet.

Exam

	OD	OS
Visual acuity	20/20	20/40
Intraocular pressure (IOP) (mm Hg)	12	10
Sclera/conjunctiva	Within normal limits (WNL)	No ciliary injection.
Cornea	WNL	Diffuse mutton fat keratic precipitate (KP) on the inferior half of corneal endothelium
Anterior chamber (AC)	WNL	2+ flare, 2+ cell
Iris	WNL	One Koeppe nodule on the pupillary margin (Fig. 29.2)
Lens	Clear	Clear
Vitreous cavity	WNL	2+ vitritis
Retina/optic nerve	WNL	Mild perivasculitis extending to the periphery

Questions to Ask

- When you had pneumonia, were you evaluated for an underlying systemic disease?
- Have you had infections other than in your lungs?

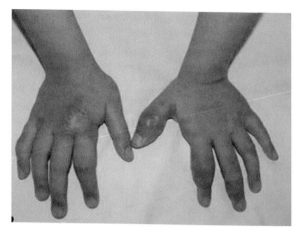

Fig. 29.1 Cutaneous erythematous, plaquelike, and scaly lesions on both hands. (From Artac H, Bozkurt B, Talim B, Reisli I Sarcoid-like granulomas in common variable immunodeficiency. *Rheumatol Int.* 2009;30: 109–112.)

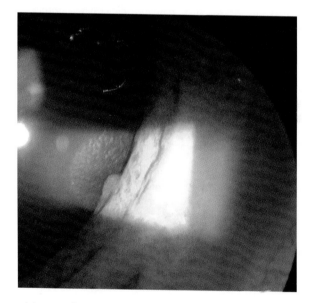

Fig. 29.2 Koeppe nodule on pupillary margin.

- Have you been examined by an eye doctor for anterior uveitis associated with oligoarthritis (i.e., juvenile idiopathic arthritis [JIA])?
- Have you detected any swollen lymph nodes on your neck, upper chest, or groin?

During her hospitalization for pneumonia, the patient was noted to have hypogammaglobulinemia and reduced B lymphocytes in her blood. Additionally, previous vaccinations for tetanus and diphtheria were determined to be nonprotective. Since then, she has had recurrent episodes of otitis media that required treatment with systemic and topical antibiotics. An eye doctor examined her within the past 6 months and did not see intraocular inflammation in either eye. Her mother has noticed some swollen lymph nodes in the patient's neck and groin.

Assessment

- Granulomatous panuveitis OS, associated with multiorgan involvement (lung, ear, skin, and lymph nodes)

Differential Diagnosis

- Systemic immune deficiency disorder
- Sarcoidosis
- Masquerade syndromes (leukemia, lymphoma)
- Infectious granulomatous uveitis (tuberculosis [TB], syphilis, herpesviruses, Lyme, borreliosis, brucellosis)
- JIA and uveitis

Working Diagnosis

- Granulomatous panuveitis OS, with multiorgan involvement (lung, ear, skin, lymph nodes) secondary to a systemic immune deficiency disorder (common variable immunodeficiency [CVID])

Testing

- Laboratory evaluation:
  - Hypogammaglobulinemia (IgG, IgA, IgM, IgE)
  - Complete blood count (CBC), erythrocyte sedimentation rate (ESR), antinuclear antibodies (ANA), antineutrophil cytoplasmic antibodies (ANCA), rheumatoid factor, antistreptolysin O (ASO)
  - Lymphocyte profile
  - Decreased CD20 count; otherwise, normal lymphocyte profile
- Computed tomography (CT) chest: no signs of lymphadenopathy or nodular opacities
- Biopsy of cutaneous lesion: noncaseating granulomas, with fibrinoid collagen degeneration surrounded by histiocytes and leukocytes

Management

- Uveitis was treated with topical corticosteroid (e.g., prednisolone acetate suspension 1%, OS, every 4 to 6 hours [q4–6h]) and cycloplegia (cyclopentolate hydrochloride 0.5%, 1 gtt, twice a day [BID] OS)
- CVID symptoms treated with intravenous (IV) immunoglobulin infusions, ibuprofen, and prophylactic antibiotics
- Consultation with the following services: dermatology, rheumatology, and infectious disease
- Follow up 1 week after hospital discharge

Key Points

- CVID is a syndrome characterized by various degrees of hypogammaglobulinemia. Autoimmunity is common with a sarcoid-like disorder affecting many different organ systems (skin, bowel, lymph nodes, lungs, liver, kidney bone marrow, and central nervous system [CNS]).

- JIA is the most common cause of anterior uveitis in children and is only rarely associated with panuveitis. The differential diagnosis of pediatric panuveitis includes Behçet disease, Vogt—Koyanagi—Harada syndrome, Lyme disease, cat scratch disease, masquerade syndromes (leukemia, lymphoma, retinoblastoma), sarcoidosis, Jabs/Blau syndrome, and tubulointerstitial nephritis and uveitis (TINU).

- Children are a challenging group of patients because it is difficult to elicit history and that contributes to a delay in diagnosis and treatment, where structural damage has already occurred. Thus early implementation of aggressive medical treatment is frequently required.

- Endogenous syndromes that are most prevalent in children and associated with ocular disease include JIA, Kawasaki syndrome, Jabs/Blau syndrome, and TINU.

- Childhood uveitis is usually chronic or recurrent and difficult to control. Treatment is complicated because of possible growth retardation with the use of corticosteroids and susceptibility to amblyopia in the pediatric population. Despite a lower incidence of uveitis in children, the rate of visual loss is worse than in adults.

- JIA-associated uveitis comprises up to 47% of pediatric uveitis, with both intermediate uveitis and panuveitis contributing around 20% each. The most common causes of pediatric uveitis based on anatomic classification are JIA (anterior uveitis), pars planitis (intermediate uveitis), and *Toxoplasma* retinochoroiditis (posterior uveitis).

CHAPTER 30

Sarcoidosis

Henry J. Kaplan

History of Present Illness

A 34-year-old African American female complains of decreasing vision in both eyes (OU) over the past year, with no previous history of ocular disease. She denies ocular redness, pain, or photophobia. However, she does complain of a dry mouth and mild dyspnea when walking up four flights of stairs. Her past history is otherwise unremarkable.

Exam

	OD	OS
Visual acuity	20/60	20/40
Intraocular pressure (IOP) (mm Hg)	12	10
Sclera/conjunctiva	No injection. Solitary nodular granuloma in inferior fornix	No injection
Cornea	Multifocal keratic precipitates (MF KP) (Fig. 30.1), with interstitial keratitis inferiorly	Diffuse MF KP with mild interstitial keratitis
Anterior chamber (AC)	2+ flare, 3+ cell	2+ flare, 2+ cell
Iris	Posterior synechiae intermittently for 360 degrees Anterior synechiae from 4:00 to 7:00	Posterior synechiae at 3:00 and 7:30
Lens	3+ PSC	1+ PSC
Vitreous cavity	3+ vitritis with string of pearls	2+ snowball opacities
Retina/optic nerve	Granulomas on optic nerve head (Fig. 30.2), with retinal periphlebitis and candle wax drippings (Fig. 30.3)	Mild swelling of optic nerve head with periphlebitis

Questions to Ask

- Did you notice a sudden change in vision or did it develop gradually (insidiously)?
- What did you notice first: your change in vision or your dry mouth/dyspnea?
- Have you noticed any plaquelike skin lesions on your face?
- Have you noticed any problem with walking, muscle weakness, paresthesia, or any other sign of central nervous system (CNS) disease?
- Have you detected any swollen lymph nodes on your neck, upper chest, or groin?

Vision OU worsened gradually over the past year. She stated that visual acuity (VA) changes occurred first, and it was not until recently that her other complaints developed. There are plaquelike lesions on both eyelids. Her gait is slightly unsteady but otherwise she has not noticed a change

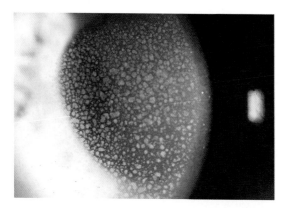

Fig. 30.1 Mutton fat KPs diffusely distributed over corneal endothelium.

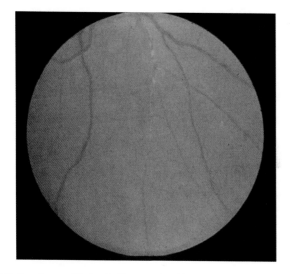

Fig. 30.2 Periphlebitis (candle wax drippings) without periarteritis.

in muscle weakness, paresthesia, or any other neurologic problem. She has not noticed any swollen lymph nodes on her neck, upper chest, or groin.

Assessment

- Granulomatous panuveitis OU, with secondary complications, including conjunctival granuloma, posterior subcapsular cataract (PSC), vitritis, perivasculitis, and optic nerve granuloma, right eye greater than left eye (OD > OS)

Differential Diagnosis

- Ocular sarcoidosis

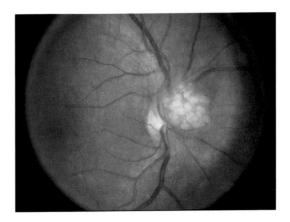

Fig. 30.3   Optic disc granuloma OD.

- Other causes of granulomatous uveitis (tuberculosis [TB], syphilis, herpesviruses, Vogt–Koyanagi–Harada syndrome, leukemia, lymphoma, Hodgkin disease, brucellosis)
- Metastatic carcinoma

Working Diagnosis

- Ocular sarcoidosis OU, OD > OS

Testing

- Biopsy of conjunctival granuloma, OD
- Histology revealed noncaseating granulomas.
- Pulmonary imaging (x-ray, if negative computed tomography [CT] scan)
  - Ninety percent or more of systemic sarcoidosis patients have thoracic disease, so it is the most useful test unless histologic biopsy can confirm the diagnosis.
  - Bilateral hilar lymphadenopathy present on chest x-ray.

Management

- Oral prednisone (0.75 mg/kg), as well as a topical corticosteroid (e.g., prednisolone acetate suspension 1%) every 4 hours (q4h) OU while awake. Corticosteroids are the mainstay of treatment for both ocular and systemic disease.
- Topical cyclopentolate hydrochloride 0.5%, 1 qtt, OU twice a day to four times a day (BID to QID)
- Follow up in 2 weeks

Follow-up

The patient returns 2 weeks later. VA has only changed slightly (20/50 OD, 20/30 OS); however, mutton fat (MF) keratic precipitates (KPs) are starting to resolve, retinal perivasculitis is much less, and no change in optic nerve granuloma in either eye.

- Start slow taper of oral prednisone, decrease topical prednisolone acetate to QID, and discontinue topical cycloplegia.
- Return appointment in 2 weeks.

Key Points

- Sarcoidosis is a multisystem inflammatory disease characterized by noncaseating granulomas in involved tissues, primarily presenting as bilateral hilar lymphadenopathy and/or pulmonary parenchymal disease.
- Diagnosis of ocular sarcoidosis, without other organ involvement, is difficult. Anterior chamber (AC) paracentesis of the aqueous humor and identification of multinucleated giant cells is strongly suggestive of the diagnosis.
- Similarly, serum angiotensin-converting enzyme (ACE), lysozyme, hypercalcemia/hypercalciuria, and gallium-67 scans are not diagnostic but can be helpful ancillary tests.
- Ocular involvement is common, second only to pulmonary disease, and may present more than a year before systemic disease.
- Ocular disease has an insidious onset and is a common presentation for granulomatous panuveitis.
- Corticosteroids are the mainstay of therapy and can be administered topically, periocularly, intravitreally, or systemically to resolve the complications of intraocular inflammation.
- Chronic ocular inflammation can result in complications involving the anterior segment (anterior/posterior synechiae, trabeculitis, PSC cataract), vitreous (vitritis, string of pearls), and posterior segment (cystoid macular edema (CME), perivasculitis, candle wax drippings, granulomatous infiltration of choroid and optic nerve).

CHAPTER 31

Punctate Inner Choroidopathy (PIC)

Henry J. Kaplan

History of Present Illness

A 39-year-old woman with no significant past medical history presents to the eye clinic for the first time complaining of blurred central vision right eye (OD), with photopsias and a central blind spot (scotoma) of 1 week duration.

Exam

	OD	OS
Visual acuity	20/60	20/20
Intraocular pressure (IOP)	11	10
Sclera/conjunctiva	Within normal limits (WNL)	WNL
Cornea	Clear	Clear
AC	No cell or flare	No cell or flare
Iris	WNL	WNL
Lens	Mild nuclear sclerosis	Mild nuclear sclerosis
Vitreous cavity	No cells	No cells
Retina/optic nerve	Normal optic nerve. Several punctate chorioretinal lesions within the arcades and paramacular (Fig. 31.1)	Normal optic nerve. No punctate chorioretinal lesions within the arcades

Questions to Ask

- Have you had any recent infection or systemic illness?
- Have you had an episode like this before in either eye?
- Are you near-sighted and have you had any corrective surgery for near-sightedness?
- Do you have metamorphopsia in your left eye (OS)?

She has no recent respiratory infection or systemic illness. She does not recall having an episode like this in either eye. She does not wear glasses because she had laser in situ keratomileusis (LASIK) surgery, but she was moderately myopic (−4.00) both eyes (OU). There is no distortion or metamorphopsia in either eye.

Assessment

- Multifocal punctate chorioretinal lesions, OD, with presumed focal chorioretinitis OD

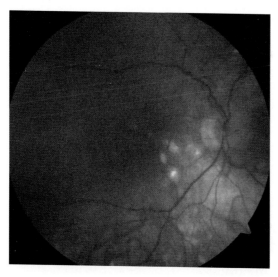

Fig. 31.1   Several punctate chorioretinal lesions within the arcades and paramacular area OD.

Differential Diagnosis

- Punctate inner choroidopathy (PIC)
- Multifocal choroiditis with panuveitis (MFCPU)
- Multifocal choroiditis with subretinal fibrosis (MFC-subretinal fibrosis)
- Multiple evanescent white dot syndrome (MEWDS)
- Sarcoidosis

Working Diagnosis

- PIC, OU, with focal chorioretinitis OD

Testing

- The presentation of punctate chorioretinal scars, ≤ {1/4} of disc diameter in size, within the vascular arcades and without vitritis or anterior chamber (AC) inflammation is diagnostic of PIC. Confirmatory tests such as spectral domain optical coherence tomography (SD-OCT) and fluorescein angiography (FA) should be performed to rule out the presence of a choroidal neovascularization (CNV) complex within the macula and to identify the presence of chorioretinitis, OD. Fundus autofluorescence (FAF) can also be helpful in documenting the progression of the disease, as hypofluorescent spots are an indicator of RPE death or absence, whereas hyperfluorescent spots are an indicator of increased lipofuscin.
- FAF (Fig. 31.2)
- SD-OCT (Fig. 31.3)
- FA/indocyanine green (ICG) (Fig. 31.4A and B)

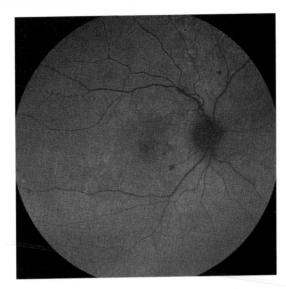

Fig. 31.2 Fundus autofluorescence of a patient with PIC demonstrating multiple hypoautofluorescent lesions (inactive disease).

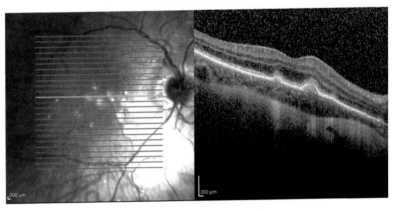

Fig. 31.3 SD-OCT demonstrating stage 3 lesions forming a chorioretinal hump beneath the RPE with moderate reflectivity breaking through the outer retinal layers.

Management

- No immediate treatment is provided because most patients with PIC and without CNV have excellent visual outcomes without intervention. However, if visual acuity (VA) remains decreased and CNV is absent, a trial with corticosteroid injection can be considered.

Follow-up

The patient is seen at 2 weeks and monthly thereafter with a rapid improvement in VA to 20/25 and the admonition to check her eyes weekly with an Amsler grid. Six months later, she returns with a complaint of decreased VA and metamorphopsia OD. She still has no symptoms OS.

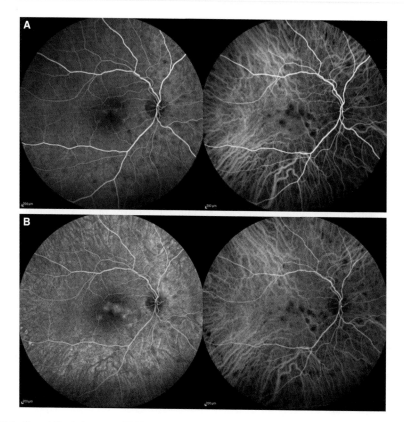

Fig. 31.4   (A and B) arteriovenous (AV) (*top*) and late phase (*bottom*) FA/ICG demonstrating hyperfluorescent lesions on FA and hypocyanescent lesions on ICG.

Follow-up Examination

VA decreased to 20/60 OD with metamorphopsia on Amsler grid, and OS remains 20/20. On examination there is a dirty gray submacular membrane with subretinal blood OD, unchanged examination OS.

Follow-up Assessment

The patient has developed a CNV membrane OD, which is responsible for decreased vision, metamorphopsia, and fundus appearance. Approximately 40% of eyes with PIC will develop this complication and is the reason patients are given an Amsler grid for weekly examination of their eyes.

Working Diagnosis 2

- CNV, OD secondary to PIC

Management

- CNV in PIC, and most forms of uveitis, can be successfully treated with an intravitreal injection of anti—vascular endothelial growth factor (VEGF) medication, such as bevacizumab.

The patient is followed every 4 to 6 weeks, and if the neovascularization has not resolved or has recurred, the injection is repeated.

Follow-up

The patient returns 2 weeks after the anti-VEGF intravitreal injection with improved VA to 20/30 and resolution of metamorphopsia OD.

Key Points

- PIC is a multifocal chorioretinitis that usually is confined within the vascular arcades and is not associated with vitritis or AC inflammation. There are some specialists who believe that PIC, MFCPU, and panuveitis with subretinal fibrosis are different manifestations of the same disease process. However, because the etiology of these three diseases is unknown, it would seem preferable to characterize them as originally described until a definitive etiology is established.
- Although most patients with PIC present with a complaint of unilateral vision problems, it is not uncommon to find characteristic focal chorioretinal scars in the other eye within the vascular arcades, although the patient has not noticed any symptoms.
- Whereas acute posterior multifocal placoid pigment epitheliopathy (APMPPE) and MEWDS will frequently be associated with a viral prodrome or systemic illness, PIC is not.
- The preponderance of patients are women, Caucasian, and moderately myopic (-4D average). However, the reason for this triad is unknown.
- CNV in PIC occurs anterior to the retinal pigment epithelium (RPE), so that surgical removal of neovascularization within the macula in this disease had a favorable prognosis before the advent of anti-VEGF medical therapy. In contrast, in age-related macular degeneration where the membrane is beneath the RPE, as well as possibly above it, the prognosis was guarded.
- Active inflammation in a parafoveal PIC lesion without CNV causing decreased vision warrants antiinflammatory intervention with corticosteroids.

CHAPTER 32

Acute Posterior Multifocal Placoid Pigment Epitheliopathy (APMPPE)

Henry J. Kaplan

History of Present Illness

A 21-year-old college student was studying for finals in May and noticed a sudden decrease in vision in both eyes (OU). He had never experienced visual problems before and recently finished studying for the Medical College Admission Test (MCAT), so he wondered whether his symptoms were the result of stress. He is athletic and on the college basketball team.

Exam

	OD	OS
Visual acuity	20/80	20/100
Intraocular pressure (IOP) (mm Hg)	10	11
Sclera/conjunctiva	Clear. No injection	Clear. No injection
Cornea	Clear	Clear
Anterior chamber (AC)	No cell or flare	No cell or flare
Iris	Normal	Normal
Lens	Clear	Clear
Vitreous cavity	No vitreous cells	No vitreous cells
Retina/optic nerve	Multiple yellowish, flat, creamy-colored placoid lesions in the posterior pole (Fig. 32.1). Normal optic nerve	Retinal lesions similar to those OD

Questions to Ask

- Have you had pain, redness, or floaters in either eye?
- Have you had any illness within the past 6 to 8 weeks?
- Did you experience transient hearing loss at the time of the flu?

He denies a history of pain, redness, or floaters in either eye. However, about 4 weeks ago he had the flu but has improved considerably. He had meningismus (stiff neck), slight hearing impairment, and occasional headaches while ill. However, they have almost totally resolved.

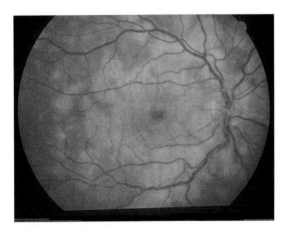

Fig. 32.1 Multiple yellow, creamy-colored placoid lesions, flat in posterior pole, OD. (This image was originally published in the Retina Image Bank website. Authors: Henry J Kaplan, Niloofar Piri. Title: Acute Posterior Multifocal Placoid Pigment Epitheliopathy. Retina Image Bank. Year; 2013. Image Number.4995 © the American Society of Retina Specialists.)

Assessment

- White dot syndrome, with loss of central vision, OU

Differential Diagnosis

- Acute posterior multifocal placoid pigment epitheliopathy (APMPPE)
- Serpiginous chorioretinitis
- Relentless placoid chorioretinitis
- Persistent placoid maculopathy
- Choroidal vasculitis (lupus, polyarteritis nodosa)

Working Diagnosis

- APMPPE, OU

Testing

- Diagnosis is made based on the appearance of the retinal lesions and course of the disease. Laboratory testing is only indicated when signs of central nervous system (CNS) involvement are present.
- Fluorescein angiography (FA): hyperfluorescence of placoid lesions in the early phase, with staining in the late phase (Fig. 32.2)
- Spectral domain optical coherence tomography (SD-OCT): disruption of the ellipsoid layer in the outer retina, with hyperreflectivity from the placoid lesions (Fig. 32.3)
- Optical coherence tomography angiography (OCTA): patchy areas of choriocapillaris ischemia associated with clinical lesions (Fig. 32.4)

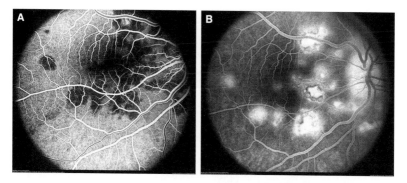

Fig. 32.2 (A) Early arteriovenous (AV) phase fundus fluorescein angiography (FFA) demonstrates multiple hypofluorescent placoid patches. (B). Late phase angiogram demonstrates hyperfluorescent lesions. (These images were originally published in the Retina Image Bank website. Authors: Henry J Kaplan, Niloofar Piri. Title: Acute Posterior Multifocal Placoid Pigment Epitheliopathy, Fluorescein angiography. Retina Image Bank. Year; 2013. Image Number.4994, 5012 © the American Society of Retina Specialists.)

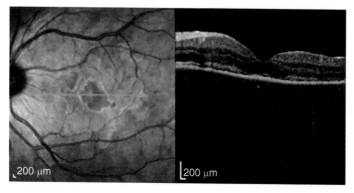

Fig. 32.3 SD-OCT demonstrating disruption of the ellipsoid layer in the outer retina, with hyperreflectivity from the placoid lesions

Management

- APMPPE is usually self-limiting and nonrecurrent, so no treatment is generally provided. However, if the patient is severely handicapped, a trial of oral prednisone is a reasonable alternative.
- The patient is scheduled to return in 2 and 6 weeks to ensure that vision has not further deteriorated. If vision does not improve or deteriorates by 6 weeks, consideration of oral prednisone is reasonable.

Follow-up

Vision gradually improves by 2 weeks and is now 20/30 right eye (OD) and 20/40 left eye (OS). Over the ensuing 6 weeks, some new placoid lesions develop, but other lesions resolve with a hypopigmented center and pigment clumping on the periphery. All lesions are posterior to the equator.

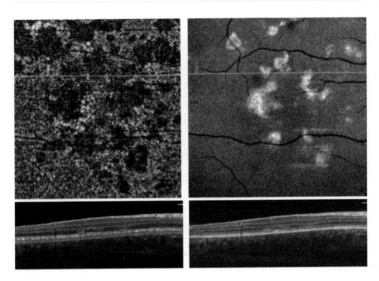

Fig. 32.4 OCTA segmentation of choriocapillaris demonstrates decreased flow in area corresponding to retinal lesions on FAF. (Image credit: Michael A Klufas, Nopasak Phasukkijwatana, Nicholas A Lafe, et al. Optical Coherence Tomography Angiography Reveals Choriocapillaris Flow Reduction in Placoid Chorioretinitis. *Ophthalmol Retina.* 2017;1:77-91.)

Key Points

- A viral prodrome may be associated with the development of APMPEE, but is not a necessary antecedent. Cerebral vasculitis has been associated with APMPEE, and neurologic evaluation with a lumbar puncture (i.e., for cerebrospinal fluid [CSF] pleocytosis), should be strongly considered with persistent signs of CNS involvement.
- Predilection for healthy young adults, affecting men and women equally, peak occurrence between ages of 20 and 40. It has primarily been observed in Caucasians, but can present in dark-pigmented racial groups.
- Visual prognosis is generally good (20/25 to 20/40), although involvement of the central macula usually results in residual complaints from the patient. Recurrences of the disease are unusual.
- Most cases are bilateral, but unilateral cases can occur. Patients may complain of photopsia, as well as central or paracentral scotomas.
- The pathogenesis of APMPPE is unknown, and so it is characterized as an autoimmune disease. However, several systemic conditions have been associated with this disease, including erythema nodosum, sarcoidosis, tuberculosis (TB), Lyme disease, and mumps.

CHAPTER 33

Multiple Evanescent White Dot Syndrome (MEWDS)

Henry J. Kaplan

History of Present Illness

A 25-year-old woman developed a "flulike" illness 4 weeks ago. In the past 48 hours she suddenly developed painless loss of vision in the left eye (OS) without redness or photophobia. She noticed a small blind spot and shimmering lights (photopsias) in her temporal visual field. The night before her loss of vision, she attended a party and snorted cocaine for the first time.

Exam

	OD	OS
Visual acuity	20/20	20/80
Intraocular pressure (IOP) (mm Hg)	11	10
Sclera/conjunctiva	Clear. No injection	Clear. No injection
Cornea	Clear	Clear
Anterior chamber (AC)	No cell or flare	No cell or flare
Iris	Normal	Normal
Lens	Clear	Clear
Vitreous cavity	Clear	Trace vitreous cells
Retina/optic nerve	Normal	Small white dots, deep in retina (Fig. 33.1A), with hyperemia, trace optic disc edema, and foveal granularity (Fig. 33.1B)

Questions to Ask

- Have you had sudden visual loss in either eye before now?
- Have you fully recovered from the flu—namely, do you still have malaise, lethargy, or tiredness?
- Have you been diagnosed with a blood or bone marrow disorder in the past?
- Are you being treated for any systemic disease affecting other organs?

Her answer to each question is "no," except although she has recovered from the flu, she still has mild malaise.

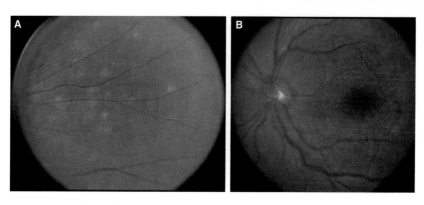

Fig. 33.1 (A) Temporal paramacular retina with white dots, OS. (B) Foveal granularity, hyperemia, and trace optic disc edema, OS.

Assessment

- White dot syndrome OS

Differential Diagnosis

- Multiple evanescent white dot syndrome (MEWDS)
- Punctate inner choroidopathy (PIC)
- Multifocal choroiditis (MFC)
- Lymphoma or other bone marrow disorder
- Sarcoidosis
- Infectious retinitis
- Central/branch retinal artery occlusion secondary to cocaine use

Working Diagnosis

- MEWDS with trace optic disc edema, OS

Testing

Diagnosis of the white dot syndromes is usually based on the classic fundus appearance. Thus although the differential diagnosis suggests other possible causes, laboratory testing is usually confined to ocular functional and imaging studies. Snorting of cocaine can cause unilateral central/branch retinal artery occlusion, which can result in severe visual loss, but the fundus appearance in this patient is not consistent with this diagnosis.

- Humphrey visual field (HVF): enlarged blind spot, OS; normal right eye (OD)
- Fluorescein angiography (FA): late retinal punctate staining, frequently in a wreathlike pattern, OS (Fig. 33.2)
- Indocyanine green chorioangiography (ICGA): multiple prominent foci of choroidal nonperfusion
- Spectral domain optical computed tomography (SD-OCT): disruption of the ellipsoid layer in the fovea and hyperreflective multifocal debris, OS (Fig. 33.3)

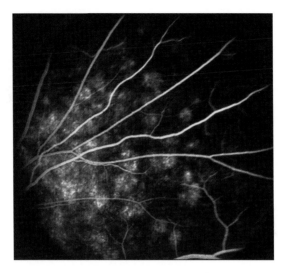

Fig. 33.2   Wreathlike pattern of hyperfluorescence in late arteriovenous (AV) phase.

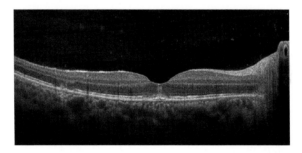

Fig. 33.3   SD-OCT demonstrating disruption of ellipsoid zone and hyperreflective debris corresponding to deep retinal white spots. (From Vânia Lages, Alessandro Mantovani, Marina Papadia, Carl P Herbort MEWDS is a true primary choriocapillaritis and basic mechanisms do not seem to differ from other choriocapillaritis entities. *J Curr Ophthalmol.* 2018;30:281–286.)

Management

- MEWDS is a self-limited disease, so no treatment is indicated. If there is persistent or worsening loss of vision, a diagnostic laboratory evaluation should be considered.
- Patient is scheduled to return in 1 month.

Follow-up

- One month later the patient's visual acuity (VA) has gradually improved and is now 20/30. The white dots in the retina have faded and optic disc edema has resolved.
- She still notices a temporal scotoma and flashing lights (photopsias), but they have not increased.

Key Points

- A key characteristic of MEWDS is that it occurs in the young, has a female predominance, usually presents unilaterally, and may have a viral prodrome. Anterior chamber (AC) inflammation may be observed but is mild. Vitritis is seen in ≈ 50% of cases.
- Unless the patient is seen in the acute phase of the disease, the multiple white dots in the retina will have disappeared; thus the name of the disease includes "evanescent." Recurrences of the disease are unusual, as is involvement of the other eye (i.e., bilateral disease).
- Visual prognosis is good even with recurrences, unless there is the rare development of choroidal neovascularization (CNV).
- A targeted workup to rule out treatable infectious or inflammatory diseases such as syphilis, tuberculosis (TB), and sarcoidosis should be considered if the natural history of the disease is unusual.
- Very rare association of MEWDS with acute zonal occult outer retinopathy (AZOOR), as well as vaccination, has been reported.

CHAPTER 34

Serpiginous Choroidits

Henry J. Kaplan

History of Present Illness

A 68-year-old man presents with 2-week history of painless unilateral loss of vision in the left eye (OS). He noticed a paracentral scotoma OS, and while hunting with a shotgun just realized that he has no central vision right eye (OD). He denies photophobia, photopsia, or floaters in either eye.

Exam

	OD	OS
Visual acuity	5/400	20/40
Intraocular pressure (IOP) (mm Hg)	11	11
Sclera/conjunctiva	Clear. No injection	Clear. No injection
Cornea	Clear	Clear
Anterior chamber (AC)	No cell or flare	No cell or flare
Iris	Normal	Normal
Lens	Clear	Clear
Vitreous cavity	Clear. No cells	Trace cells
Retina/optic nerve	See Fig. 34.1. Serpiginous chorioretinal scars originating from optic disc and extending to midperipheral retina.	See Fig. 34.2. A chorioretinal scar within the macula and extending along the superotemporal (ST) arcade. Creamy subretinal lesions are noticed at the inner margin.

Questions to Ask

- Has your vision been tested within the past few years?
- What is your general health? Have you been diagnosed with a systemic disease?
- Have you had ocular trauma to either eye that required surgery or visit to an emergency room?
- Have you traveled to an area of the country with a history of fungal disease?

His visual acuity (VA) was not tested within the past few years, and he did not notice any visual problem until recently. He denies a history of a systemic or autoimmune disease. There is no history of ocular trauma to either eye that required surgery or a visit to an emergency room. He has lived in the Ohio Valley most of his life and occasionally traveled to the Southwest United States.

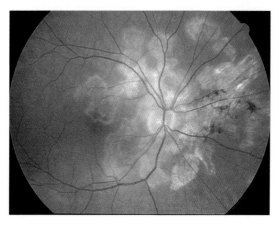

Fig. 34.1 Gray-white, serpentine, deep chorioretinal scars extending from the optic nerve centrifugally, including the fovea. Notice RPE hyperplasia nasally. (This image was originally published in the Retina Image Bank website. Authors Henry J Kaplan, Niloofar Piri. Title. Serpiginous choroiditis. Retina Image Bank. Year; 2013 Image Number. 4883 © the American Society of Retina Specialists.)

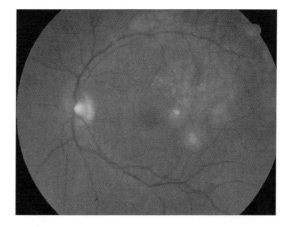

Fig. 34.2 Serpentine chorioretinal lesion originating along the superotemporal arcade and extending to the macula with creamy subretinal lesions at the margin temporal to the fovea, suggestive of active disease.

Assessment

- Chorioretinitis, remote OD and acute OS, unknown etiology

Differential Diagnosis

- Acute posterior multifocal placoid pigment epitheliopathy (APMPPE)
- Relentless placoid chorioretinitis
- Persistent placoid maculopathy

- Infectious retinitis (tuberculosis [TB], outer-layer retinal toxoplasmosis, syphilis)
- Presumed ocular histoplasmosis syndrome (POHS)
- Multifocal choroiditis (MFC)
- Sarcoid choroiditis

Working Diagnosis

- Serpiginous choroiditis, both eyes (OU)—remote OD, acute OS
  - A bilateral asymmetric disease that affects healthy patients from the second to seventh decade and presents with unilateral loss of vision and characteristic peripapillary serpiginous chorioretinal lesions. Diagnosis is made by the typical clinical appearance and history.

Testing

- Laboratory results: Venereal Disease Research Laboratory/rapid plasma reagin (VDRL/RPR), fluorescent treponemal antibody absorption (FTA-ABS), QuantiFERON—TB Gold In-Tube test (QFT-GIT), and chest x-ray are all normal.
- Fundus fluorescein angiography (FFA) (Fig. 34.3) to identify the active edge of the acute lesion and to rule out choroidal neovascularization (CNV), which may develop adjacent to the active edge of the lesion.
- Other tests are not necessary to establish the diagnosis but are useful in documenting the anatomic status of the retina and choroid in this disease (e.g., spectral domain optical coherence tomography [SD-OCT], optical coherence tomography angiogram [OCTA], indocyanine green chorioangiography [ICGA], fundus autofluorescence [FAF])

Management

- Triple immunomodulatory therapy (IMT) is the mainstay of treatment, with prednisone, cyclosporine, and azathioprine used most frequently in the acute phase of the disease. After complete resolution of the acute phase, chronic therapy with an immunosuppressive drug (e.g., azathioprine, methotrexate, or mycophenolate mofetil) should be continued to prevent recurrent disease. Tumor necrosis factor-alpha (TNF-α) inhibitors may be

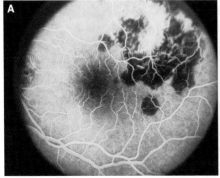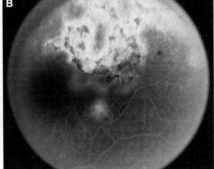

Fig. 34.3 Fluorescein angiography of the same eye in early (A) and late arteriovenous (AV) phase (B), demonstrating a late increase in hyperfluorescence with indistinct borders (leakage) at the margin of the lesion suggestive of active disease.

considered if there is no history of exposure to TB, blood testing for TB is negative, and the patient objects to conventional immune suppression.

- Follow up in 2 weeks and monthly thereafter, with tapering and discontinuation of systemic prednisone and cyclosporine, with maintenance of a chronic IMT regimen, as mentioned earlier.

Follow-up Care

Acute chorioretinitis OS starts to resolve at 2 weeks and by 3 months is totally inactive while on chronic IMT.

Two years after initial presentation, the patient returns with a sudden change in VA OS. The patient's chronic IMT was changed by rheumatology to methotrexate with discontinuation of azathioprine.

Working Diagnosis

Recurrent serpiginous choroiditis, OS—rule out CNV

Testing

- FFA: To demarcate the extent of choroiditis and to rule out CNV OS. Subfoveal CNV is observed on fluorescein angiography (FA) with extension of the border of chorioretinitis.

Management

- Patient is treated with anti–vascular endothelial growth factor (VEGF) intravitreal injections to resolve CNV and restarted on original chronic IMT treatment regimen.
- Follow up in 1 month and monthly thereafter.

Follow-up

- The patient returns with resolution of CNV at 1 month and is maintained on chronic IMT. If CNV returns, repeat intravitreal anti-VEGF therapy will be administered.

Key Points

- Serpiginous choroidopathy (SC) is a rare, chronic, progressive, asymmetric, bilateral inflammatory disease involving the retinal pigment epithelium (RPE), choriocapillaris, and choroid. It is characterized by irregular, gray-white or yellowish subretinal infiltrates that have a serpentine pattern frequently originating from the optic disc. Occasionally isolated lesions begin elsewhere in the retina.
- Because the lesions are painless and associated with very little inflammation in the anterior chamber (AC) or vitreous cavity, patients will often present only when the second eye is involved and have end-stage SC in the contralateral eye.
- Initiation of triple therapy and then chronic IMT, before the loss of central vision, can result in very good visual results and suppression of recurrent disease.
- Tuberculous SC can resemble idiopathic SC confined to the macula, but is associated with more vitritis, and multifocal retinal lesions are usually seen in the far periphery. Diagnostic evidence of TB infection is required, and antituberculosis therapy should be implemented.

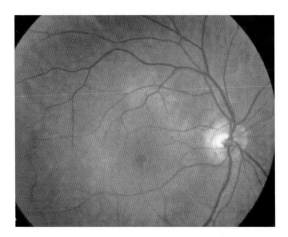

Fig. 34.4 Fundus photograph of a patient with persistent placoid maculopathy demonstrating white, deep, plaquelike lesion in the posterior pole. He had a similar lesion in the left eye. (From Pamela R Golchet, Lee M Jampol, David Wilson, Lawrence A Yannuzzi, Michael Ober, Edward Stroh Persistent placoid maculopathy: a new clinical entity. *Ophthalmology*. 2007;114[8]:1530–1540.)

■ Persistent placoid maculopathy is a bilateral, symmetric disease affecting elderly patients. In contrast to SC, patients develop decreased vision OU, with photopsias. White plaquelike retinal lesions (Fig. 34.4) involving the fovea resemble macular SC, because they are not contiguous with the optic disc. Central VA is initially preserved, although decreased, but visual prognosis is poor because of recurrent CNV. The effect of IMT on disease prognosis is not known.

■ Relentless (ampiginous) placoid chorioretinitis and APMPPE should also be considered in the differential diagnosis.

CHAPTER 35

Relentless (Ampiginous) Placoid Chorioretinitis

Henry J. Kaplan

History of Present Illness

A 62-year-old man noticed difficulty shooting his rifle when looking through the mount with his left eye (OS) 1 week ago. Over the next few days he observed floaters and paracentral scotomas OS. Since then he has been testing his vision and noticed that similar changes have occurred in the right eye (OD). He had no history of systemic illness and was otherwise in good health.

Exam

	OD	OS
Visual acuity	20/23	20/84
Intraocular pressure (IOP) (mm Hg)	10	11
Sclera/conjunctiva	Clear. No injection	Clear. No injection
Cornea	Rare nongranulomatous (NG) keratic precipitates (KPs)	Rare NG KPs
Anterior chamber (AC)	1+ cell, trace flare	1+ cell, trace flare
Iris	Normal	Normal
Lens	Clear	Clear
Vitreous cavity	Trace vitreous cells	Trace vitreous cells
Retina/optic nerve	Similar to OS	See Fig. 35.1. Creamy white lesions in outer retina <{1/2} disc area extending to periphery, with more than 50 lesions throughout the fundus

Questions to Ask

- Have you had acute visual loss in either eye before?
- Have you experienced a flulike illness with malaise, lethargy, or tiredness?
- Have you been diagnosed with a blood or bone marrow disorder in the past?
- Are you being treated for any systemic disease affecting other organs?

The patient denies a previous history of acute visual loss, as well as any prodromal illness. He recently underwent a complete annual examination and is in good health with normal complete blood count (CBC) and urinalysis.

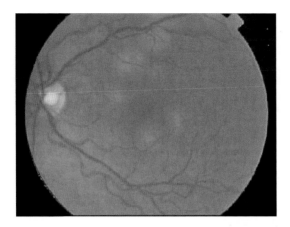

Fig. 35.1 Creamy white spots in outer retina, <{1/2} disc area, in posterior pole, OS. (Image credit: Mirza RG, Jampol LM. Relentless placoid chorioretinitis. *Int Ophthalmol Clin*. 2012;52(4):237–242.)

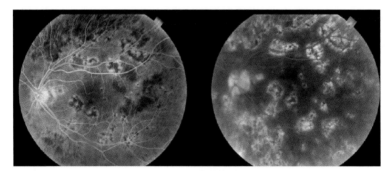

Fig. 35.2 Early fluorescein angiography (FA) after creamy white spots have progressed demonstrates hypofluorescent lesions, especially in the center. Late FA demonstrates hyperfluorescence resulting from staining of the lesions. (Image credit: Mirza RG, Jampol LM. Relentless placoid chorioretinitis. *Int Ophthalmol Clin*. 2012;52(4):237–242.)

Assessment

- White dot syndrome, both eyes (OU), with lesions distributed throughout the retina. Over the ensuing weeks, some of the lesions enlarged and others resolved (Fig. 35.2).

Differential Diagnosis

- Acute posterior multifocal placoid pigment epitheliopathy (APMPPE)
- Serpiginous choroiditis
- Persistent placoid maculopathy (PPM)
- Relentless placoid maculopathy
- Multifocal choroiditis (MFC; idiopathic, hematologic, syphilis, sarcoidosis, tuberculosis [TB])

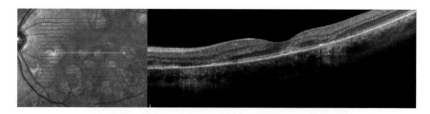

Fig. 35.3 SD-OCT demonstrates subfoveal ellipsoid zone irregularity associated with hyperreflectivity in the outer retina associated with active lesions. Nasal outer layer disruption is related to older atrophied lesions. (Image credit: Michael A Klufas, Nopasak Phasukkijwatana, Nicholas A Iafe, Pradeep S Prasad, Aniruddha Agarwal, Vishali Gupta, Waseem Ansari, Francesco Pichi, Sunil Srivastava, K Bailey Freund, SriniVas R Sadda, David Sarraf. Optical Coherence Tomography Angiography Reveals Choriocapillaris Flow Reduction in Placoid Chorioretinitis. *Ophthalmol Retina.* 2017.)

Working Diagnosis

- Relentless placoid chorioretinitis, OU

Testing

- Diagnosis is made on clinical fundus presentation and course. Laboratory evaluation is only of value in excluding some of the entities of MFC if there are signs or symptoms of systemic disease. Ruling out TB in endemic areas should be done using either the TB skin test or QuantiFERON-TB Gold Test.
- Fundus fluorescein angiography (FFA) shows early hypofluorescence and late staining of the lesions (see Fig. 35.2)
- Spectral domain optical coherence tomography (SD-OCT): acute lesions reveal disruption of the ellipsoid layer and retinal pigment epithelium (RPE) with outer retinal hyperreflectivity (Fig. 35.3)
- Optical coherence tomography angiogram (OCTA): multifocal areas of inner choroidal ischemia associated with acute retinal lesions (Fig. 35.4)

Management

- Immunomodulatory therapy (IMT) with systemic corticosteroids and immunosuppressive agents assist in preventing progression of the retinal lesions and recurrent episodes. However, tapering of systemic corticosteroids and immunosuppressive medications is frequently associated with recurrent disease. Recent observations with adalimumab (Humira), a human anti–tumor necrosis factor-alpha monoclonal antibody, suggest it may be more effective than conventional IMT. The prognosis for retention of central visual acuity (VA) is dependent on the location of lesions, but may be good.
- The patient is started on prednisone (0.75 mg/kg) and azathioprine (1–2 mg/kg) and asked to return every 2 weeks over the ensuing 2 months.

Follow-up

- Prednisone is tapered at 2 weeks and discontinued slowly while being maintained on azathioprine, with possible addition of Humira if recurrent disease is noted.
- The patient is scheduled to return every 3 months because relapse of the disease is common, as well as to continue monitoring IMT (Fig. 35.5).

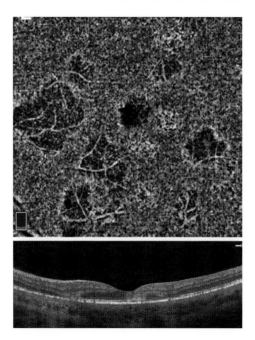

Fig. 35.4 OCTA at choriocapillaris level demonstrates decreased flow in active lesions. (Image credit: Michael A Klufas, Nopasak Phasukkijwatana, Nicholas A Iafe, Pradeep S Prasad, Aniruddha Agarwal, Vishali Gupta, Waseem Ansari, Francesco Pichi, Sunil Srivastava, K Bailey Freund, SriniVas R Sadda, David Sarraf. Optical Coherence Tomography Angiography Reveals Choriocapillaris Flow Reduction in Placoid Chorioretinitis. *Ophthalmol Retina*. 2017.)

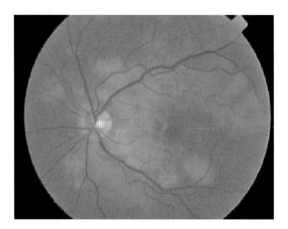

Fig. 35.5 Creamy white spots in outer retina, increasing in size and extending to the equator and periphery, after several weeks, OS. Please notice development of pigmented chorioretinal atrophy. (Image credit: Mirza RG, Jampol LM. Relentless placoid chorioretinits. *Int Ophthalmol Clin*. 2012;52[4]: 237–242.)

Key Points

- Acute bilateral retinal lesions are one of the features that helps differentiate this disease from serpiginous choroiditis.
- Configuration of the retinal lesions, with continued progression of the disease over time, distinguishes this disease from APMPPE.
- Diagnostic testing to rule out TB is important, particularly in endemic areas or with unilateral presentation.
- Development and growth of new retinal lesions over the next 24 months are common, as well as relapses after periods of apparent quiescence. However, visual prognosis is generally good in contrast to serpiginous choroiditis.
- PPM is an outer retinal chorioretinitis variant that resembles macular serpiginous chorioretinitis, as well as relentless placoid chorioretinitis. The whitish plaquelike lesions in PPM have a jigsaw pattern, occur in both eyes symmetrically, and over time may be associated with choroidal neovascularization (CNV). Otherwise, prognosis for retention of central vision is good.

CHAPTER 36

Uveitis with Subretinal Fibrosis Syndrome (USF)

Henry J. Kaplan

History of Present Illness

A 33-year-old woman with no significant past medical history presents to the eye clinic complaining of slowly progressive decreased vision over the past 6 months. She notes that it first started in her left eye (OS) with mild sensitivity to light, followed by blurred vision. She has not noticed similar symptoms in her right eye (OD). Because her vision has gotten progressively worse, she decided to see an eye doctor. She has worn glasses since early childhood and knows that she is myopic.

Exam

	OD	OS
Visual acuity	20/20	20/400
Intraocular pressure (IOP)	13	10
Sclera/conjunctiva	Within normal limits (WNL)	Episcleral injection with mild conjunctival hyperemia
Cornea	WNL	Few nongranulomatous (NG) KP
Anterior chamber (AC)	WNL	1+ cell, 1+ flare
Iris	WNL	No posterior synechiae
Lens	Clear	Clear
Vitreous cavity	WNL	1+ vitreous cells
Retina/optic nerve		Multiple small (50–250 µ), round, discrete, yellowish lesions with indistinct borders (Fig. 36.1)

Questions to Ask

- Do you have any other ocular complaints or symptoms?
- How nearsighted are you?
- Have you had any recent viral illnesses within the past year?

She does notice multiple scotomas, occasional photopsias and floaters in her OS, and has no problem with her OD. Her myopia has not progressed, and she is about −4.00 D both eyes (OU). No major illnesses in the past year, including viral infections.

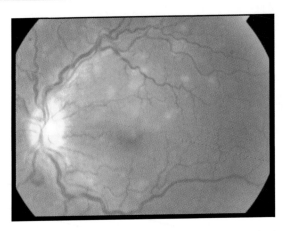

Fig. 36.1 Fundus photograph OS demonstrating multiple creamy small lesions in the posterior pole with indistinct margins.

Assessment

- White dot syndrome (WDS), OS, with mild panuveitis and multifocal choroiditis (MFC)

Differential Diagnosis

- Multifocal choroiditis with panuveitis (MFC-PU)
- Acute posterior multifocal placoid pigment epitheliopathy (APMPPE)
- Sarcoidosis
- Punctate outer retinal toxoplasmosis
- Infectious retinitis (tuberculosis [TB], syphilis)
- Presumed ocular histoplasmosis syndrome
- Punctate inner choroidopathy (PIC)
- Birdshot chorioretinopathy

Working Diagnosis

- MFC-PU, OS

Testing

- The presentation of unilateral MFC-PU has an extensive differential diagnosis, and the routine laboratory tests to exclude infection and sarcoidosis were performed. The entities of WDS can be distinguished by fundus appearance and natural history.
- Fundus fluorescein angiography (FFA): (Fig. 36.2, left panel)
- Indocyanine green chorioangiography (ICGA): (Fig. 36.2, right panel)

Management

- Anterior uveitis treated with topical prednisolone acetate 1% four times a day (QID) OS with cyclopentolate 1% twice a day (BID) OS

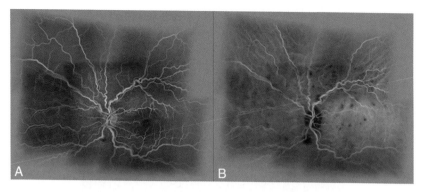

Fig. 36.2   (A) Fluorescein angiogram, late phase, OS, shows pinpoint, deep, hyperfluorescent foci. (B) ICGA, OS, demonstrates multiple hypocyanescent lesions corresponding to clinical lesions.

- Routine laboratory tests returned normal
- Follow up in 2 weeks

Follow-up

The patient returns 2 weeks later. She notes that her light sensitivity is better but that her symptoms and vision have not improved.

Follow-up Examination

The only change in examination is that OS conjunctival hyperemia, episcleritis, and anterior chamber (AC) flare and cell have resolved, with fewer keratic precipitates (KPs). Visual acuity (VA) OS has not improved, and posterior segment examination is unchanged.

Working Diagnosis 2

- Remains MFC-PU with persistent posterior segment inflammation

Follow-up Management

Topical prednisolone acetate was decreased to BID and cyclopentolate stopped. The patient was started on oral prednisone 0.75 mg/kg and asked to return in 2 weeks. Two weeks of prednisone at 0.75 to 1.0 mg/kg daily is a solid trial of oral antiinflammatory therapy. In general, lack of response in such a situation suggests two possibilities: an infectious cause or a severe inflammatory/auto-immune disease refractory to oral antiinflammatory treatment.
- Return in 2 weeks for follow-up

Follow-up

The patient returns in 2 weeks without any change in symptoms. Additionally, many of the acute lesions have enlarged and coalesced. The patient is then continued on prednisone and started on concomitant immunomodulatory therapy (IMT) with mycophenolate mofetil (CellCept). She is followed at 2- to 4-week intervals. She is not expected to have an improvement in VA because there

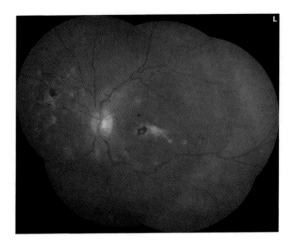

Fig. 36.3 Color fundus photograph OS of the same patient after 6 months demonstrates subretinal stellate fibrosis in the posterior pole with resulting chronic low vision. Also notice fibrosis in the area of peripheral lesions, as well as centrally.

is a subretinal scar within the fovea. It is anticipated that over the next few months she will develop stellate irregular zones of coalescent lesions with subretinal fibrosis (Fig. 36.3).

Final Diagnosis

- Uveitis with subretinal fibrosis (USF), OS

Key Points

- USF is a rare clinical entity that presents with a distinctive multifocal posterior uveitis and progresses to subretinal fibrosis. Healthy young women with myopia are most commonly involved with either acute or slowly progressive vision loss. The disease has also been referred to as *diffuse subretinal fibrosis (DSF) syndrome.*
- Although disease may be unilateral initially, over time it frequently becomes bilateral and remains asymmetric.
- Many of the acute lesions enlarge and coalesce, with subretinal pockets of fluid, before developing subretinal fibrosis. The progression to fibrosis may take many months to years to occur, eventually forming radial bands of fibrosis that extend peripherally.
- Differential diagnosis of USF is large with many autoimmune or infectious diseases included. Thus in patients refractory to therapy, underlying infections must be carefully excluded.
- Despite the use of prednisone and IMT (with antimetabolites, T-cell inhibitors, alkylating agents, and biologic agents) for many months, the disease is most often refractory to treatment, and subretinal choroidal neovascularization (CNV) may develop about fibrotic lesions within the macula.
- Thus the visual prognosis in such patients is poor, and careful follow-up is needed to treat newly developed CNV with anti–vascular endothelial growth factor (VEGF) agents.

CHAPTER 37

Birdshot Retinochoroidopathy (BRC)

Bahram Bodaghi ■ Sara Touhami ■ Dinu Stanescu ■ Adelaide Toutee

History of Present Illness

A 53-year-old Caucasian male was referred to a tertiary uveitis care unit for chronic bilateral floaters and blurred vision in both eyes (OU). He noticed the floaters for the first time over a year ago but was not worried until his vision started to drop with concomitant distorted vision, 3 weeks before the consultation. His medical history includes tonsillectomy during childhood (Figs. 37.1 to 37.3).

Exam

	OD	OS
Visual acuity	20/200	20/200
Intraocular pressure (IOP)	11	12
Sclera/conjunctiva	Quiet	Quiet
Cornea	Clear	Clear
Anterior chamber (AC)	Deep and quiet	Deep and quiet
Iris	Unremarkable	Unremarkable
Lens	Opalescent	Opalescent
Anterior vitreous	Vitritis (1+)	Vitritis (1+)

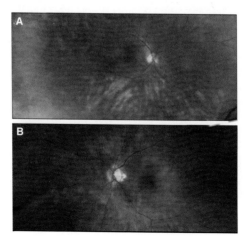

Fig. 37.1 (A and B) Fundus photographs (OD and OS) showing the presence of oval, white, and creamy chorioretinal dots (<{1/2} to {3/4} papillary diameter) at the level of the posterior pole, especially in the inferonasal peripapillary segment of the right fundus. Visualization of the fundus is mildly affected by vitritis.

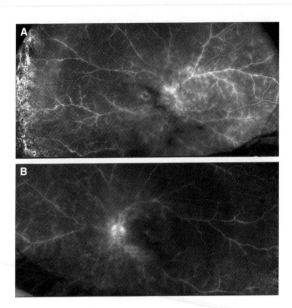

Fig. 37.2 (A and B) Fluorescein angiograms (OD and OS) show the presence of mild papillitis, periphlebitis, and diffuse capillaropathy evocative of macular edema OD > OS. No macular atrophy or optic disc damage is suspected at this stage.

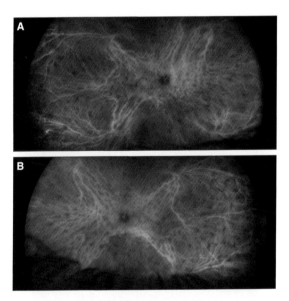

Fig. 37.3 (A and B) Indocyanine green angiograms (ICGA) (OD and OS) disclose the presence of presumably granulomatous lesions, corresponding to the white dots, in the form of hypofluorescent, round, black dots during the intermediate phase of the angiogram. Lesions are more numerous and extensive on ICGA compared with fundus photographs or fluorescein angiograms.

Questions to Ask

- Did you ever experience redness or pain in your eyes?
He responded no.
- Do you have any difficulty while driving in the dark or while performing any activities in dim light?
He responded yes.
- Do you ever see any spontaneous or flashing lights?
He answered yes.

Assessment

Bilateral vitritis, retinochoroiditis, and periphlebitis with bilateral macular edema

Differential Diagnosis

- Sarcoid-associated posterior uveitis
- Syphilitic uveitis
- Multifocal choroiditis
- Tuberculosis-associated posterior uveitis
- Less likely: Acute posterior multifocal placoid pigment epitheliopathy (APMPPE), serpiginous choroiditis, primary intraocular lymphoma, Vogt—Koyanagi—Harada disease in its late phase and sympathetic ophthalmia

Working Diagnosis

- Birdshot retinochoroidopathy (BRC): Bilateral autoimmune posterior uveitis belonging to the "white dot syndrome" spectrum of diseases.
- The anterior segment is rarely affected, explaining the absence of pain or redness.
- Floaters are related to the presence of vitritis, and the exact timing of their occurrence is often difficult to assess because of the insidious and chronic nature of the disease.
- Snowballs and snowbanks are not observed in BRC.
- Photopsia, nyctalopia, photophobia, and abnormal color vision relate to the fact that this autoimmune disease targets the retina (+ choroid, ± optic nerve).

Testing

- The diagnosis of BRC is straightforward in the presence of the classical bilateral "birdshot" white dots, especially when they are associated with bilateral mild to moderate vitritis, and periphlebitis in middle-aged, usually Caucasian individuals (females > males)
- Medical history is often unremarkable
- HLA-A29 positivity is an important clue
- Fluorescein and indocyanine green angiograms (ICGAs) are important to confirm the diagnosis, exclude the differentials, and evaluate the follow-up
- Fluorescein angiography does not show the inflammatory dots; however, it can show the presence of:
  - Papillitis

- Capillaropathy, either diffusely or in the macular region (in that case, it is usually associated with the presence of cystoid macular edema [CME])
- Periphlebitis
- Nonspecific alterations of the retinal pigment epithelium
- The birdshot dots are better seen with ICGA
  - Hypofluorescent round (black dots) lesions (usually more numerous than seen on fundoscopy or green photographs) during the early-to-intermediate phase
  - The lesions remain hypofluorescent (atrophic) or become isofluorescent (active) during the late phase
  - ICGA shows choroidal vasculitis of the posterior pole in the form of blurry hyperfluorescent choroidal vessels during the intermediate and late frames of the angiogram
- Optical coherence tomography can help identify the cause of decreased vision when present:
  - CME
  - Epiretinal membrane
  - Macular atrophy in the late stages of the disease
  - It can also show the presence of:
    - Choroidal granulomas
    - Choroidal thickening (active) or thinning in the late stages
  - Optical coherence tomography angiogram (OCTA) may be helpful even though choroidal neovascularization is rare in these cases
- Perimetry can show central or peripheral scotomas suggesting the involvement of the macula or the optic nerve
- Electrophysiology is important for follow-up and can show the following:
  - Multifocal electroretinogram (ERG) can show a decrease in the amplitudes of the N1 and P1 waves and an increase in their implicit times
  - Flicker (30 Hz) ERG often shows increased implicit times
  - Full-field ERG can become electronegative in the late stages
  - Electro-oculography can show an abnormal Arden ratio
- In all cases, check:
  - Fluorescent treponemal antibody absorption (FTA-ABS) and/or Treponema pallidum hemagglutination assay (TPHA)−Venereal Diseases Research Laboratory (TPHA-VDRL)
  - QuantiFERON and/or purified protein derivative (PPD)
  - Angiotensin-converting enzyme (ACE), lysozyme, and chest x-ray
- In doubtful cases, especially when the white dots are difficult to visualize, the diagnosis of intraocular lymphoma should always be ruled out
- Anterior chamber (AC) tap with measure of the IL6/10 ratio and brain magnetic resonance imaging (MRI) (at the very least) should be performed to rule out this life-threatening condition that may target the same age population if intraocular lymphoma is suspected

Management

- BRC is an insidious autoimmune disease that can evolve slowly towards retinal atrophy and blindness.

- Systemic steroids are almost always necessary and started at the dose of 1 mg/kg/day with progressive tapering. Pulses of methylprednisolone may be performed in severe cases.
- Systemic immunosuppressive therapy/biotherapies are frequently indicated for a minimum duration of 2 years.
- In case of unilateral or bilateral flare-ups while on systemic steroids/immunosuppressive treatment, local steroids are useful adjuncts:
  - Subtenon triamcinolone
  - Intravitreal dexamethasone
- Intravitreal fluocinolone acetonide can be proposed for more unilateral presentations, especially to prevent relapses.
- Anti—vascular endothelial growth factor (VEGF) may be used in rare cases with choroidal neovascularization.
- Vitrectomy may be proposed in case of epiretinal membranes.

Follow-up

Corticosteroids and conventional immunosuppressors failed to control macular edema and choriocapillaropathy in this case, requiring the addition of biologic agents with a rapid resolution of macular alterations and improvement of visual acuity.

Management Algorithm

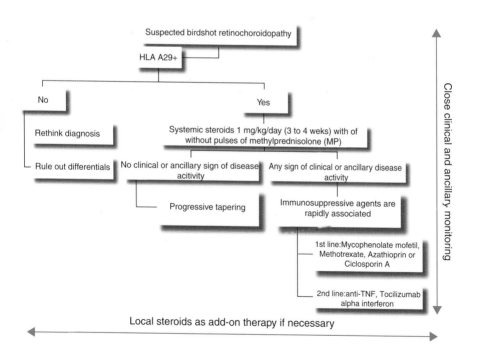

Key Points

- Birdshot retinochoroidopathy is an autoimmune posterior uveitis that targets middle-aged Caucasians of both genders
- Vitritis and periphlebitis are frequent findings
- Vision can decrease acutely/subacutely because of vitritis, macular edema, or epiretinal membrane
- Long-term preservation of visual function is attainable
- Chronic visual loss is observed in case of retinal atrophy or optic nerve involvement
- Disease progression towards retinal atrophy and blindness in the absence of treatment and close monitoring
- Spectral domain optical coherence tomography (SD-OCT) can be helpful in the diagnosis of CME, as well as its response to treatment

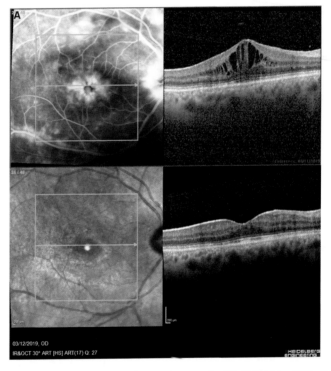

Fig. 37.4 (A and B) spectral domain-optical coherence tomography (SD-OCT) horizontal B-scan through the fovea (OD and OS) showing cystoid macular edema (*upper panel*) and its resolution after initiation of corticosteroid and biologic agents.*

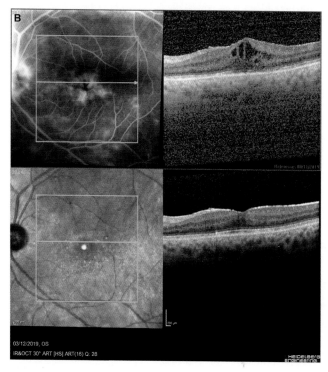

Fig. 37.4 (Continued)

- Monitoring should not rely solely on clinical grounds and OCT, but also on a set of criteria such as 30 Hz flicker ERG implicit times, visual field (VF), and angiograms (Fig. 37.4).
- Initial treatment relies on systemic steroids with progressive tapering
- Systemic immunosuppressive agents (or biologics) are almost systematically used during the course of the disease
- Local steroids can be used for unilateral flare-ups or in case of intolerance to systemic strategies when necessary

CHAPTER 38

Autoimmune Retinopathy

Weilin Chan ■ Lucia Sobrin

History of Present Illness

A 63-year-old woman presents with small light flashes in both eyes (OU) that interfere with her ability to see. The flashes have different color patterns. She especially has difficulty seeing in bright lighting.

Exam

	OD	OS
Visual acuity	20/25	20/25
Intraocular pressure (IOP)	19	19
Sclera/conjunctiva	Normal	Normal
Cornea	Normal	Normal
Anterior chamber (AC)	Normal	Normal
Iris	Normal	Normal
Lens	1+ nuclear sclerosis	1+ nuclear sclerosis
Vitreous	Normal	Normal
Dilated Fundus Examination (DFE)	See Fig. 38.1A	See Fig. 38.1B

Because the fundus examination was unremarkable aside from mild vessel attenuation, autofluorescence imaging (Fig. 38.2) and optical coherence tomography (OCT) of the macula (not shown) were pursued. OCT was within normal limits OU.

Questions to Ask

- Do you or does anyone in your family have a history of cancer?
- Do you have a family history of retinal disease?
- Do you have a history of liver disease?
- Have you ever had bariatric surgery?
- Are you currently on any medications?

The patient is currently on levothyroxine for hypothyroidism and cetirizine for seasonal allergies. Her mother has a history of breast cancer and father of gastric cancer. She answers no to all other questions.

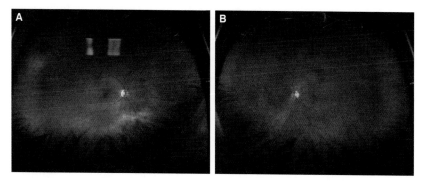

Fig. 38.1 Fundus photographs of the right (A) and left (B) eyes showing clear media and mild vessel attenuation.

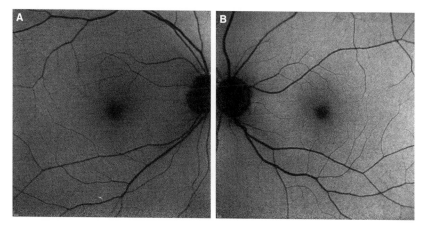

Fig. 38.2 Autofluorescence photographs of the right (A) and left (B) eyes.

Assessment

- Occult retinopathy OU

Differential Diagnosis

- Retinal toxicity from medications
- Vitamin A deficiency
- Autoimmune retinopathy (AIR)
  - Nonparaneoplastic AIR
  - Cancer-associated retinopathy
- Inherited retinal degeneration
- Acute zonal occult outer retinopathy (AZOOR)

Further Testing

- Visual field testing (Fig. 38.3)

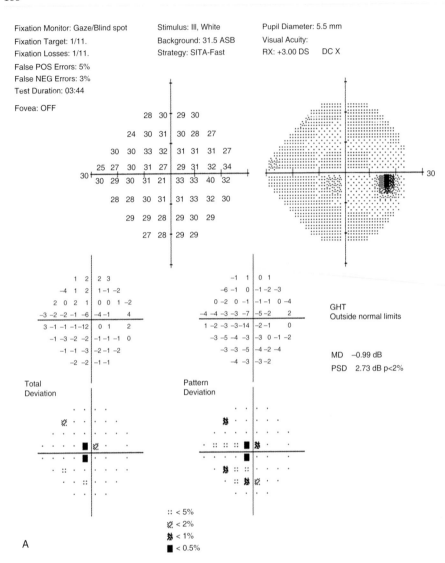

Fig. 38.3 Humphrey visual fields of the right (A) and left eye (B) show central scotomas OU.

- Multifocal electroretinogram (mfERG, Fig. 38.4)
- Full-field electroretinogram (ERG)—all amplitudes significantly reduced OU

Working Diagnosis

- AIR vs. cancer-associated retinopathy

Testing

- In patients with an unexplained retinopathy documented with ERG, antiretinal antibodies are obtained to help establish the diagnosis of AIR. Antiretinal antibodies must be

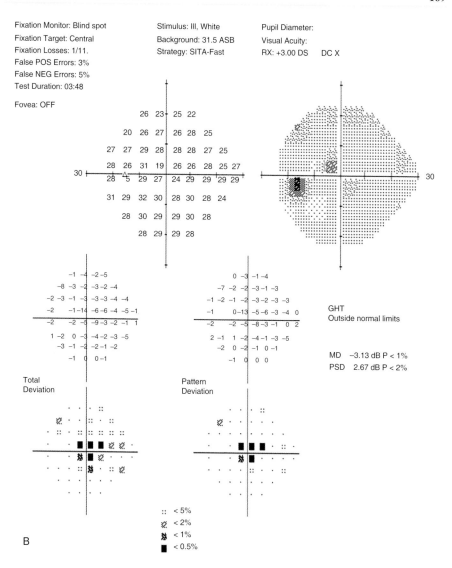

Fixation Monitor: Blind spot
Fixation Target: Central
Fixation Losses: 1/11.
False POS Errors: 3%
False NEG Errors: 5%
Test Duration: 03:48

Fovea: OFF

Stimulus: III, White
Background: 31.5 ASB
Strategy: SITA-Fast

Pupil Diameter:
Visual Acuity:
RX: +3.00 DS   DC X

GHT
Outside normal limits

MD   −3.13 dB P < 1%
PSD   2.67 dB P < 2%

Total Deviation

Pattern Deviation

:: < 5%
⊠ < 2%
❋ < 1%
■ < 0.5%

B

Fig. 38.3   (Continued).

interpreted cautiously within the context of the entire clinical picture. Antiretinal antibodies can be positive in people without any eye disease, so positive antiretinal antibodies do not establish the diagnosis on their own. This patient had antiretinal antibodies against 29-kDa and 92-kDa proteins by Western blot, and immunohistochemistry was positive for moderate staining of the photoreceptor cell layer and outer nuclear layer.

- In patients with AIR, an investigation for malignancy must be performed, as a small percentage of patients with AIR develop this disease as a paraneoplastic response to a cancer. The workup should be guided by the primary care physician and/or a medical oncologist.
- This patient did not have any detectable cancer on pelvic ultrasound; colonoscopy; abdominal ultrasound; and computed tomography (CT) scan of the chest, abdomen, and pelvis.

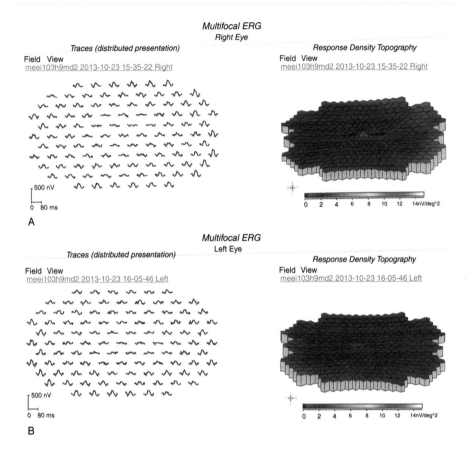

Fig. 38.4 Multifocal electroretinograms (*ERG*) of the right (A) and left eye (B) show markedly reduced responses OU.

- This patient's case was reviewed by an inherited retinal degeneration disease specialist, who felt this was unlikely to be an inherited retinal degeneration given the late onset, preservation of excellent visual acuities, and lack of structural abnormalities on OCT (not shown). She did not recommend genetic testing.

Management

This patient was treated initially with periocular steroid injections and oral methotrexate without response. She received combination rituximab and cyclophosphamide for 1 year and since then has been receiving monthly intravenous immunoglobulin (IVIg) infusions.

Follow-up

After 1 year on IVIg, vision was 20/32 right eye (OD) and 20/25 left eye (OS). Her visual field and ERG remained stable as well.

Diagnostic Algorithm

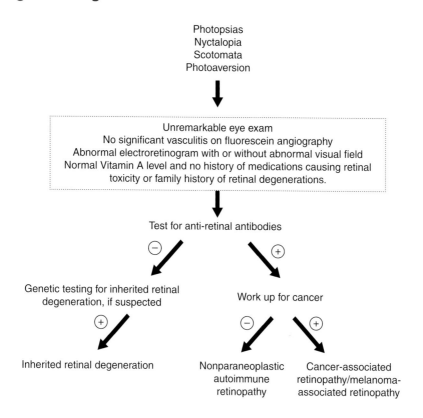

Key Points

- Antiretinal antibodies can be present in normal controls and in patients with diseases on the differential diagnosis for AIR.
- Antirecoverin and anti-enolase are the antiretinal antibodies for which there is the most evidence for pathogenicity, but they are not completely specific to the diagnosis of AIR.
- It is important to rule out inherited retinal degenerations, medication toxicity, vitamin A deficiency, and occult posterior uveitis before giving the diagnosis of AIR.
- When testing for antigens in AIR, there are two main tests. Western blots provide information on the size of the antibody, but identification of the specific antigen requires additional testing. Immunohistochemistry indicates what layer of the retina is being targeted by the antibody and can help identify the specific antigen.
- Immunomodulatory treatments can be used to preserve function. Although there are only case series to guide initial management choice, there is emerging evidence that rituximab and IVIg are efficacious in AIR.

CHAPTER 39

Melanoma-Associated Retinopathy

Tomas S. Aleman

History of Present Illness

A 30-year-old male with a history of melanoma presents for the first time to the eye clinic complaining of some distortion of images in the left eye (OS). He noticed that in his OS he now sees "through a screen of colored squiggly lines and white dots." It was hard for the patient to look at dark backgrounds. Initially, these symptoms were intermittent and then became constant within a week of onset.

Exam

	OD	OS
Visual acuity	20/25+	20/20
Intraocular pressure (IOP)	14	14
Sclera/conjunctiva	White and quiet	White and quiet
Cornea	Clear	Clear
Anterior chamber (AC)	Deep and quiet	Deep and quiet
Iris	Unremarkable	Unremarkable
Lens	Clear	Clear
Anterior vitreous	2+ cell	2+ cell
Dilated Fundus Examination (DFE)	See Fig. 39.1	

Given the history of nyctalopia in the setting of a normal fundus, electroretinogram (ERG) is pursued (Fig. 39.2).

Questions to Ask

- Are you sure this is a new symptom?
- Is there a family history of eye or vision problems?
- Are you otherwise healthy?

The patient was sure this was of acute onset, and there was no family history of retinal degenerations. He had presented a month and a half prior with a left neck node. Fine needle aspiration was positive for melanoma of unknown primary site. One month before presentation he underwent bulky left posterior triangle lymphadenopathy followed by left radical neck dissection and parotidectomy. He had metastatic melanoma involving 3 of 12 lymph nodes. Treatment had not yet been initiated at the time of presentation with visual symptoms. There were no other intercurrent illnesses. He had no history of autoimmune disease.

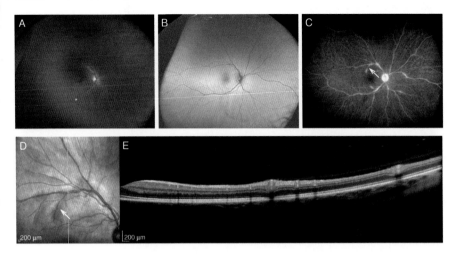

Fig. 39.1 (A) Ultrawide-field fundus photograph of the right eye showing clear media and normal appearance of the vessels and a flat, small, choroidal nevus inferiorly (*asterisk*). (B) Normal short-wavelength autofluorescence imaging. (C) Fluorescein angiogram (FA) 7 minutes after administration of contrast showing mild perivascular staining/trace leakage (*arrow*) of vessels within the arcades. (D) Near infrared reflectance shows hyporeflectance along vessels (arrow) that were abnormal on FA. (E) Spectral domain optical coherence image extending 9 mm from the foveal center into the superior near midperiphery is within normal limits. The clinical picture is nearly the same for the left eye.

Assessment

Acute inner retinal dysfunction of the on pathway associated with mild signs of posterior uveitis.

Differential Diagnosis

- Non-paraneoplastic autoimmune retinopathy (npAIR)
- Cancer-associated retinopathy (CAR)
- Melanoma-associated retinopathy (MAR)
- Metastatic melanoma
- Congenital stationary night blindness
- Less likely: Syphilis, Lyme-associated, tuberculous, and multiple sclerosis (MS)—associated intermediate uveitis

Working Diagnosis

- MAR

Testing

- In patients with a classic presentation of MAR, such as this one, it is desirable to obtain an autoimmune panel and, for completion, order the necessary laboratory tests for infectious uveitis. There is no need to undergo genetic testing in an acute presentation, although the clinical findings (with the exception of the inflammatory signs) are

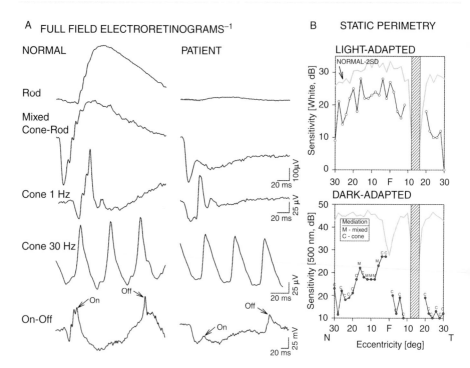

Fig. 39.2 (A) Full-field electroretinograms (ERGs) from the right eye of the patient compared with a normal subject. ERGs are dramatically abnormal with reduced rod-mediated responses, a negative configuration ERG to the (much larger a-wave compared to the b-wave), an abnormal waveform shape for cone-mediated responses, and reduced "on" pathway signal on long-duration on–off ERGs. (B) Horizontal sensitivity profiles measured with achromatic, light-adapted (*top panel*) and dark-adapted, chromatic (500 nm), automatic static perimetry in the patient compared with the normal range (*gray line* = mean −2 SD). Dark-adapted photoreceptor mediation estimated with two-color (500 nm and 650 nm) dark-adapted perimetry is shown above the dark-adapted sensitivity profile (*M* = mixed rod and cone mediation; *C* = cone mediation). The gap in the dark-adapted, rod-mediated sensitivity profile corresponds to the rod-free region near fixation. *Hatched bar*: blind spot. There is a dramatic loss of rod-mediated sensitivities mainly. Sensitivities are mediated by cone photoreceptors for most of the locations. The functional picture is nearly the same for the left eye.

indistinguishable from certain forms of congenital stationary night blindness. The vitreal and vascular inflammation is atypical in MAR but has been previously reported.
- Typical cases should have retinal autoimmune profiling. The patient showed moderate immunohistochemistry staining of some segment of photoreceptor cells in the human retina. He was also positive for autoantibodies against 21 kDa, 34 kDa, and 60 kDa proteins.

Management

- There is no established treatment for MAR.
- Treating the underlying tumor with surgery, chemotherapy, radiation, or immunotherapy are all options, as managed by oncology.
- This patient's malignancy was treated with ipilimumab after the onset of visual symptoms.
- Systemic steroids were deferred and just topical steroids started.
- Follow up in 1 month then extend gradually to twice a year or if symptoms recur.

Follow-up

The patient reports nearly complete resolution of his symptoms. Vision remains at 20/20 both eyes (OU). There was improvement in cellularity and retinal vasculitis. ERG and perimetry did not improve significantly. No further treatment was necessary.

Key Points

- Patients with acute onset of visual symptoms with minimal findings such as this case should be suspected of carrying an autoimmune retinopathy.
- Retinal imaging, including fluorescein angiography (FA), is indicated, as well as full-field. ERG and in some cases multifocal ERG.
- If there is no history of cancer, full screening should take place and periodic surveillance instituted.
- Some patients can be monitored without therapy.
- More severe disease requires immunosuppression.
- Vitrectomy with a sample of the vitreous may be indicated if there is suspicion for metastatic disease or lymphoma.
- As in this case, the mainstay of treatment is treating the underlying tumor.
- For MAR itself, various forms of systemic immunomodulatory therapy have been tried: corticosteroids, plasmapheresis, and intravenous immunoglobulin (IVIg).
- Local treatment with sub-Tenon's triamcinolone 40 mg may also be attempted.

CHAPTER 40

Hemorrhagic Occlusive Retinal Vasculitis

Dean Eliott ■ Kareem Moussa

History of Present Illness

A 70-year-old man with a history of hypertension, hyperlipidemia, and emphysema presented to an optometrist with sudden loss of vision in the left eye (OS) 2 weeks after seemingly uncomplicated cataract surgery. Uncorrected visual acuity was 20/20 1 day after cataract surgery. The sudden loss of vision occurred over a 10-minute period while eating dinner. He presented to an optometrist, who suspected central retinal vein occlusion and then referred him to the retina clinic for further evaluation.

Exam

	OD	OS
Visual acuity	20/20	Hand motion
Intraocular pressure (IOP)	12	14
Sclera/conjunctiva	White and quiet	White and quiet
Cornea	Clear	Clear
Anterior chamber (AC)	Deep and quiet	Deep and quiet
Iris	Unremarkable	Unremarkable
Lens	Well-positioned posterior chamber intraocular lens	Well-positioned posterior chamber intraocular lens
Anterior vitreous	Clear	Clear
Dilated Fundus Examination (DFE)	Normal	See Fig. 40.1A

Questions to Ask

- Do you have eye pain?
- Did you receive intraocular antibiotics at the time of cataract surgery?

He reported no eye pain. Review of records showed he received intracameral vancomycin 1 mg/0.1 mL at the end of uncomplicated cataract surgery.

Assessment

- Postoperative hemorrhagic occlusive retinal vasculitis (HORV) OS

Differential Diagnosis

- Vancomycin-associated HORV
- Less likely: Postoperative infectious endophthalmitis; central retinal vein occlusion; syphilis-, tuberculosis-, or sarcoid-associated uveitis; antineutrophil cytoplasmic antibodies (ANCA)—associated vasculitis

Working Diagnosis

- Vancomycin-associated HORV

Testing

- Fluorescein angiography is necessary to confirm occlusive retinal vasculitis (see Fig. 40.1B).
- Optical coherence tomography (OCT) frequently shows macular edema and variable degrees of inner retinal hyperreflectivity (Fig. 40.2).

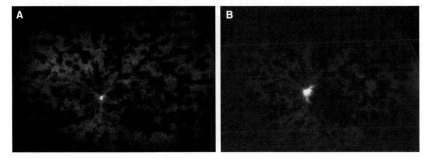

Fig. 40.1 (A) Wide-field color fundus photograph of the left eye shows clear media, arteriolar attenuation, and diffuse retinal hemorrhages. (B) Late-phase fluorescein angiogram of the left eye showing staining of the optic disc, occlusive retinal vasculitis, and blockage due to dense retinal hemorrhages.

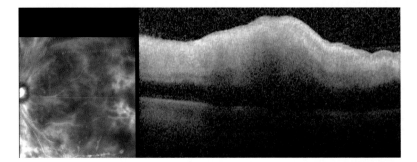

Fig. 40.2 Spectral domain optical coherence tomography of the left eye shows retinal thickening and hyperreflectivity consistent with dense intraretinal hemorrhage, macular edema, and inner retinal ischemia.

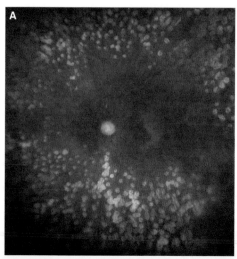

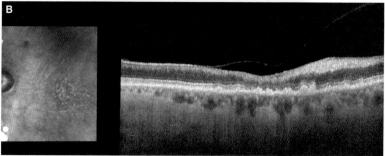

Fig. 40.3 (A) Fundus photograph of the left eye shows clear media, optic nerve pallor, arteriolar sclerosis, epiretinal membrane, resolution of retinal hemorrhages, and PRP scars. (B) Optical coherence tomography of the left eye shows an epiretinal membrane, resolution of macular edema, inner retinal thinning, and drusenoid subretinal pigment epithelium changes.

- To rule out syphilis and tuberculosis, obtain:
  - Fluorescent treponemal antibody absorption (FTA-ABS), rapid plasma reagin (RPR)
  - QuantiFERON or purified protein derivative (PPD)
- Consider obtaining ANCA to rule out ANCA-associated vasculitis and a chest x-ray to evaluate for possible sarcoidosis.

Management

- Intravitreal bevacizumab injection
- Follow up in 4 weeks

Follow-up

The patient reported no change in vision. Visual acuity remained hand motion. Dilated examination was unchanged. OCT showed persistent retinal thickening and hyperreflectivity. FTA-ABS, RPR, QuantiFERON Gold, and ANCA were negative.

He continued to receive intravitreal bevacizumab injections every 4 to 6 weeks, with gradual improvement in macular edema and retinal hemorrhages. Nine months after initial presentation, the retinal hemorrhages had resolved, allowing panretinal photocoagulation (PRP) to be performed.

Two years after initial presentation, visual acuity remained hand motion (Fig. 40.3).

Key Points

- HORV is a rare condition that has been reported after cataract surgery in eyes that received intracameral vancomycin.
- The onset of HORV is subacute, usually presenting between day 1 and 14 with painless loss of vision. Mild to moderate inflammation of the anterior chamber (AC) and vitreous can occur. Characteristic features include an occlusive retinal vasculitis and diffuse retinal hemorrhages.
- Fluorescein angiography is necessary to confirm occlusive retinal vasculitis. OCT frequently shows macular edema and hyperreflectivity of the inner retina consistent with inner retinal ischemia.
- Infectious endophthalmitis should always be considered in a postoperative eye with ocular inflammation, even in the absence of pain; the absence of severe intraocular inflammatory cells, however, makes HORV a more likely diagnosis.
- Intravitreal anti–vascular endothelial growth factor (VEGF) injections should be considered for macular edema. Local and systemic corticosteroids can also be administered as an adjunctive treatment.
- Anti-VEGF injections and/or PRP should be considered as prophylaxis for the development of neovascular glaucoma, a common complication of HORV.

CHAPTER 41

Syphilitic Posterior Placoid Chorioretinitis

Ashleigh L. Levison ▪ Eduardo Uchiyama ▪ Bobeck S. Modjtahedi

History of Present Illness

A 62-year-old Caucasian male presents with 3 days of painless vision loss in the left eye (OS).

Past Medical History

Human immunodeficiency virus (HIV) on antiretrovirals

Examination Findings

Exam

	OD	OS
Visual acuity	20/20	Count fingers
Intraocular pressure	12	13
Pupils	5 mm → 3 mm, no APD	5 mm → 3 mm, no APD
External	Normal	Normal
Lids/lashes	Normal	
Conjunctiva/sclera	White and quiet	White and quiet
Cornea	Clear	Clear
Anterior chamber	Deep and quiet	Deep and quiet
Iris	Round, reactive, no atrophy, no lesions	Round, reactive, no atrophy, no lesions
Lens	Mild nuclear sclerosis	Mild nuclear sclerosis
Vitreous	No vitreous cell/haze	No vitreous cell/haze
Dilated Fundus Examination (DFE)	See Fig. 41.1A	See Fig. 41.1B and C

Given the disc edema right eye (OD) and chorioretinal lesion OS, fluorescein angiography and optical coherence tomography were pursued (Figs. 41.2 and 41.3).

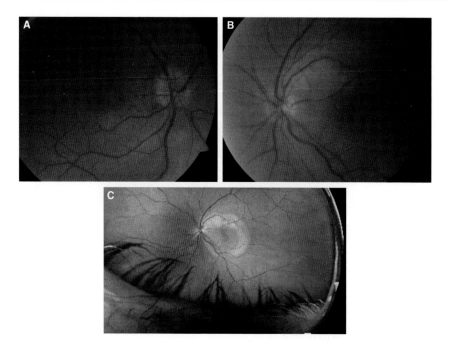

Fig. 41.1 (A) Color fundus photograph of the right eye shows mild disc edema. (B) Standard color fundus photograph and (C) wide-field photograph demonstrate a large posterior area of chorioretinitis.

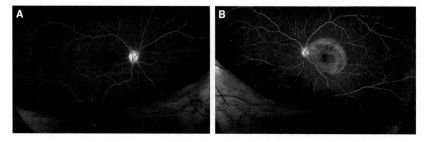

Fig. 41.2 (A) Fluorescein angiogram of the right eye shows disc leakage. (B) A mild-to-late frame fluorescein angiography (FA) of the left eye shows mild disc leakage and leakage within the macula.

Questions to Ask

- Any prior episodes of eye redness, floaters, or loss of vision?
- Any history of oral or genital ulcerations, joint pain, rashes, gastrointestinal distress, or sexually transmitted disease?
- Any history of illicit drug use, including intravenous drug use?
- Have there been any exposures to tuberculosis or at-risk individuals for tuberculosis?

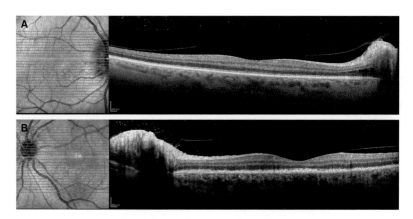

Fig. 41.3 (A) Optical coherence tomography (OCT) of the right eye shows nasal thickening around the nerve. (B) OCT of the left eye shows patchy outer retinal layers and retinal pigment epithelium.

Assessment

- Disc edema OD, chorioretinitis OS

Differential Diagnosis

- Syphilis
- Sarcoidosis
- Tuberculosis
- Endogenous infectious chorioretinitis
- Toxoplasmosis (primary toxoplasmosis in the absence of an old chorioretinal scar)
- Less likely: viral retinitis (progressive outer retinal necrosis)

Testing

- The main concerns in an HIV patient with chorioretinitis are infectious, starting with syphilis on the differential diagnosis and including toxoplasmosis and viral etiologies. Endogenous endophthalmitis should be considered, especially in those with risk factors such as recent hospitalization or intravenous drug use.
- *Treponema pallidum* (syphilis) screening cascade (treponemal antibody test that is followed by a rapid plasma reagin [RPR] if positive)
- QuantiFERON Gold (preferred given convenience) or purified protein derivative (PPD)
- Chest imaging (chest x-ray or spiral chest computed tomography [CT] with contrast), angiotensin-converting enzyme (ACE), and lysozyme for sarcoidosis

Management

- Observe closely. Await results of testing.

Follow-up

The patient returns a few days later. Testing returned with syphilis immunoglobulin G (IgG) >8 and RPR of 1:512.

Diagnosis

- Syphilitic papillitis OD, acute syphilitic posterior placoid chorioretinitis OS

Management

- Infectious disease consultation with initiation of intravenous (IV) penicillin
- Lumbar puncture (LP) with plan to initiate corticosteroids once antibiotic coverage was started

Further Follow-up

One day after initiation of penicillin IV, the patient reported worsening of vision. His right eye developed chorioretinitis, and vision dropped to 20/40. Prednisone 40 mg daily was started, followed by a slow taper. Vision improved to 20/40 OS at the time of final follow-up with resolution of chorioretinitis. Vision OD returned to 20/20.

Diagnostic Algorithm for Ocular Syphilis

- Syphilis is an important public health challenge and a re-emerging epidemic. The Centers for Disease Control and Prevention has a recommended syphilis testing cascade that ophthalmologists should be familiar with. This testing recommendation is different from what has been followed in the past (See Diagnostic Algorithm for Ocular Syphilis).
- RPR can be negative in the presence of active syphilis
  - Negative RPR in remote infection even without treatment

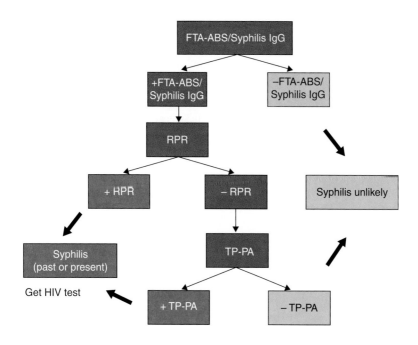

- The Prozone Phenomenon, a false-negative response resulting from high RPR titers
- HIV-positive patients can have delayed seropositivity and rarely have false negatives of both the treponemal and nontreponemal tests
- Treponemal tests (fluorescent treponemal antibody absorption [FTA-ABS], *Treponema pallidum* particle agglutination [TP-PA], syphilis IgG, or *Treponema pallidum* antibodies) should be used to screen for syphilis in patients with ocular inflammation
- Some clinicians order both treponemal and nontreponemal tests simultaneously for the sake of convenience

Key Points

- After diagnosis is confirmed with serology, the authors' recommendations are to obtain an HIV test (if status is not known) and perform an LP in coordination with an infectious diseases specialist to have a baseline cerebrospinal fluid (CSF) Venereal Disease Research Laboratory (VDRL) and cell count. If CSF results are normal, there is no need to repeat an LP in the future. If CSF results are abnormal, repeat LP should be conducted a few months after treatment to assess efficacy.
- Consider intraocular fluid sampling for polymerase chain reaction (PCR) testing for human simplex virus (HSV), varicella zoster virus (VZV), cytomegalovirus (CMV), and toxoplasmosis (prioritize based on clinical suspicion of each condition). Anterior chamber (AC) samples are typically sufficient, less so for toxoplasmosis.
- The current recommendations are to treat ocular syphilis using neurosyphilis protocols (i.e., IV penicillin 3 to 4 million units every 4 hours [q4h] for 14 days), regardless of CSF results.
- Oral prednisone can be added after penicillin is started to manage Jarisch–Herxheimer reaction and to improve intraocular inflammation if needed.

CHAPTER 42

Syphilitic Uveitis and Outer Retinopathy

Henry J. Kaplan

History of Present Illness

A 28-year-old Caucasian man with complains of mild redness, floaters, photophobia, and blurred vision in both eyes (OU) that began 2 weeks ago. He previously had excellent visual acuity (VA) with a mild myopic correction. He mentions that he has lost 20 pounds over the past 2 months and has malaise and weakness.

Exam

	OD	OS
Visual acuity	20/40	20/30
Intraocular pressure (IOP) (mm Hg)	9	8
	Purple-red skin lesions on lower lid (Fig. 42.1). Mild ciliary flush.	No skin lesions on lids. Mild ciliary flush.
Cornea	Nongranulomatous keratic precipitate (KP) in Arlts triangle	Nongranulomatous KP in Arlts triangle
Anterior chamber (AC)	1+ flare and 1+ cells	1+ flare and 1+ cells
Iris	No posterior synechiae. Argyll Robinson pupil	No posterior synechiae Argyll Robinson pupil
Lens	Clear	Clear
Vitreous cavity	1+ vitreous cells	1+ vitreous cells
Retina/optic nerve	Small white dots (<{1/4} disc diameter) scattered throughout the posterior and peripheral retina (Fig. 42.1A and B)	Small white dots (<{1/4} disc diameter) scattered throughout the posterior and peripheral retina. Optic disc edema

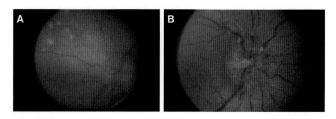

Fig. 42.1 (A) Diffuse, well-circumscribed white dots throughout the outer retina. (B) Optic disc edema OD with perivascular infiltrates and hyperemia.

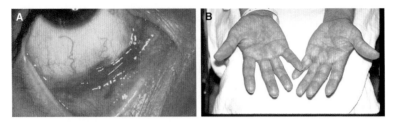

Fig. 42.2 (A) Chronic subconjunctival hemorrhage in the left lower cul-de sac suspicious for Kaposi sarcoma. (B) Chronic rash on the palms of both hands.

Questions to Ask

- Have you been diagnosed with a sexually transmitted disease (STD)?
- Have you used intravenous (IV) drugs or had sex with high-risk partners?
- Do you have any skin lesions?
- Have you been tested for infection with acquired immunodeficiency virus (AIDS)?

He responds that no, he has not been diagnosed with an STD, and he denies IV drug use, but he is a man who has sex with other men (MSM). He recently noticed a subconjunctival hemorrhage inside his left lower eyelid, which has been present for over 2 months (Fig. 42.2A), and he has been bothered by a rash on his hands for over 3 months (Fig. 42.2B).

Assessment

- Nongranulomatous (NG) panuveitis with chorioretinitis, OU, with Kaposi sarcoma of right lower lid (RLL)
- Systemic malaise and weight loss, possibly secondary to HIV infection

Differential Diagnosis

- Syphilis
- Viral retinitis (herpes simplex virus [HSV], cytomegalovirus [CMV], or varicella zoster virus [VZV])
- Tuberculosis
- Primary intraocular lymphoma or bone marrow disorder
- Sarcoidosis
- White dot syndrome (acute posterior multifocal placoid pigment epitheliopathy [APMPPE])
- Acute zonal occult outer retinopathy (AZOOR)—see "Key Points"

Working Diagnosis

- Infectious panuveitis and chorioretinitis, OU, possibly secondary to AIDS

Testing

See Figs. 42.3 and 42.4.

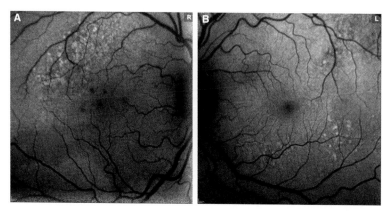

Fig. 42.3 Fundus autofluorescence (FAF) imaging demonstrating multiple hyperfluorescent dots in outer retina of posterior pole OU, as well as few hypofluorescent perifoveal foci OD.

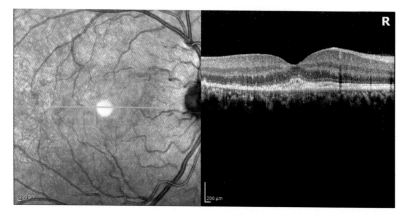

Fig. 42.4 Spectral domain optical coherence tomography (SD-OCT) imaging OD demonstrating outer retinal irregularity with disruption of ellipsoid zone temporally, as well as granular hyperreflective deposits subfoveally.

Systemic Workup

- CBC — leukopenia with CD4+ T-cell count = 120 (normal = 500 to 1500)
- HIV serology (+)
- *Treponema palladium* testing — Venereal Disease Research Laboratory (VDRL) (+), fluorescent treponemal antibody absorption (FTA-ABS) (+)
- Lumbar puncture — VDRL (+)

Management

- Topical corticosteroids and cycloplegia to control mild anterior uveitis and resolve symptoms.

- Presence of acute syphilitic chorioretinitis implies neurosyphilis, which was confirmed by a positive cerebrospinal fluid (CSF) VDRL test. Therefore treatment with aqueous penicillin G for 10 to 14 days was started.
- Patient scheduled to return at 2 weeks to ophthalmology and referral to the AIDS clinic.

Follow-up

- Upon return visit, anterior chamber (AC) inflammation had resolved and chorioretinitis showed improvement. VA improved from 20/40 right eye (OD) to 20/30 and 20/30 left eye (OS) to 20/25.
- Topical cyclopentolate was discontinued. Topical prednisolone acetate was tapered.
- Patient was scheduled to return in 1 month.

Key Points

- Penicillin is the preferred treatment option for syphilis, so that true penicillin allergies can warrant desensitization, although alternative antibiotic regimens are available (e.g., doxycycline or tetracycline). Infectious diseases consultation is warranted in all such cases. Intravitreal treatments have been described, although are rarely used. Corticosteroids can be used adjunctively but often are not necessary because the treatment response to antimicrobials is quite sufficient. Failure of primary treatment or evidence of tertiary disease, such as ocular complications, mandates further evaluation of CSF.
- The clinical presentation of ocular disease with either secondary or tertiary syphilis is diverse, including iritis, chorioretinitis, vitritis, and panuveitis. The most common form of syphilitic uveitis is anterior uveitis (iritis, iridocyclitis) and may manifest as either a granulomatous or nongranulomatous inflammation.
- Secondary syphilis can present as a chronic rash on either the palms of the hands or the soles of the feet. Tertiary syphilis can demonstrate the Argyll Robertson pupil, namely light near dissociation (i.e., the pupil responds poorly to light but briskly to near-point accommodation).
- CD4+ T-cell count <200 cells/mm^3 suggests a diagnosis of AIDS, with a count of <50 frequently associated with CMV retinitis. In patients with HIV, juxtapapillary placoid lesions, yellow to gray in color, are observed and termed *syphilitic posterior placoid chorioretinitis.*
- Cutaneous Kaposi sarcoma can be a presenting sign of AIDS.
- AZOOR affects young adults in the second to fourth decade. It is characterized by an outer retinopathy, as demonstrated by optical coherence tomography (OCT) and electroretinography, usually in the absence of overt lesions on fundus examination. Patients complain of photophobia, photopsias, and a dense scotoma, which can be either unilateral or bilateral. Narrow retinal vessels and depigmentation of the retinal pigment epithelium (RPE) develops, corresponding to zones of visual field loss that are often contiguous to the optic disc. There is a sharp demarcation between abnormal and normal retina.

CHAPTER 43

Tuberculous Uveitis

Henry J. Kaplan

History of Present Illness

A 25-year-old man noticed the vision in his left eye (OS) became blurry 2 weeks ago and is associated with a productive cough. His appetite has been poor recently, and he has lost 20 pounds in the past 2 months.

Exam

	OD	OS
Visual acuity	20/25	20/100
Intraocular pressure (IOP)	11	7
Sclera/conjunctiva	Within normal limits (WNL)	Clear, no injection
Cornea	Clear	Multiple multifocal (MF) keratic precipitates (KPs) on corneal endothelium
Anterior chamber (AC)	WNL	3+ flare and 3+ cell
Iris	WNL	Intermittent posterior synechiae, Koeppe iris nodules on pupillary margin (Fig. 43.1)
Lens	Clear	Clear
Vitreous cavity	Clear	2+ vitreous cell
Retina/optic nerve		Choroidal mass in posterior pole (Fig. 43.2), with retinal vasculitis and perivascular sheathing. Mild optic disc swelling at temporal margin

Questions to Ask

- Have you had blurry vision in either eye before?
- Why have you been losing weight? Is your appetite good?
- Have you been diagnosed with a systemic illness?
- What medications are you taking?
- Have you been exposed to anyone with a contagious disease?

He has not had blurry vision before. His appetite is poor, which he attributes to his recent chest infection. He is gay, and 2 years ago he was diagnosed positive for human immunodeficiency virus (HIV). He is currently on highly active antiretroviral therapy (HAART), and about 1 month ago visited a friend who had recently been diagnosed with pneumonia.

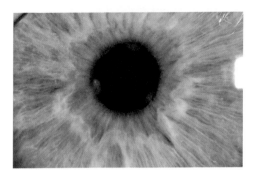

Fig. 43.1   Koeppe nodules at pupillary margin. (Courtesy of Emmet Cunnigham, MD, PhD.)

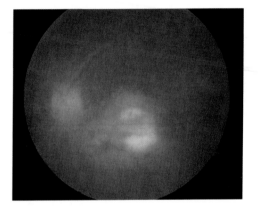

Fig. 43.2   Choroidal tuberculoma in posterior pole, associated with perivascular sheathing, OS. (This image was originally published in Retina Image Bank website. Author: Theodore Lenge. Title: TB granuloma. Retina Image Bank. Year 2017; Image Number 27463. © the American Society of Retina Specialists.)

Assessment

- Likely infectious uveitis/choroiditis/perivasculitis, OS, associated with a pulmonary infection

Differential Diagnosis

- Tuberculosis (TB)
- Brucellosis
- Syphilis
- Sarcoidosis
- Vogt–Koyanagi–Harada syndrome
- Bone marrow dysplasia (leukemia, lymphoma, Hodgkin disease)
- Metastatic carcinoma

Working Diagnosis

- Granulomatous tuberculous uveitis with choroidal tuberculoma, OS

Testing

- HIV+ men have an increased risk of secondary infection with many pathogens. History of pneumonia strongly suggests TB. Although *Pneumocystis carinii* pneumonia (PCP) is a common complication in acquired immunodeficiency syndrome (AIDS) patients without prophylactic therapy, intraocular inflammation is usually absent or mild.
- Laboratory evaluation:
  - QuantiFERON TB Gold Test: positive
  - Fluorescent treponemal antibody absorption (FTA-ABS) and rapid plasma reagin (RPR): both negative
- Computed tomography (CT) scan of chest: confirms diagnosis of bilateral pneumonia with a cavity in the left upper lobe
- Polymerase chain reaction (PCR) test of sputum: positive for TB

Management

- With a proven diagnosis of pulmonary TB and a presumed choroidal tuberculoma OS, anti-TB therapy was started. Topical prednisolone acetate 1% every 4 hours (q4h) and cyclopentolate 1% three times a day (TID) OS were given for his granulomatous anterior uveitis; periocular triamcinolone acetate 40 mg was injected in the sub-Tenon space OS for his posterior uveitis.
- Infectious diseases consult to identify the appropriate TB regimen and follow-up for pneumonitis.
- Follow up in 2 weeks.

Follow-up

On return visit there is no change in visual acuity (VA). Anterior chamber (AC) inflammation was resolving, so topical prednisolone was tapered and cyclopentolate stopped. An anti-TB four-drug regimen was started: isoniazid, rifampin, pyrazinamide, and ethambutol. Once the TB isolate is known to be fully susceptible, ethambutol will be discontinued. Oral prednisone 0.75 mg/kg to prevent progression of the posterior retinal lesions and subretinal fibrosis was also started. After 2 to 4 weeks immunomodulatory therapy (IMT) will replace prednisone to avoid complications associated with high-dose maintenance systemic corticosteroids.

Key Points

- *Mycobacterium tuberculosis* has been in decline as a cause of uveitis since the early twentieth century. In Wood series at Johns Hopkins University reported in 1944, over half of the patients with uveitis were thought to be due to *M. tuberculosis*.
- Although infectious inflammation of every structure within the eye has been associated with *M. tuberculosis*, uveitis is the most common ocular manifestation. It is thought to spread to the eye by hematogenous spread from a distant focus of infection, such as the lung.
- Known risk factors for TB infection include close contact with infected individuals, HIV infection, and other forms of immunocompromise. TB is endemic in many areas of the world, and individuals from these countries should be considered at high risk of infection. Eight countries in 2017 accounted for two-thirds of new cases of TB: India, China, Indonesia, Philippines, Pakistan, Nigeria, Bangladesh, and South Africa.
- Choroiditis caused by TB may present as serpiginous-like choroiditis, and thus treatment with corticosteroids and/or IMT without anti-TB medications may exacerbate the disease.

- An inflammatory retinal periphlebitis leading to ischemia, neovascularization, and traction retinal membranes called *Eales disease* has been thought to be associated with TB infection.
- Ocular manifestations presumed to originate from TB can arise from acute infection, such as pulmonary TB, or from latent infection without evidence of pulmonary involvement.
- Tuberculin skin testing with purified protein derivative (PPD) of *M. tuberculosis* and QuantiFERON TB Gold Test are the two most important diagnostic tests.
- Current anti-TB medications are effective against most strains of *Mycobacterium*; thus if TB is promptly diagnosed and treated, a cure follows in most cases.

CHAPTER 44

Diffuse Unilateral Subacute Neuroretinitis (DUSN)

Henry J. Kaplan

History of Present Illness

A 56-year-old man presents with a paracentral blind spot and floaters right eye (OD), but no ocular pain, for about 4 weeks. He first noticed the blind spot while hunting in Michigan and closing his left eye (OS). He has been in excellent health and enjoys hunting, fishing, and swimming in the outdoors. He does not recall being bitten by an insect or tick this fall while hunting deer.

Exam

	OD	OS
Visual acuity	20/60	20/20
Intraocular pressure (IOP) (mm Hg)	10	9
Sclera/conjunctiva	Clear. No injection	Clear. No injection
Cornea	Clear	Clear
Anterior chamber (AC)	No cell or flare	No cell or flare
Iris	No relative afferent pupillary defect (RAPD)	Normal
Lens	Clear	Clear
Vitreous cavity	2+ vitritis	Clear
Retina/optic nerve	White worm within the macula (Fig. 44.1)	Normal

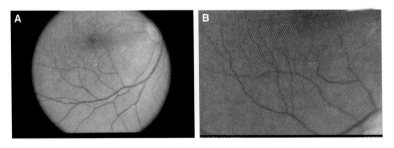

Fig. 44.1 (*Left panel*) Live white subretinal nematode within the vascular arcades (OD), which migrated over time (*right panel*).

Questions to Ask

- Have you been in the woods within the past 3 months hunting or swimming in rivers?
- Do you eat the animals that you have hunted?
- Have you eaten steak tartare or other raw meat in the past?
- Do you have unprotected sex with women or men?
- Have you traveled to the tropics within the past 6 months?

He has been hunting in Michigan for the past 3 months during the fall deer season and was successful in bringing down a white-tailed deer as part of a deer culling program in Ann Arbor. He does not usually eat game, but he and a few friends had a cookout at the end of the day. He has not had unprotected sex with either gender and has never been to the tropics.

Assessment

- Posterior uveitis with chorioretinitis, OD

Differential Diagnosis

- Infectious chorioretinitis (nematode, parasite)
- Unlikely: syphilis, sarcoidosis

Working Diagnosis

- Diffuse unilateral subacute neuroretinitis (DUSN), OD

Testing

- Laboratory testing: normal complete blood count (CBC) with mild eosinophilia
- Visual field (VF): paracentral blind spot, OD
- Fluorescein angiography (FA): diffuse degeneration of retinal pigment epithelium (RPE) and peripapillary capillary dye leakage, OD

Management

- Laser photocoagulation was performed on the live worm, who initially moved but was subsequently surrounded by laser spots and directly photocoagulated.
- Return appointment in 1 week.

Follow-up

- At the 1-week appointment, clinical examination OD was unchanged but there was no increase in intraocular inflammation.
- At 1 month, VA improved to 20/40 and mild vitritis resolved.

Key Points

- Early stage: mild optic nerve edema, mild vitritis, optic disc edema, and clustered yellow-gray-white lesions (Fig. 44.2). Late stage: optic nerve atrophy, retinal arteriolar narrowing, increased internal limiting membrane reflex, subretinal tunnels, diffuse RPE degeneration, and afferent pupillary defect (Fig. 44.3).

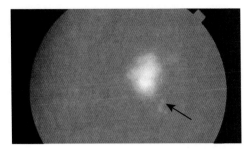

Fig. 44.2   Live white nematode (*black arrow*) associated with an inflammatory reaction in the early stages of DUSN and faint subretinal tracks.

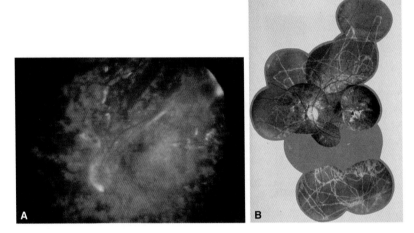

Fig. 44.3   End stage of DUSN with wipe-out syndrome.

- The most common nematodes associated with DUSN are *Baylisascaris procyonis* (a parasite of raccoons and skunks, often found in the Midwestern United States), *Ancylostoma caninum* (a dog hookworm found in the southeastern United States and Brazil), *Gnathostoma spinigerum* (found in raw or undercooked fish and meat in India), *Strongyloides stercoralis*, and *Brugia malayi*.
- The nematode eggs are ingested after they have been shed from carriers such as dogs or raccoons. The nematode may also invade cutaneously and migrate hematogenously over the course of months and reside in the fundus for years.
- The focal chorioretinal white spots in the fundus are presumably an immune response to the secretions of the worm.
- Electroretinography (ERG): Although the a:b ratio can be normal in the early stages, b-wave depression becomes proportional to retinal involvement, with the inner retina more profoundly affected than the outer retina.
- Indocyanine green chorioangiography (ICGA): Hypofluorescent spots (black dots) correspond to choroidal infiltration and inflammation.
- Antihelminthic therapy (e.g., albendazole) may be useful adjunctively when laser treatment alone does not kill the worm. Oral corticosteroids will help decrease inflammatory responses in the eye.

CHAPTER 45

Exudative Retinal Detachment

Harpal S. Sandhu

History of Present Illness (HPI)

A 42-year-old man with no significant past ocular or medical history complains of progressively decreased vision in his right eye (OD) over the last 1 to 2 months. He says he can only see a small sliver of the world out of the bottom portion of the right eye. He denies problems in the left eye (OS).

Exam

	OD	OS
Vision	Count fingers (CF) 3'	20/20
Intraocular pressure (IOP)	8	15
Lids and lashes:	Normal	Normal
Sclera/conjunctiva:	White and quiet	White and quiet
Cornea:	Clear	Clear
Anterior chamber (AC)	3+ cell 2+ flare	Deep and quiet
Iris	Nearly 360-degree synechiae	Flat
	Small pupil	
Lens	Clear	Clear
Anterior vitreous	+Haze, unclear grade	Clear
Dilated fundus examination (DFE):	No view	Normal

B scan ultrasound is pursued because there is no view of the fundus (Fig. 45.1).

Questions to Ask

- Do you have any history of eye problems?
- Have you ever had surgery on either eye or trauma to either eye?
- Have you traveled outside the country recently?
- Do you practice safe sex?
- Have you started any new medications recently or been ill in the last few months?
- Do you have any joint pain, back pain, new skin rashes, problems with bowel movements, or oral or genital ulcers?

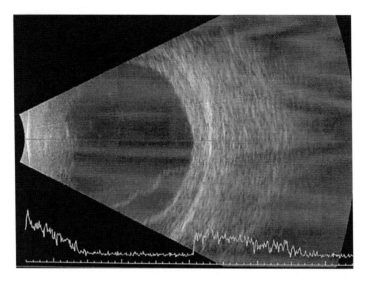

Fig. 45.1   B scan of the right eye shows an inferior retinal detachment extending to the optic nerve and diffuse choroidal thickening.

The patient denies any history of eye problems, eye surgery, or trauma. He reaffirms that he is healthy and has not been on any new medications. He has had low-back pain for 2 years but works in a warehouse and has always attributed it to his labor.

Assessment

- Panuveitis OD
- Retinal detachment OD, likely exudative

Differential Diagnosis

- Sarcoidosis
- Idiopathic
- HLA-B27—associated uveitis
- Syphilis
- Less likely: other infectious causes of panuveitis with serous detachment, such as tuberculosis and toxoplasmosis, or primary or secondary intraocular lymphoma

Working Diagnosis

- Noninfectious panuveitis, but with need to rule out infectious etiologies before using intensive corticosteroid therapy

Testing

- B scan as noted earlier

■ Check HLA-B27, angiotensin-converting enzyme (ACE), lysozyme, chest x-ray, fluorescent treponemal antibody absorption (FTA-ABS), rapid plasma reagin (RPR), purified protein derivative (PPD) or QuantiFERON, and toxoplasma serologies

Management

■ Start prednisolone acetate 1% every 2 hours (q2h) OD and cyclopentolate 1% three times a day (TID) OD
■ Await results of testing
■ Follow up in 1 week

Follow-up

HPI

The patient returns a week later. He says his vision is maybe slightly better, but he does not really notice a consistent change. All testing is negative aside from positive HLA-B27.

Exam

	OD	OS
Vision	CF 3′	20/20
IOP	10	15
Lids and lashes:	Normal	
Sclera/conjunctiva:	White and quiet	
Cornea:	Clear	
AC:	1+ cell 2+ flare	
Iris:	Nearly 360-degree synechiae	
Lens:	Clear	
Anterior vitreous:	+Haze	
DFE:	No view	

Management

■ Start prednisone 60 mg by mouth (PO) daily
■ Continue topical corticosteroids and cycloplegic

Follow-up #2

After 2 weeks of prednisone 60 mg PO daily, vision improved to 20/400, intraocular pressure (IOP) has increased to 12, and the anterior chamber (AC) inflammation has resolved. However, the retinal detachment remains unchanged.

Management

■ Increase prednisone to 100 mg PO daily for an additional 2 weeks
■ Taper topical corticosteroids

Follow-up #3

It is now 2 months after his initial presentation. His improvement plateaued after the first week, and vision was always in the 20/200 to 20/400 range. Sub-Tenon's triamcinolone was injected without any improvement after discontinuation of oral prednisone. Methylprednisolone 1000 mg intravenous (IV) × 3 days was administered with minimal change in the retinal detachment. Today, vision is 20/300 OD, IOP 20, and the examination and B scan are unchanged. The retinal detachment has not progressed superiorly.

Management

- The patient initially improved with corticosteroids, but improvement has plateaued even with intensive systemic and local corticosteroid therapy. It is highly unlikely that any other medical therapy will have a beneficial effect. It is possible that the retinal detachment is rhegmatogenous, but in that case one would have expected the extent of the retinal detachment to progressively increase and vision to worsen, which it has not.
- Proceed to vitrectomy with internal drainage of subretinal fluid.

Follow-up #4

The surgery was uneventful. No retinal breaks were identified intraoperatively. Highly viscous sub-retinal fluid was drained and the retina flattened appropriately. Three months postoperatively, the superior visual field had partly improved, visual acuity had improved to 20/100, and there were numerous pigmentary changes throughout the macula and inferior periphery.

Key Points

- Although HLA-B27 is classically associated with acute anterior uveitis, it can present with a broad spectrum of findings, including chronic anterior and intermediate uveitis, panuveitis, and serous/exudative retinal detachment.
- Medical therapy is first-line treatment for presumed inflammatory exudative retinal detachment. Surgical treatment should be reserved for refractory cases.
- Vogt—Koyanagi—Harada disease, sympathetic ophthalmia, and posterior scleritis are prominent causes of exudative retinal detachment. The first two are distinctive for their bilaterality, and the latter for having pain as a prominent feature, which essentially ruled them out in this case.
- On initial presentation, a thorough scleral depressed examination should be performed to ensure no retinal breaks are present and confirm that the retinal detachment is truly serous/exudative. In cases such as this, where a small pupil and/or media opacities preclude a view of the fundus, shifting fluid on B scan when the patient is positioned supine versus erect is strongly suggestive of an exudative retinal detachment.
- Unlike rhegmatogenous retinal detachment, in which a macula-involving retinal detachment lasting several months would have a poor visual prognosis, exudative retinal detachments involving the macula tend to have better visual outcomes.

CHAPTER 46

Endogenous Endophthalmitis

Harpal S. Sandhu ■ Aristomenis Thanos

History of Present Illness

The coronary care unit has consulted ophthalmology regarding a 46-year-old male inpatient who complains of decreased vision in his right eye (OD). He has had a protracted course in the hospital. He presented 2 weeks ago with ST-elevation myocardial infarction complicated by cardiogenic shock. He underwent emergent coronary artery stenting of the left anterior descending artery. He has been on multiple vasopressors and had an aortic balloon pump placed. He was on mechanical ventilation earlier in his course, but was extubated a few days ago. He was also febrile last week and has been treated for ventilator-associated pneumonia.

He notes that he started to see floating spots in his OD about 3 or 4 days ago. These have gradually been increasing, and he says his vision is now blurry in that eye. He denies pain or any problems with his left eye (OS). His only past ocular history is mild myopia.

Questions to Ask the Primary Team

- What clinical data are available regarding the patient's infection (e.g., culture results and sensitivities)?
- What antimicrobials was he or is he on?
- Is his clinical course improving?

The following information is gathered from a review of the patient's chart and discussion with the intensive care unit (ICU) team. The patient had a ventilator-associated pneumonia from which he is recovering. Blood cultures have all been negative. 1,3-β-D-glucan was positive. The patient is no longer febrile, is hemodynamically stable, and his oxygen requirement is decreasing. He was started on broad-spectrum antimicrobials last week, specifically vancomycin, piperacillin–tazobactam, and voriconazole.

Exam

	OD	OS
Vision	J12	J3
	(20/125 distance equivalent)	(20/30 distance equivalent)
Intraocular pressure (IOP)	14	15

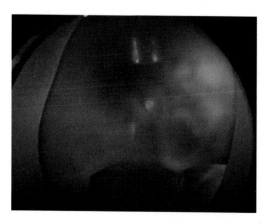

Fig. 46.1   Color wide-field fundus photograph of the right eye shows hazy media, consistent with diffuse vitritis, with particularly dense vitreous haze nasally. There appears to be a bright, yellow-white lesion in the superonasal fundus posterior to the dense haze. Note: The opacity inferiorly is a photographic artifact (gloved finger retracting the lower eyelid).

Penlight Exam

	OD	OS
Lids and lashes:	Normal	Normal
Sclera/conjunctiva:	White and quiet	White and quiet
Cornea:	Clear	Clear
Anterior chamber (AC):	Deep and quiet	Deep and quiet
Iris:	Flat	Flat
Lens:	Clear	Clear

Dilated fundus examination (DFE) (See Fig. 46.1)

Nerve:	Pink, sharp, cup-to-disc (c/d) 0.3
Macula:	Multiple fluffy, white chorioretinal lesions
Vessels:	Normal caliber and course
Periphery:	A few scattered white, fluffy chorioretinal lesions

Assessment

- Chorioretinitis with vitritis OD, multifocal chorioretinitis OS.
- The patient has been systemically toxic, has had multiple indwelling pieces of hardware, and has had a recent infection with an unknown organism; hence treatment with broad-spectrum antimicrobials, including an antifungal. 1-3-β-D-glucan was also positive, which is a nonspecific marker of fungal infection. The examination is consistent with an infectious chorioretinitis in both eyes (OU) of endogenous origin, given the history. In particular, the white fluffy lesions are suggestive of *Candida* infection. The vitritis OD in the absence of severe anterior chamber (AC) inflammation (in general, only severe

inflammation will be detected by a bedside examination with a penlight) means that the patient has an early endophthalmitis OD.

Differential Diagnosis

- Fungal endogenous endophthalmitis OD and chorioretinitis OS
- Bacterial endogenous endophthalmitis OD and chorioretinitis OS

Management

- Tap the vitreous and send for Gram stain, culture, and polymerase chain reaction (PCR), if available
- Inject broad-spectrum antimicrobials OD: vancomycin 1 mg/0.1 mL, ceftazidime 2.25/0.1 mL, voriconazole 100 μg/0.1 mL
- Recommend to the ICU team that they continue all antimicrobials for now, and likely antifungal treatment, for a minimum of 6 weeks

Follow-up

The patient is seen the following day and then multiple times over the next 6 weeks. The vitreous haze steadily cleared in the right eye, and the fundus lesions in the left eye steadily regressed. PCR was not available, and cultures did not grow any organisms. Because there was no growth, all three antimicrobials were continued for 6 weeks: vancomycin and ceftazidime via a peripherally inserted central catheter and voriconazole orally. The patient is then seen 8 weeks status post tap and inject procedure.

Exam

	OD	OS
Vision	20/25	20/20
IOP	16	15
Lids and lashes:	Normal	Normal
Sclera/conjunctiva:	White and quiet	White and quiet
Cornea:	Clear	Clear
AC:	Deep and quiet	Deep and quiet
Iris:	Flat	Flat
Lens:	Clear	Clear

DFE (See Fig. 46.2)

Nerve:	Pink, sharp, c/d 0.3
Macula:	Multiple hypopigmented, atrophic spots in place of prior lesions
Vessels:	Normal caliber and course
Periphery:	A few hypopigmented, atrophic spots

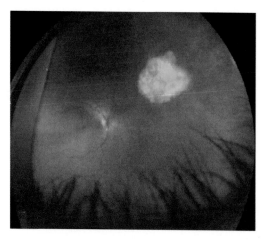

Fig. 46.2 Wide-field color fundus photo shows clear media, normal macula, nerve, and vessels and a large area of atrophy of the retina and retinal pigment epithelium (RPE) superonasally. Large atrophic lesions like this can be indicative of a resolved subretinal abscess.

Key Points

- Endogenous, infectious chorioretinitis is a well-known complication of fungemia. As such, a dilated eye examination is recommended on all fungemic patients, even if asymptomatic, by the Infectious Diseases Society of America (IDSA).
- Chorioretinitis alone can be treated initially with just systemic therapy and close follow-up. Therapy should be continued for at least 6 weeks and until all lesions have fully regressed.
- Cases without positive cultures present a therapeutic challenge. Although the examination in this case was suggestive of a fungal origin, bacterial seeding, although less common, can also present as a nonspecific chorioretinitis. Therefore the safest course is to cover broadly for gram-positive bacteria, gram-negative bacteria, and fungi, just as the primary medical team was doing systemically. It is helpful to look through all antibiotics that an inpatient has been on during his or her course in order to better understand what organisms the primary team has suspected, even if there is no definitive culture evidence. If and when cultures or PCR of intraocular fluids is positive, treatment can be narrowed.
- It is not uncommon for there to be a mild, local vitritis just over the chorioretinal lesions. In such cases, the patient does not have a frank endophthalmitis, and first-line treatment can again be systemic therapy. However, very close follow-up is necessary, and there should be a low threshold for intravitreal injection antimicrobials.
- Bacteria and fungi can both cause subretinal abscesses. *Nocardia* and *Aspergillus* are among the most common organisms reported to cause subretinal abscesses. Candida looks distinctly different and more often presents with smaller, multifocal lesions that are fluffy and white (Fig. 46.3).
- Vitreoretinal surgery with injection of intravitreal antibiotics may be considered in select cases of subretinal abscess. However, there is a high incidence of proliferative vitreoretinopathy, especially with surgical approaches to drain the abscess intraocularly.

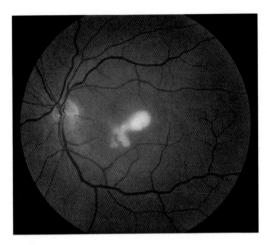

Fig. 46.3 Color fundus photograph of the macula of the left eye shows a representative case of *Candida* chorioretinitis without endophthalmitis in an intravenous drug user. There is a bright, fluffy, yellow-white lesion in the central macula at the level of the retina with fainter, deeper lesions immediately adjacent to it. Endogenous Endophthalmitis: Bacterial and Fungal, Ajay E. Kuriyan, Stephen G. Schwartz, Janet L. Davis and Harry W. Flynn, Ryan's Retina, 90, 1700–1708, 6th edition, Elsevier. Fig 90.3. (Case courtesy of Jeffrey K. Moore, MD.)

- Although most cases of endogenous endophthalmitis occur in the inpatient setting, ambulatory outpatients can also present with the disease. Especially vulnerable populations include intravenous drug users, patients on total parental nutrition, and other patients with indwelling hardware.
- Liver function tests must be periodically checked in patients on extended courses of azole antifungals.

CHAPTER 47

Acute Retinal Necrosis (ARN)

Eduardo Uchiyama ■ Bobeck S. Modjtahedi

History of Present Illness

A 38-year-old black Haitian male presented with worsening vision and floaters in his right eye (OD) for the past 2 weeks. The day before symptoms started, the patient felt a foreign body sensation while cutting lumber. He was evaluated by an outside physician, who started the patient on difluprednate drops without improvement.

Exam

	OD	OS
Visual acuity	20/200+ 1 sc PH no improvement	20/20 sc
Intraocular pressure	17	13
Pupils	7 mm → 5 mm, + afferent pupillary defect (APD)	7 mm → 4 mm
External	Normal	Normal
Lids/lashes	Normal	
Conjunctiva/sclera	White and quiet, lids everted, and no foreign bodies	White and quiet
Cornea	Granulomatous keratic precipitates (KP)	Clear
Anterior chamber	3+ cell with fibrin	Deep and quiet
Iris	Posterior synechiae, no atrophy, no lesions	Round, reactive, no atrophy, no lesions
Lens	Pigment on anterior lens surface	Clear
Vitreous	2+ vitreous haze	No vitreous cell or haze
Dilated fundus examination (DFE)	Figs. 47.1A and B	Fig. 47.2

Questions to Ask

- Any prior episodes of eye redness, floaters, or loss of vision?
- Any history of oral or genital ulcerations, joint pain, rashes, gastrointestinal distress, or sexually transmitted disease?
- Any history of illicit drug use, including intravenous drug use?
- Have there been any exposures to tuberculosis or at-risk individuals for tuberculosis?

The patient answers no to all of these questions.

Assessment

- Panuveitis with peripheral retinitis OD

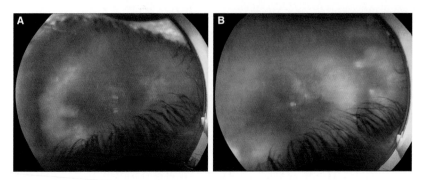

Fig. 47.1   (A and B) Color wide-field fundus photograph of the right eye demonstrates hazy view to the posterior segment secondary to vitritis. The peripheral retina demonstrates confluent areas of retinitis.

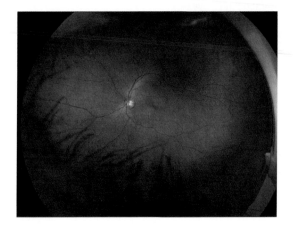

Fig. 47.2   Left eye is within normal limits.

Differential Diagnosis

- Acute retinal necrosis (necrotizing herpetic retinitis)
- Posttraumatic endophthalmitis
- Sarcoid uveitis
- Syphilitic uveitis
- Toxoplasmosis
- Behçet disease
- Less likely: Tuberculous uveitis

Working Diagnosis

- Acute retinal necrosis

Testing

In patients presenting with panuveitis, check:
- *Treponema pallidum* (syphilis) screening cascade (treponemal antibody test that is followed by a rapid plasma reagin [RPR] if positive)

- QuantiFERON Gold (preferred, given convenience) or purified protein derivative (PPD)
- Chest imaging (chest x-ray or chest computed tomography [CT] with contrast), angiotensin-converting enzyme (ACE), and lysozyme can also be considered to evaluate for sarcoidosis.
- In patients with concurrent retinitis, send intraocular fluid sample for polymerase chain reaction (PCR) testing for herpes simplex virus (HSV), varicella zoster virus (VZV), cytomegalovirus (CMV), and toxoplasmosis (prioritize based on clinical suspicion of each condition). Anterior chamber (AC) samples are typically sufficient except for toxoplasmosis.

Management

- AC fluid sent for PCR to check for viral deoxyribonucleic acid (DNA) (HSV, VZV, and CMV)
- Oral valacyclovir 1000 mg two tablets three a day (TID) by mouth (alternative: intravenous acyclovir 10 to 15 mg/kg divided every 8 hours [q8h] × 5 to 10 days with transition to oral therapy such as 800 mg five times daily acyclovir thereafter)
- Intravitreal foscarnet 1.2 to 2.4 mg in 0.1 mL (alternative: ganciclovir 400 μg–4 mg in 0.1 mL)
- Difluprednate 0.05% 1 gtt four times a day (QID) OD
- Atropine 1% twice a day (BID) OD

Follow-up

PCR was positive for VZV. All other testing was negative. The patient developed a retinal detachment with large retinal breaks. He underwent a scleral buckle and pars plana vitrectomy with placement of silicone oil. The retinitis regressed, and the patient was started on 60 mg of oral prednisone, which was eventually tapered down to 10 mg over the next 6 weeks. Valacyclovir was decreased to 1000 mg TID after 2 weeks and then kept on that dose for 3 months. The patient was maintained at 1000 mg every day as prophylaxis, with creatinine checked every 6 months. On last follow-up, the patient's vision was 20/100 in the presence of a 1+ nuclear sclerotic cataract (Fig. 47.3).

Key Points

- Acute retinal necrosis is a highly aggressive, potentially devastating, infectious panuveitis with retinitis that necessitates aggressive treatment, as in this case. It can be caused by HSV-1, HSV-2, and VZV.

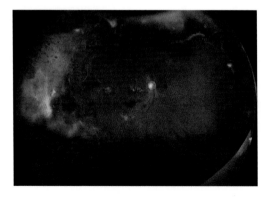

Fig. 47.3 Color wide-field fundus photograph of the right eye shows that the retina is attached 360 degrees. Necrotic retina in the temporal periphery is nicely supported by the scleral buckle.

- In addition to the diagnostic testing suggested earlier, other tests should be tailored to specific clinical findings (e.g., test for toxoplasmosis if there is focal retinitis and an old scar) or history (e.g., consider endophthalmitis in recently hospitalized patients or those with intravenous drug use).
- Aspirin by mouth (PO) has been used to prevent vascular occlusions, a complication of acute retinal necrosis, but it is unclear if this is effective.
- Retinal detachment is another serious complication of acute retinal necrosis and unfortunately is fairly common.
- Laser demarcation around the necrotic retina as prophylaxis for retinal detachment is controversial. Although it may barricade the necrotic tissue, the laser treatment itself can produce retinal holes and detachment in fragile tissue.
- One can consider silicone oil removal after 6 months, but patients remain at high risk for redetachment from small breaks. Alternatively, the oil can remain in the eye indefinitely if it is not causing any complications (e.g., glaucoma or corneal decompensation from migration into the AC).
- Intravenous foscarnet and intravenous cidofovir can be attempted in patients whose disease is refractory to the previous management strategies. The latter drug carries significant risks, including ocular hypotony and nephrotoxicity.
- Many experts recommend lifelong antiviral treatment to protect the contralateral eye.

CHAPTER 48

Progressive Outer Retinal Necrosis (PORN)

Henry J. Kaplan

History of Present Illness (HPI)

A 24-year-old jazz musician noticed poor vision, both eyes (OU), about 3 months ago. He has not been feeling well recently, but attributed that to his odd hours of work and little sleep. He has no history of vision problems, although he was hit in his left eye (OS) as a child and required stitches to close his skin wound. His weight has recently decreased even though his appetite has not changed and he admitted to iv drug use.

Exam

	OD	OS
Visual acuity	20/60	20/400
Intraocular pressure (IOP) (mm Hg)	12	11
Sclera/conjunctiva	Clear. No injection	Clear. No injection
Cornea	Clear	Clear
Anterior chamber (AC)	No cell or flare	No cell or flare
Iris	Within normal limits (WNL) – no posterior synechiae	WNL – no posterior synechiae
Lens	Clear	Clear
Vitreous cavity	Trace vitreous cells	Trace vitreous cells
Retina/optic nerve	Multifocal retinal whitening/necrosis of outer retina (Fig. 48.1)	Multifocal retinal whitening/necrosis of outer retina; mottling of RPE; pallor of optic nerve (Fig. 48.2)

Questions to Ask

- Has your vision changed in the past month?
- Have you seen a doctor recently to find out why you have not been feeling well?
- Because you work in jazz clubs, did you ever participate in drug use or unprotected sex with women and/or men?
- Do you have redness, pain, photophobia, or floaters in either eye?

The patient reports that he started to notice changes in vision 3 months ago, but only recently has it gotten so bad that he is having difficulty reading music sheets. He has an appointment to see a family doctor in 2 weeks but has not sought medical care until now. Occasionally, he injects heroin intravenously (IV) and does have unprotected sex with several of the women waitresses and women bartenders. He reports his eyes feel fine except that the vision is blurred, particularly in the OS. He reports no pain, redness, light sensitivity, or floaters in either eye.

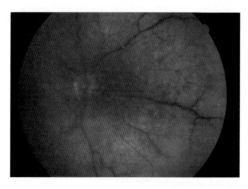

Fig. 48.1 Disseminated multifocal retinal whitening/necrosis of outer retina, with minimal retinal vasculitis (mud-cracking appearance, given sparing of the retinal vasculature), OD.

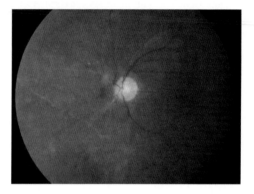

Fig. 48.2 Pigmentary clumping of retinal pigment epithelium (RPE), subretinal fibrotic bands, and atrophy of optic nerve, OS.

Assessment

- Diffuse retinitis, OU, with atrophy of optic nerve OS possibly associated with acquired immunodeficiency syndrome (AIDS)

Differential Diagnosis

- Cytomegalovirus (CMV) retinitis
- Syphilitic retinitis
- Ocular lymphoma or other bone marrow disorder
- Sarcoidosis

Working Diagnosis

- Progressive outer retinal necrosis (PORN), OU, with retrobulbar atrophy of optic nerve OS associated with AIDS

Testing

- Complete blood count (CBC): marked lymphopenia with CD4+ T-cell count = 46

- Human immunodeficiency virus (HIV) testing blood: + HIV antigen (p24) and antibodies
- Polymerase chain reaction (PCR) testing vitreous: + varicella zoster virus (VZV)
- Goldmann Witmer coefficient (GWC) vitreous: anti-VZV immunoglobulin G (IgG) 1:32

Management

- Combination IV antiviral therapy (e.g., acyclovir and/or foscarnet and ganciclovir) with intravitreal (IVIT) injection of antivirals was started immediately.
- Infectious diseases consulted to manage HIV infection and AIDS
- Patient hospitalized for 48 hours and to continue treatment as an outpatient

Follow-up

- Scheduled to return weekly for IVIT injection of antivirals. Unfortunately, combined IVIT and oral antiviral medications did not halt the progression of disease. Visual acuity (VA) decreased to light perception (LP) right eye (OD) and no light perception (NLP) OS.

Key Points

- VZV is a member of the herpesviruses family, which includes herpes simplex virus 1 (HSV-1) and 2 (HSV-2). After primary infection, these viruses become latent and reside in sensory ganglia, such as the trigeminal ganglion.
- Infection in early childhood presents as varicella (chickenpox). After establishment of latency, recurrent disease can present as cutaneous herpes zoster (shingles) or ocular herpes zoster (herpes zoster ophthalmicus).
- PORN is a severe, rapidly progressive retinitis of the outer retina and is frequently refractory to medical therapy. However, combined systemic and IVIT antiviral medications can occasionally halt disease progression. Nevertheless, visual prognosis remains poor because of confluent, necrotic retina and retrobulbar optic nerve damage.
- There is a relative paucity of intraocular inflammation with PORN because most patients present with advanced AIDS and CD4+ T-cell counts ≤50. Involvement of the optic nerve is common and contributes to the poor visual prognosis.
- Retinal detachment is common, and prophylactic laser barricade posterior to affected areas may decrease the incidence. However, once a retinal detachment develops, pars plana vitrectomy with silicone oil instillation is required.
- PORN can also present initially with intraretinal multifocal whitening and progression of the lesions observed (Fig. 48.3A and B).

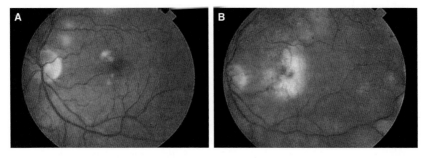

Fig. 48.3 (A) Early presentation of PORN as multifocal outer retinal whitening in posterior pole. (B) Progression of the disease with coalescence of the lesions.

CHAPTER 49

Toxoplasmosis

Harpal S. Sandhu

History of Present Illness

A 27-year-old woman with no significant past ocular history or medical history complains of new floaters in the left eye (OS) for 3 days. She states her vision is also blurred in this eye. She has no complaints in the other eye.

Exam

	OD	OS
Vision:	20/20	20/30−
Intraocular pressure (IOP):	11	19
Lids and lashes:	Normal	Normal
Sclera/conjunctiva:	White and quiet	White and quiet
Cornea:	Clear	Clear
Anterior chamber (AC):	Deep and quiet	1+ cells
Iris:	Flat	Flat
Lens:	Clear	Clear
Anterior vitreous:	Clear	1+ anterior vitreous cells

Dilated fundus examination (DFE) (See Fig. 49.1)

Nerve:	Cup-to-disc (c/d) 0.2, pink, sharp
Macula:	Normal
Vessels:	Normal caliber and course
Periphery:	Unremarkable

Further Questions to Ask

- Have you ever experienced anything like this before?
- Do you live with any pets?
- Have you traveled internationally recently?
- Have you eaten any uncooked or poorly cooked meat recently?
- Do you have any problems with your immune system?

She did used to live with a cat at one time. Otherwise, she answers no to the questions.

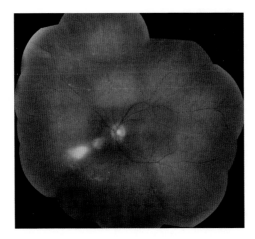

Fig. 49.1 Color fundus photograph of the left eye shows a partially hyperpigmented scar inferonasal to the nerve with a bright white lesion, with hazy borders at the level of the retina adjacent to the scar, consistent with active retinitis. There are multiple yellow-white perivascular plaques and several small vitreous opacities.

Assessment

- Focal retinochoroiditis with panuveitis and retinal vasculitis OS
- Evidence of prior retinochoroiditis OS

Differential Diagnosis

- Toxoplasmic retinochoroiditis
- Syphilis
- Herpetic retinitis
- Sarcoidosis
- Less likely: Behçet disease

Working Diagnosis

- Toxoplasmic retinochoroiditis

Testing

- Toxoplasma serologies

Management

- Start trimethoprim—sulfamethoxazole (TMP-SMX) one double-strength tablet by mouth (PO) twice a day (BID)
- Start prednisone 1 mg/kg PO daily starting 2 days later
- Follow up in 1 week

Follow-up

You see the patient a little over a week later. She notes her vision and floaters are improving. Vision is 20/25 OS, anterior chamber (AC) cells have resolved, and vitreous opacification has improved. Toxoplasma immunoglobulin M (IgM) returned negative, immunoglobulin G (IgG) positive at 1:256.

Management

- Continue TMP-SMX
- Taper prednisone by 10 mg each week
- Follow up in 2 to 3 weeks

Management Algorithm

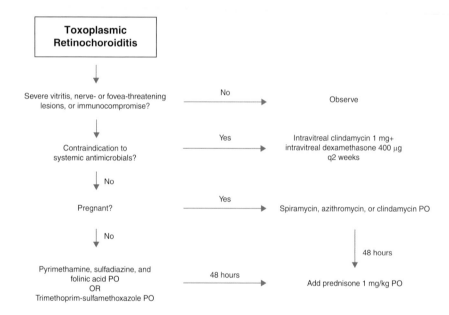

Key Points

- Toxoplasmosis is one of the most common causes of posterior uveitis worldwide and has a particularly high prevalence in South America and the tropics.
- Active retinochoroiditis adjacent to a hyperpigmented scar is strongly suggestive of acquired toxoplasmic retinochoroiditis. Vitritis is typically dense (in contrast to the mild vitritis in this case), producing the classic "headlight in the fog" presentation.
- The distinctive perivascular plaques (Kyrieleis plaques) featured in this case are not very sensitive for toxoplasmosis but are somewhat specific for the disease. They can linger for months to even years after acute episodes of reactivation and thus do not imply active disease. They have also been seen in rare cases of syphilitic and herpetic retinitis.

- Congenital toxoplasmosis has a significantly different fundus appearance, manifesting with large macular scars, usually bilaterally.
- Cats and their feces, as well as ingestion of undercooked meat, are risk factors for the disease.
- Not all flares have to be treated. Dense vitritis, optic nerve–threatening lesions, fovea-threatening lesions, and immunocompromise are classic indications for treatment.
- There are multiple different options for treatment, including local or systemic routes, and multiple different antiparasitic agents. There has been some suggestion that classic therapy (pyrimethamine and sulfadiazine) is the most efficacious and should be used in severe cases, but this is not definitive.
- Antiparasitic therapy should be continued as long as the patient is on corticosteroids. Acute flares typically resolve in 3 to 6 weeks.
- Some patients with frequent recurrences may benefit from chronic antiparasitic therapy (e.g., TMP-SMX every other day)

CHAPTER 50

Severe, Atypical Toxoplasmosis

Harpal S. Sandhu ■ Albert M. Maguire

History of Present Illness (HPI)

A 64-year-old man presents complaining of decreased vision in his right eye (OD). He is positive for human immunodeficiency virus (HIV) and has a history of cytomegalovirus (CMV) retinitis, left eye (OS), complicated by recurrent retinal detachment and ultimately phthisis bulbi OS.

Exam

	OD	OS
Vision:	20/40	No light perception (NLP)
Intraocular pressure (IOP):	22	4
Lids and lashes:	Normal	Ptotic left upper lid
Sclera/conjunctiva:	White and quiet	Trace injection, shrunken globe
Cornea:	Clear	2+ stromal edema, band keratopathy
Anterior chamber (AC):	Deep and quiet	Shallow
Iris:	Flat	Flat
Lens:	2+ nuclear sclerosis (NS)	4+ brunescent NS
Anterior vitreous:	Clear	No view
Dilated fundus examination (DFE):	See Fig. 50.1	No view OS

Questions to Ask

- How long has this been going on for?
- Is there any pain?
- Have you had recent illnesses or hospitalizations?
- Are you taking your HIV medications? What is your current CD4 count?
- When was the last time you saw an infectious diseases doctor?

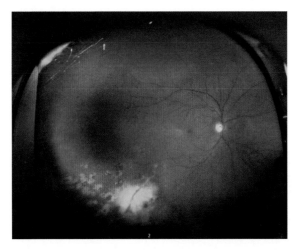

Fig. 50.1 Color wide-field photograph of the right eye shows a creamy, white-yellow lesion inferotemporally, vascular sheathing within the lesion and proximal to it, pigmented chorioretinal scars inferotemporally, and vitreous debris inferiorly. There was no vitritis. B scan OS: shrunken, disorganized globe.

He responds that his vision has been declining for a few weeks. There is no pain. He has HIV medications at home but hates taking pills and takes them "when I feel like it." He has not seen his infectious diseases doctor in about a year.

Assessment

- Focal retinitis OD with adjacent retinal vasculitis
- Phthisis bulbi OS secondary to CMV retinitis complicated by retinal detachment

Differential Diagnosis

- CMV retinitis
- Atypical toxoplasmosis
- Other herpetic retinitis (herpes simplex virus [HSV], varicella zoster virus [VZV])
- Syphilis

Working Diagnosis

- CMV retinitis OD
- Although the patient's exact immune status is unknown, he has HIV and admits noncompliance with highly active antiretroviral therapy (HAART). One can safely assume that he is immunocompromised. He is monocular and has already lost the left eye to CMV retinitis. He now presents with decreased vision and active retinitis without vitritis or anterior chamber (AC) reaction in the right eye. Although the lack of hemorrhages in the right eye and the unusual morphology of the retinitis lesion are atypical for CMV, he is at high risk of CMV in this eye.

Management

- Start valganciclovir 900 mg by mouth (PO) twice a day (BID)
- Check CD4 count
- Restart home HAART medications
- Follow up in 1 week

Follow-up

HPI

The patient misses his 1-week follow-up appointment but returns at 2 weeks saying his vision is no better. If anything, it seems worse. He still has no pain and no new symptoms. He insists that he has been taking his valganciclovir regularly, as he does not want to go blind.

Exam

	OD	OS
Vision	20/60	NLP
IOP	21	4
SLE: Stable OU from presentation.		
DFE:	See Fig. 50.2	No view

CD4 count: Toxoplasma IgM negative 94 cells/μL

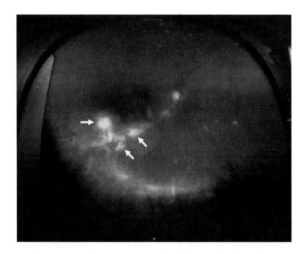

Fig. 50.2 Color wide-field photograph of the right eye shows that the retinitis is now multifocal with multiple new, more posterior lesions (*white arrows*). There is also more vascular sheathing nasally and a mild vitritis with layering of vitreous debris inferiorly. The green spots superiorly are artifacts of the wide-field fundus camera. (Modified from Sandhu HS, Maguire AM. Atypical retinitis in the setting of prior cytomegalovirus retinitis. *JAMA Ophthalmol.* 2016;134[6]:709–710.)

Assessment

- Worsening retinitis OD despite ganciclovir therapy.
- The patient's condition has worsened despite being on valganciclovir. Although there are strains of CMV that are resistant to the drug, valganciclovir is generally an effective treatment. Moreover, CMV retinitis progresses slowly, and one would not expect a distinct worsening of the disease over just 2 weeks. Thus a misdiagnosis must be considered. Given the presence of a pigmented scar adjacent to the active retinitis, atypical toxoplasmosis should be higher on the differential.

Differential Diagnosis

- Atypical toxoplasmosis
- CMV retinitis resistant to valganciclovir
- Refractory or resistant herpetic retinitis (HSV, VZV)
- Syphilitic retinitis

Working Diagnosis

- Atypical toxoplasmosis

Management

- Trial of antitoxoplasmic therapy as a diagnostic and therapeutic maneuver. Inject clindamycin 1 mg/0.1 cc intravitreally
- Check serum anti–*Toxoplasmosis gondii* serologies
- Check rapid plasma reagin (RPR), fluorescent treponemal antibody absorption (FTA-ABS)
- Follow up in 1 week

Follow-up #2 (3 Weeks Post-presentation)

HPI

The patient reports hating the injection but is relieved that his vision seems a bit better.

Exam

	OD	OS
Vision	20/50	NLP
IOP	10	5
SLE: Stable OU from last examination, small temporal subconjunctival hemorrhage OD		
DFE:	See Fig. 50.3	No view

Toxoplasma IgM negative, toxoplasma IgG 1:1024, RPR negative, FTA-ABS negative.

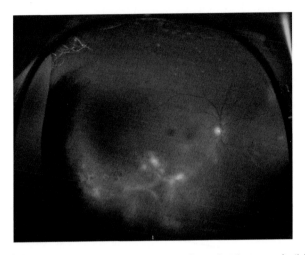

Fig. 50.3 Color wide-field fundus photograph of the right eye shows that the areas of retinitis along the inferior arcade are beginning to regress. There are a few new intraretinal hemorrhages after the injection.

Assessment

- Multifocal retinitis OD, improving after local antitoxoplasmic therapy

Final Diagnosis

- Atypical toxoplasmosis OD

Key Points

- Toxoplasmosis can present quite differently in the immunocompromised patient than it does in the immunocompetent one. It is more likely to have larger and/or multifocal lesions, little to no vitritis, and no pigmented scars indicative of prior active infection.
- Its presentation can thus mimic forms of herpetic retinitis. Treating for herpetic disease first, as in this case, is reasonable, but the diagnosis must be reconsidered if the patient does not respond appropriately.
- Risk factors include typical causes of immunocompromise, such as chemotherapy, HIV, and immunosuppressive therapy. Interestingly, elderly age has also been identified as a risk factor in some studies.
- Although polymerase chain reaction (PCR) is usually an instructive test in diagnostic dilemmas and could be considered here, the yield is low in these cases because toxoplasma can remain relatively confined to the retina and choroid.
- Although positive serum immunoglobulin G (IgG) generally only confirms previous exposure, very high titers or a large increase in titers from baseline is suggestive of an active infection.
- In cases where all testing has been unhelpful, clinical response to empiric treatments, such as intravitreal clindamycin for toxoplasmosis, may be the only nonsurgical means by which to make the diagnosis. Severe cases without a clear diagnosis, even after multiple empiric treatments, may warrant diagnostic vitrectomy with or without chorioretinal biopsy.
- Much like CMV retinitis, these patients are also at risk of rhegmatogenous retinal detachment, the treatment for which is pars plana vitrectomy with silicone oil tamponade due to the propensity for multiple retinal breaks and microbreaks.
- See Chapter 45 for a more detailed discussion of treatment options for toxoplasmosis.

CHAPTER 51

Toxocariasis

Henry J. Kaplan

History of Present Illness

It is the beginning of the school year for first graders. An eye examination is required, and a 6-year-old girl has best corrected visual acuity (VA) 20/20 right eye (OD) and 20/80 left eye (OS). She is otherwise is in good health. Her mother has noticed that she does not see objects or people coming from either side. She has no history of trauma to either eye. However, she likes to play in the sandbox in a park near her house.

Exam

	OD	OS
Visual acuity	20/20	20/80
Intraocular pressure (IOP) (mm Hg)	9	8
Sclera/ conjunctiva	Clear. No injection	Clear. No injection
Cornea	Clear	Clear
Anterior chamber (AC)	No cell or flare	No cell or flare
Iris	Within normal limits (WNL) – no posterior synechiae	WNL – no posterior synechiae
Lens	Clear	Clear
Vitreous cavity	Clear	No vitreous cells
Retina/optic nerve	Normal optic nerve, posterior and peripheral retina	Tractional band extending from the optic nerve to the center of the macula with a localized tractional retinal detachment in the posterior pole (Fig. 51.1)

Questions to Ask

- Has your daughter ever complained of not seeing well in her OS?
- Has she ever had redness, pain, or light sensitivity in her OS?
- Do you have any pets at home?
- Does she play in a sandbox where dogs also are occasionally seen?

The patient has not complained of not seeing well in her OS, nor has she had redness, pain, or light sensitivity in either eye. The family has two golden retrievers at home who are now 4 and 5 years old. The family frequently goes to the local public park, which has a sandbox, and many dogs are roaming around the park with their owners.

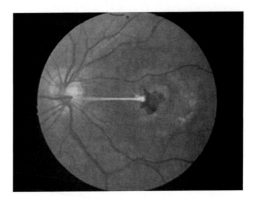

Fig. 51.1 Tractional fold extending from the optic nerve to an epiretinal membrane causing a localized neurosensory retinal detachment in the center of macula, OS.

Assessment

- Posterior retina granuloma with a tractional fold extending to the optic disc and macular pucker secondary to an epiretinal membrane, OS

Differential Diagnosis

- Toxocariasis
- Retinoblastoma
- Retinopathy of prematurity
- Persistent hyperplastic primary vitreous/persistent fetal vasculature
- Coats disease

Working Diagnosis

- Toxocariasis with a peripheral granuloma, tractional retinal fold extending posteriorly, and macular pucker, OS

Testing

- Enzyme-linked immunosorbent assay (ELISA) *Toxocara* titer: +1:16

Management

- Pars plana vitrectomy to relieve traction on the retina and to remove the epiretinal membrane within the macula should be considered.
- Without significant intraocular inflammation, neither topical nor systemic corticosteroids need to be administered preoperatively.

Follow-up

- Return postoperative appointments 1 day, 1 week, and 1 month.
- Referral to a pediatric ophthalmologist after her 1-month postoperative visit to begin amblyopia therapy OS.

Key Points

- Toxocariasis is a rare infection caused by the dog roundworms *Toxocara canis* and *Toxocara cati* and is usually found in young children. Infection frequently occurs in children from playing in a sandbox that has been frequented by a dog with the infection. In puppies 2 to 6 months old, the prevalence of *T. canis* has been reported to be over 80%; in dogs older than 1 year this number drops to 20%.

- Presentations typically include posterior uveitis with symptoms and signs such as reduced vision, photophobia, floaters, and leukocoria. Three forms of ocular toxocariasis are a peripheral retinal granuloma (Fig. 51.2), a posterior pole granuloma (Fig. 51.3), and chronic endophthalmitis. The posterior pole granuloma usually presents with a hazy vitreous and an ill-defined posterior pole whitish mass with traction bands to the surrounding retina. Chronic endophthalmitis presents as a dense vitritis, frequently associated with a retinal detachment, sometimes presenting with leukocoria (Fig. 51.4). The acute stage of endophthalmitis may present with a granulomatous iritis and hypopyon.

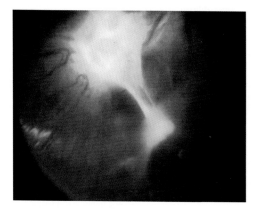

Fig. 51.2 Localized white peripheral granuloma with a traction band extending posteriorly to the optic nerve, OS.

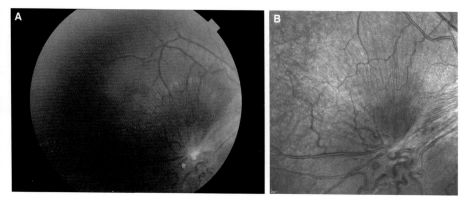

Fig. 51.3 (A) Fundus photograph of a patient with *Toxocara* granuloma adjacent to the inferior arcade, with dragging of the macula and secondary epiretinal membrane formation, OD. (B) Infrared reflectance imaging of the same patient.

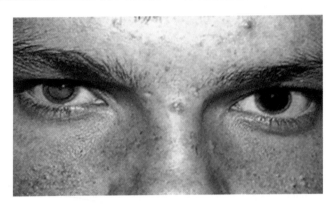

Fig. 51.4 Leukocoria OD secondary to chronic endophthalmitis resulting from toxocariasis.

- After ingestion, the eggs mature into larvae and reach systemic circulation via the gut. The larvae can infect many organs, including the heart, liver, brain, muscle, lungs, and eyes. When it infects different tissues, it is called *visceral larva migrans*. Reactive inflammatory processes lead to the organism's encapsulation and the formation of eosinophilic granulomas.
- Ocular toxocariasis is unilateral in 90% of cases and typically presents as posterior uveitis in three different subtypes: chronic endophthalmitis (25%), central posterior granuloma (25% to 46%), and peripheral granuloma (20% to 40%). The most common sign associated with ocular toxocariasis is vitritis in over 90% of patients. Other presenting signs include leukocoria, ocular injection, and strabismus.
- Management includes quieting inflammation and repairing vitreoretinal sequelae. Severe inflammation may be treated with topical corticosteroids, cycloplegics, and systemic corticosteroids. There usually is no role for antihelminthics like thiabendazole or diethylcarbamazine. Surgical intervention is indicated to relieve retinal traction, macular pucker, or dense vitreous opacities that interfere with the visual axis.

CHAPTER 52

Systemic Lupus Erythematosus with Retinal Vasculitis

Aleksandra Radosavljevic ▦ Jelena Karadzic ▦ Manfred Zierhut

History of Present Illness

A 36-year-old female presented with complaints of blurred vision in both eyes (OU). In 1990, at the age of 15, she had developed butterfly-shaped skin lesions on the face; treatment was unspecific. In 1993, swelling and pain of the knee and small joints of both hands occurred. She was now found positive for antinuclear antibodies (ANA) leading to the diagnosis of systemic lupus erythematosus (SLE). She was treated with prednisone 10 to 20 mg per day for years.

In 1998 she had developed proteinuria leading to the diagnosis of lupus nephritis. She had developed arterial hypertension and moderate anemia (both were controlled with medications). Additional immunosuppressive treatment was initiated with Resochin, azathioprine, and pulsed cyclophosphamide, but the patient either did not tolerate the medication or it was inefficient.

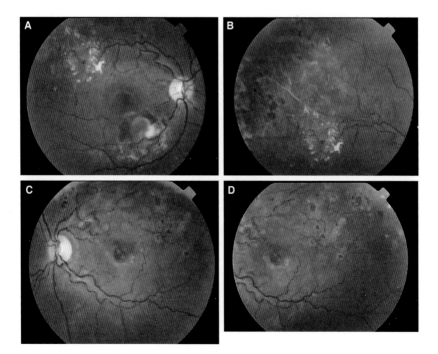

Fig. 52.1 Fundus photo of the right (A and B) and the left eye (C and D) in 2005: Large areas of ischemic retina with small intraretinal hemorrhages and lipid exudates.

Finally, mycophenolate mofetil was introduced and continued for the next 4 years. This improved the patient's condition.

In 2005, 1 year after she stopped mycophenolate in remission, she was found to have large areas of retinal ischemia, occlusive retinal vasculitis, and retinal neovascularization elsewhere (NVE) in the temporal retina (Figs. 52.1 and 52.2). Laser photocoagulation of the ischemic areas was performed. In 2011 she needed peritoneal dialysis due to terminal renal insufficiency. Systemic treatment included prednisone 20 mg daily, which caused moderate osteoporosis and cataracts in both eyes. She had one episode of peritonitis in 2012 (due to *Klebsiella*).

At the first examination in our clinic, she complained about deterioration of vision. Optical coherence tomography (OCT) revealed macular edema OU and a chorioretinal scar in the left macula. The patient received sub-Tenon triamcinolone injections bilaterally, and macular edema resolved. Due to retinal ischemia, laser photocoagulation was performed.

Exam

	OD	OS
Visual acuity	20/25	20/250
Intraocular pressure (IOP)	14	14
Sclera/conjunctiva	Clear, no hyperemia	Clear, no hyperemia
Cornea	Clear	Clear
Anterior chamber (AC)	Deep, no cells, no flare	Deep, no cells, no flare
Iris	Unremarkable	Unremarkable
Lens	Posterior subcapsular cataract	Posterior subcapsular cataract
Anterior vitreous	Clear	Clear
Fundus	Occlusive retinal vasculitis in superotemporal retina with old inactive NVE and chorioretinal scars after laser photocoagulation. Macular edema and large pigmented chorioretinal scar below the macula	Occlusive retinal vasculitis in superotemporal retina and chorioretinal scars after laser photocoagulation. Macular edema

Questions to Ask

- Have you ever had any problems with sugar levels, excessive thirst, urination, night sweats, or loss of body mass?
- Have you ever had any numbness, tingling, weakness on one side of the body, or bowel or bladder problems? Is there any history of neurologic disorders in the family?
- Have you had any cough, lung problems, or episodes of fever?
- Have you noticed any recent ticks or tick bites on your body?
- Have you ever had a cat scratch?
- Do you have a travel history?

She answers no to all of the questions.

Assessment

Occlusive retinal vasculitis (arteritis) OU, macular edema

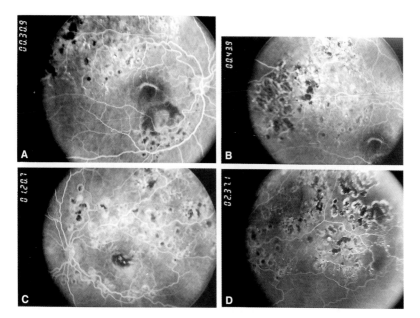

Fig. 52.2 Fluorescein angiography (FA) of the right (A and B) and the left eye (C and D) in 2005: In the right eye beneath the inferior vascular arcade, hyperfluorescent choroidal neovascularization (CNV) was observed.

Differential Diagnosis

- SLE vasculitis
- Sarcoid vasculitis
- Multiple sclerosis (MS)—associated retinal vasculitis
- Less likely: Lyme-associated, cat scratch disease—associated, or tuberculous retinal vasculitis

Working Diagnosis

Occlusive retinal vasculitis (arteritis), OU

Testing

- In patients with a medical history of lupus-related renal insufficiency, the workup includes urinalysis with microscopy (proteinuria, hematuria), basic biochemistry with ESR, C-reactive protein (CRP), serum creatinine, ANA, anti—double-stranded deoxyribonucleic acid (DNA) antibodies, anti-Ro/SSA antibodies, anti-SSB (La) antibodies, anticardiolipin antibodies, anti-B2 glycoprotein antibodies, lupus anticoagulant, complement levels, circulating immune complexes, neurologic investigation for neurolupus (nuclear magnetic resonance [NMR] of the brain, if neurologic review of systems is positive).
- For atypical cases, check:
  - Angiotensin-converting enzyme (ACE), lysozyme, soluble IL-2 receptors
  - QuantiFERON gold test or purified protein derivative (PPD), antineutrophil cytoplasmic antibodies (c-ANCA)
  - Fluorescent treponemal antibody absorption (FTA-ABS), rapid plasma reagin (RPR)
  - Lyme antibodies with Western blot

- *Bartonella* antibodies
- Neurologic investigation for MS or vasculitis of the brain

Management

- Systemic prednisone 1 mg/kg for 1 week then slowly taper by 10 mg every week to 20 mg, then further reduction by 2.5 mg every week to 10 mg. Then very slow taper depending on the activity of uveitis.
- In severe cases, immediate addition of an immunosuppressive drug is necessary.
- Local treatment: topical nonsteroidal antiinflammatory drug (NSAID) three to four times per day and sub-Tenon or intravitreal steroid injections for macular edema.
- Intravitreal anti−vascular endothelial growth factor (VEGF) for choroidal neovascularization (CNV). Anti-VEGF may be used as additional therapy for severe cases of retinal neovascularization (NVE or NVD—neovascularization of the optic disc) in occlusive retinal vasculitis.
- Follow up in 2 weeks.

Follow-up

Since 2013, the patient was negative for ANA, anti−double-stranded DNA (anti-dsDNA) antibodies, anti-Ro/SSA antibodies, anti-myeloperoxidase (anti-MPO) antibodies, anticardiolipin antibodies, and anti-B2 glycoprotein antibodies and had a normal range of C3 and C4 complement components. Circulating immune complexes were detected occasionally (maximum level in 2014 was 0.600). Since 2016, the patient was planned for renal transplantation but could not perform it due to physical distress and frequent systemic infections (including skin abscesses). Arterial hypertension and anemia responded well to medical treatment. In 2018, the patient had developed congestive cardiomyopathy with pleural effusion, which has been punctured (punctate was sterile and QuantiFERON Gold Test was negative). She also developed an abscess of the skin in the gluteal region and was treated with antibiotics. Under this treatment, the patient was stable.

Regarding the ophthalmologic findings, in 2013 the patient had exudative retinal detachment (Fig. 52.3) in the right eye (OD), which resolved after an increased dose of steroids (prednisone

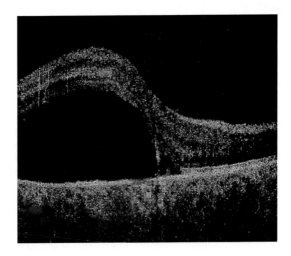

Fig. 52.3   OCT of the right eye in 2013: Exudative retinal detachment in the temporal retina.

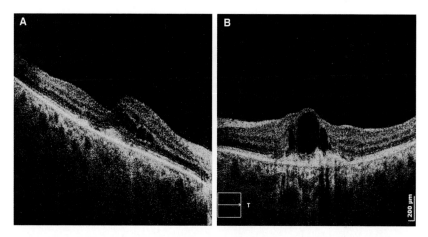

Fig. 52.4 (A and B) OCT of both eyes in 2016: Bilateral macular edema and CNV.

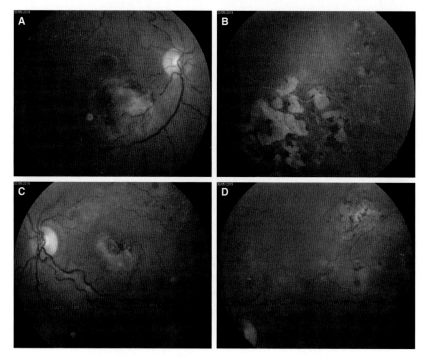

Fig. 52.5 Fundus photo of the right (A and B) and the left eye (C and D) in 2019: In the mid-periphery chorioretinal scars after panretinal laser photocoagulation. Ischemic areas with occluded blood vessels in superotemporal retina. Below the right macula and in the left macula, chorioretinal scars with subretinal fibrosis (left macula).

1 mg/kg). In 2016, a decrease in visual acuity (VA) occurred (OD 20/30 and left eye [OS] 20/250) and active CNV with cystoid macular edema (CME) was documented in both eyes (Fig. 52.4). The patient received sub-Tenon triamcinolone injections OU, after which reduction of intraretinal fluid occurred but was not complete in the OS. Therefore an intravitreal anti-VEGF agent was

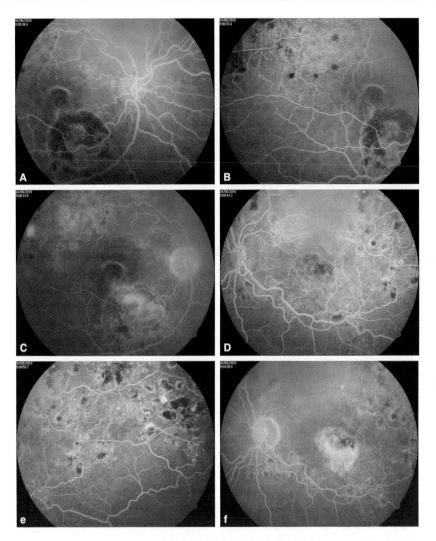

Fig. 52.6 FA of the right (A–C) and the left eye (D–F) in 2019: Findings include mid-periphery hypofluorescent chorioretinal scars after panretinal laser photocoagulation and ischemic areas in the superotemporal retina with NVE. Bolow the right macula and in the left macula, early hypofluorescent lesions with later hyperfluorescence and leakage (CNV).

given in the OS and fluid resorbed. Also, mycophenolate mofetil was reintroduced along with prednisone 10 mg. After 3 months, VA in the OD was 20/25 and 20/200 in the OS. In 2019, progression of cataract in both eyes was detectable (OD 20/30, OS 20/250). The final fundus photographs (Fig. 52.5), fluorescein angiography (FA) (Fig. 52.6), OCT, and OCT angiography (OCTA) (Fig. 52.7) are shown.

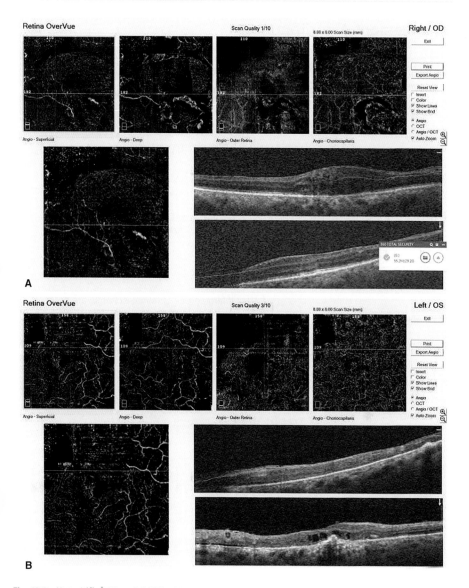

Fig. 52.7 (A and B) OCT and OCTA of both eyes: Cystoid macular edema and CNV OU, OD > OS (lens opacities reduced the picture quality).

Management Algorithm

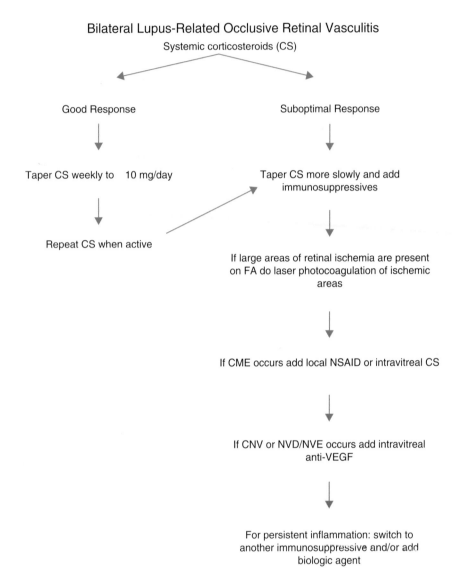

Bilateral Lupus-Related Occlusive Retinal Vasculitis
Systemic corticosteroids (CS)

Good Response

Suboptimal Response

Taper CS weekly to 10 mg/day

Taper CS more slowly and add immunosuppressives

Repeat CS when active

If large areas of retinal ischemia are present on FA do laser photocoagulation of ischemic areas

If CME occurs add local NSAID or intravitreal CS

If CNV or NVD/NVE occurs add intravitreal anti-VEGF

For persistent inflammation: switch to another immunosuppressive and/or add biologic agent

Key Points

- Lupus-related uveitis most commonly presents with occlusive retinal vasculitis, but many other ocular manifestations have been reported, such as hypertensive retinopathy, dry eye, superficial punctate keratitis, episcleritis, scleritis, discoid lupus of the eyelids, choroidal vasculitis with exudative retinal detachment, optic neuritis or ischemic optic neuropathy, and orbital pseudotumor.

- In most cases, lupus nephritis has a progressive course, and if not treated the prognosis is poor.
- Often SLE-related vasculitis is asymmetric in ocular disease.
- More severe cases require additional systemic immunosuppressive treatment.
- Vascular occlusions (central retinal artery, central retinal vein, branch retinal vein, anterior ischemic optic neuropathy), macular edema, CNV, and NVD/NVE with vitreous hemorrhage are the most common causes of vision loss in these patients.

CHAPTER 53

Cytomegalovirus (CMV) Retinitis

Henry J. Kaplan

History of Present Illness

Cc: Weight loss over the past 3 months, with onset of floaters OU over the past 6 weeks

A 38-year-old man presents in the emergency department (ED) with blurred vision in the right eye (OD) and floaters in both eyes (OU) over the past 6 weeks. He is an artist who lost 24 pounds over the past 3 months and has complained of chronic watery stools since that time. He has no history of pain, photophobia, or redness in either eye.

Exam

	OD	OS
Visual acuity	20/80	20/25
Intraocular pressure (IOP) (mm Hg)	12	10
Lids/sclera/conjunctiva	Purplish-red lesion on RLL, 0.5 mm diameter. Otherwise, within normal limits (WNL) (Fig. 53.3)	Clear. No injection
Cornea	Clear with no keratic precipitate (KP)	Clear with no KP
Anterior chamber (AC)	No flare or cell	No flare or cell
Iris	Round pupil without posterior synechiae	Round pupil without posterior synechiae
Lens	Clear	Clear
Vitreous cavity	0.5 vitreous cell	0.5 vitreous cell
Retina/optic nerve	Swollen optic nerve head with peripapillary hemorrhage, vascular sheathing along arcades and macular edema (Fig. 53.1)	Central retinal granular opacities in atrophic retina surrounded by active border of retinitis in the peripheral retina progressing posteriorly (Fig. 53.2)

Questions to Ask

- Were you evaluated for your weight loss and watery stools? If so, what tests were done?
- Have you participated in the use of intravenous (IV) drugs or unprotected sex with men or women?
- Have you had any skin lesions on your face or body that have not regressed?

He was recently hospitalized in a community hospital for weight loss and frequent diarrhea. A colon biopsy was done, and he was told that he had an infection with a fungus, cryptococcosis, and was started on IV therapy with amphotericin and another drug. He was then sent to the ED.

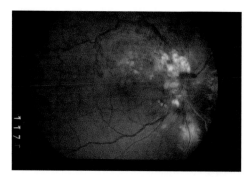

Fig. 53.1 OD: Optic nerve swelling with peripapillary hemorrhagic retinitis and white exudates extending along the vascular arcades with macular edema.

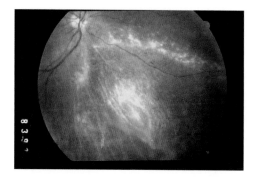

Fig. 53.2 OS: Granular active border of retinitis surrounding an atrophic retina.

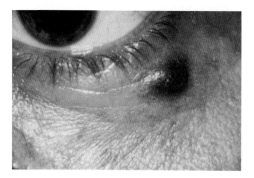

Fig. 53.3 Purple-red vascular nodular skin lesion on right lower lid (RLL) diagnosed as Kaposi sarcoma.

He has had unprotected sex with men, and he has had a little red nodule on the right lower lid for the past few months (Fig. 53.3).

Assessment

- Infectious retinitis, OU, presumably secondary to immune suppression
- Cryptococcosis enteritis

Differential Diagnosis

- Cytomegalovirus (CMV) retinitis secondary to acquired immunodeficiency syndrome (AIDS)
- Human immunodeficiency virus (HIV) retinopathy
- Causes of infectious retinitis (syphilis, herpes simplex virus [HSV], varicella zoster virus [VZV])
- *Toxoplasma* retinochoroiditis
- Fungal retinitis (e.g., *Candida*)

Working Diagnosis

- CMV retinitis and Kaposi sarcoma secondary to AIDS

Testing

- Imaging
  - See Figs. 53.4 and 53.5
- Complete blood count (CBC): leukopenia with CD4+ T-cell count ≤ 50
- HIV serology: (+), with Western blot confirmation
- *Treponema palladium* testing: Venereal Disease Research Laboratory (VDRL) (−), fluorescent treponemal antibody absorption (FTA-ABS) (−)
- Aqueous and/or vitreous paracentesis: polymerase chain reaction (PCR) testing for viral, bacterial, or fungal etiology of retinitis if progression of retinopathy while on therapy

Management

- CMV retinitis in a patient with AIDS is a clinical diagnosis. Therapy for HIV infection and CMV infection should be started immediately. Referral to infectious diseases service for initiation of highly active antiretroviral therapy (HAART) to treat HIV and improve immune status, as well as evaluation and treatment for other secondary systemic infections, such as cryptococcosis enteritis.
- Oral anti-CMV therapy with valganciclovir for both induction and maintenance therapy.
- Follow up in 2 weeks, with monthly visits thereafter to monitor regression of CMV retinitis by fundus examination.

Follow-up

At 2 weeks, no change in visual acuity (VA) or on retinal examination. However, at 1 month VA has decreased in the left eye (OS) and there is clear progression of CMV retinitis, OU.

Working Diagnosis

Progression of CMV retinitis, OU, on oral valganciclovir therapy

Management

- Intravitreal ganciclovir injections OU two times a week.

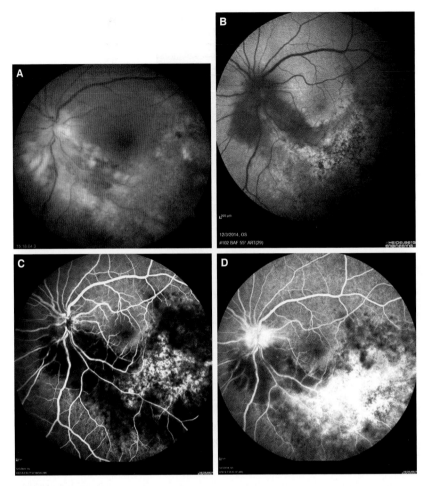

Fig. 53.4 Top row: Color photo (A) and fundus autofluorescence (FAF) (B) of a patient with CMV retinitis demonstrating both the granular and hemorrhagic form. Bottom row: (C) FA of CMV retinitis demonstrating hypofluorescent patches along the inferior vascular arcade secondary to blocking from intraretinal hemorrhages and edema, as well as granular hyperfluorescence inferotemporally. (D) Late stage of FA demonstrates leakage from optic nerve and hyperfluorescence inferotemporally from retinal pigment epithelium (RPE) window defect.

- There was noticeable improvement in his CMV retinitis after 2 weeks. He was continued on both oral and intravitreal CMV therapy.
- Follow up in 1 month.

Follow-up

One month after combined intravitreal and oral anti-CMV therapy, the retinitis halted, and the patient was continued on weekly injections for another month, with continued combined systemic anti-CMV therapy.

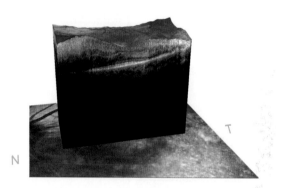

Fig. 53.5 Spectral domain optical coherence tomography (SD-OCT) of the same patient demonstrating edema and retinitis nasally, as well as outer retinal disruption (granular form) temporally.

Key Points

- CMV is a double-stranded deoxyribonucleic acid (DNA) virus in the herpesviruses family and is a ubiquitous pathogen in the general population. It rarely causes disease except in patients with a compromised immune system.
- However, CMV is one of the most common opportunistic infections affecting the eye and the leading cause of blindness in AIDS. Symptoms of early CMV retinitis are minimal because retinitis usually presents in the peripheral retina, and AIDS patients have a profound leukopenia. CD4+ T-cell counts <50 cells/mm^3 occur in most patients with CMV retinitis.
- CMV retinitis may occur in patients on HAART even with CD4+ T cells >100 cells/mm^3. Thus patients on HAART need to pay attention to any visual disturbances that develop and see an ophthalmologist shortly after their onset.
- CMV retinitis has three distinct clinical presentations: a hemorrhagic necrotizing retinitis that usually involves the arcades (catsup retinopathy); a granular indolent form in the retinal periphery, with central retinal atrophy and active borders; and a perivasculitis termed *frosted branch angiitis*.
- Patients with resolved CMV retinitis still retain latent CMV and may develop immune recovery uveitis (IRU) when their immune response recovers after HAART. The inflammation is most likely an immune response to the latent viral particles and is treated with corticosteroid therapy.
- CMV antiviral resistance: Resolution of CMV retinitis on systemic therapy is dependent on improvement in the immune status of the patient, as well as the sensitivity of CMV virus to the drug. CMV antiviral resistance testing can be used to identify nonresponsive infections, but intraocular anti-CMV therapy is an alternative approach, with intravitreal injections of ganciclovir or foscarnet, two to three times weekly for the induction phase and weekly for maintenance.
- Paracentesis and PCR testing: If the clinical presentation of retinitis changes and suggests the presence of another or different organism, aqueous humor and/or vitreous can be PCR-tested for viral, bacterial, or fungal organisms.

CHAPTER 54

Vogt-Koyanagi-Harada Disease

Harpal S. Sandhu

History of Present Illness

A 31-year-old healthy woman with no significant past medical history presents to the eye clinic for the first time complaining of progressively decreased vision over the last 2 weeks. She notes that it first started in the left eye (OS) with mild sensitivity to light, followed quickly by blurred vision. She noticed similar symptoms in the right eye (OD) a few days later. She brushed off her symptoms for the first few days, but they have been getting progressively worse.

Exam

	OD	OS
Visual acuity	20/100	20/200
Intraocular pressure (IOP)	20	22
Sclera/conjunctiva	1+ injection	1+ injection
Cornea	Clear stroma, mutton-fat keratic precipitates (KP)	Clear stroma, mutton-fat KP
Anterior chamber (AC)	2+ white cells	2+ white cells
	1+ flare	1+ flare
Iris	Unremarkable	Unremarkable
Lens	Clear	Clear
Anterior vitreous	2+ white cells	2+ white cells
Dilated fundus examination (DFE)	Fig. 54.1A	Fig. 54.1B

Questions to Ask

- Have you ever suffered a serious injury to either eye or ever had intraocular surgery?
- Have you noticed any neck stiffness, changes in your hearing, or changes in the color of your skin or hair?
- Do you have any Native American or East Asian ancestry?

She has never had any serious trauma to either eye, nor has she had surgery. She has not noticed any neck stiffness or issues with her hearing, hair, or skin. She answers that one of her grandparents was of Cherokee descent.

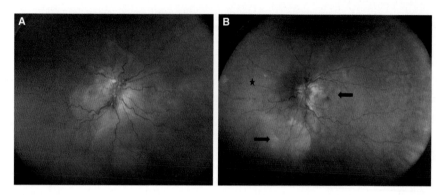

Fig. 54.1 (A) Color wide-field fundus photograph of the right eye shows massive optic nerve swelling, multiple splinter hemorrhages in the posterior pole, and multiple large blebs of retinal elevation consistent with subretinal fluid 360 degrees around the nerve, extending into the periphery. (B) Color wide-field fundus photograph of the left eye shows similar findings to the right. The areas of subretinal fluid are less bullous, but there is still a somewhat bullous area of detachment inferiorly (*right arrow*), and there are folds in the macula (*left arrow*) and fluid far nasally (*star*).

Assessment

- Panuveitis with multifocal, large serous retinal detachments both eyes (OU)

Differential Diagnosis

- Vogt–Koyanagi–Harada (VKH) syndrome
- Sympathetic ophthalmia
- Less likely: posterior scleritis, systemic leukemia/lymphoma involving the eyes

Working Diagnosis

- VKH

Testing

- The presentation of bilateral, presumably granulomatous, panuveitis with nerve swelling and multiple funduscopically obvious serous detachments is consistent only with VKH (or simply Harada syndrome if there is no systemic involvement) or sympathetic ophthalmia. The absence of a history of penetrating trauma or surgery to the eye rules out sympathetic ophthalmia, leaving only VKH. Posterior scleritis characteristically has pain, which is absent here.
- The diagnosis should be confirmed with fluorescein angiography (FA) (Fig. 54.2).
- Optical coherence tomography (OCT) is helpful not so much for diagnosis but for objective biomarkers (e.g., extent of subretinal fluid) that one can follow for signs of improvement (Fig. 54.3).

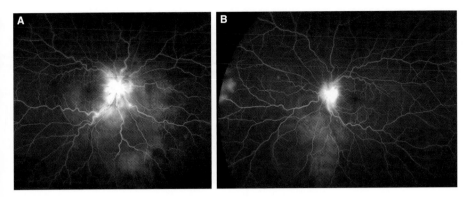

Fig. 54.2 (A) Late frame FA of the right eye shows normal retinal vasculature, massive leakage from the optic nerve, multiple pinpoint spots of hyperfluorescence, and pooling of fluorescein into the subretinal space. (B) Late frame FA of the left eye shows similar findings with prominent pooling inferiorly. There is also an area of leakage in the far nasal periphery.

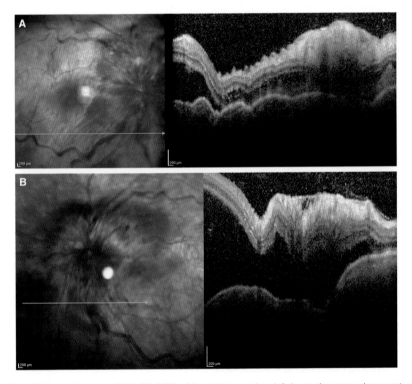

Fig. 54.3 (A) Spectral domain OCT (SD-OCT) of the right eye taken inferior to the nerve shows extensive subretinal fluid and chorioretinal folds. (B) SD-OCT of the left eye in a similar location shows massive subretinal fluid and folds.

Management

- Prednisone 100 mg by mouth (PO) daily
- Prednisolone acetate 1% every 2 hours (q2h) OU
- Check complete blood count (CBC)
- Follow up in 1 to 2 weeks

Follow-up

The patient returns 2 weeks later. She notes that her light sensitivity seems somewhat better but that she does not see any better. To make matters worse, she is having difficulty sleeping at night ever since she started the pill. She wants to stop prednisone. CBC was normal.

Exam

	OD	OS
Visual acuity	20/150	20/300 − 2
IOP	21	22
Sclera/conjunctiva	Trace injection	Trace injection
Cornea	Clear, stable KP	Clear, stable KP
AC	1/2+ white cells	1/2+ white cells
	1+ flare	1+ flare
Iris	Unremarkable	Unremarkable
Lens	Clear	Clear
Anterior vitreous	2+ white cells	2+ white cells

Fundus examination is unchanged. There is unchanged nerve swelling and similar serous detachments OU.

Follow-up Assessment

The patient has not responded despite being on high-dose prednisone for 2 weeks. The anterior inflammation is improved on frequent topical corticosteroids, but otherwise the examination is unchanged, and her vision is somewhat worse OU. Two weeks of prednisone 100 mg daily is a solid trial of oral antiinflammatory therapy. In general, lack of response in such a situation suggests two possibilities: an infectious cause mimicking VKH or a severe inflammatory/autoimmune disease refractory to typical oral antiinflammatory treatment.

Working Diagnosis 2

- Severe VKH refractory to standard oral therapy.
- The presentation is almost pathognomonic for VKH, is supported by FA, and is further supported by the patient's Native American ancestry. Maintain the original diagnosis and escalate antiinflammatory therapy.

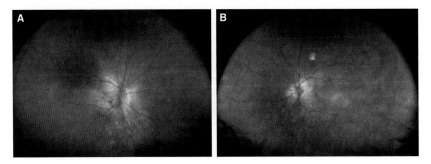

Fig. 54.4 (A) Color fundus photograph of the right eye 2 months after discharge shows persistent but improved nerve swelling and resolved serous detachment, leaving prominent pigmentary changes in their wake. (B) Color fundus photograph of the left eye shows similar findings to the right.

Management

- Admit to the hospital (or infusion center) and begin methylprednisolone 1000 mg intravenously (IV) daily for 3 to 5 days
- Discharge on prednisone 100 mg PO daily

Follow-up

The patient returns a week later noting that her vision has started to improve. Visual acuity (VA) is 20/40 OD and 20/50 OS. Some of the shallower serous detachments have resolved, and the macular detachments are significantly flatter. Prednisone was slowly tapered, and the patient was started on mycophenolate mofetil 1500 mg PO twice a day (BID) (Fig. 54.4).

Key Points

- VKH is an idiopathic, presumably autoimmune, multisystem disease characterized by poliosis, vitiligo, hearing loss, meningismus, and bilateral panuveitis. More commonly, patients present with just ocular disease (Harada syndrome).
- Sympathetic ophthalmia and VKH can be indistinguishable on examination, but a history of penetrating trauma or intraocular surgery usually allows the clinician to discriminate between them.
- VKH is much more common in patients of East Asian or Native American descent, and one should always ask about the patient's ethnic background.
- Chronic disease is characterized by depigmentation of the fundus ("sunset glow" appearance) and typically recurrent or chronic anterior uveitis, though any anatomic compartment can be involved.
- VKH typically requires initially high doses of oral corticosteroids (1 to 1.5 mg/kg PO daily) followed by tapers that are slower than those for other uveitic syndromes. Some advocate tapering prednisone to <10 mg daily over 6 to 12 months.
- A minority of VKH cases, such as here, are refractory even to prednisone 100 mg and necessitate IV methylprednisolone at mega-doses to obtain adequate control.
- Rarely, systemic leukemias metastatic to the choroid can simulate VKH and should be suspected in patients with constitutional symptoms or abnormal white blood cell counts.
- Chronic immunomodulatory therapy is usually required to manage VKH.

CHAPTER 55

Neuroretinitis

Harpal S. Sandhu

History of Present Illness (HPI)

A 36-year-old woman with no past ocular history and no significant past medical history complains of increasingly blurry vision in the right eye (OD). It started 2 weeks ago with some mild blurriness that has progressed to the point of a fuzzy gray spot in the center of her vision. The left eye (OS) seems the same as usual. In the last few days she has noticed some new floaters in the right eye as well (Fig. 55.1).

Exam

	OD	OS
Vision	20/40−	20/20
Intraocular pressure (IOP)	16	15
Lids and lashes:	Normal	Normal
Sclera/conjunctiva:	White and quiet	White and quiet
Cornea:	Clear	Clear
Anterior chamber (AC):	Deep and quiet	Deep and quiet
Iris:	Flat	Flat
Lens:	Clear	Clear
Anterior vitreous:	1+ white cells	Clear

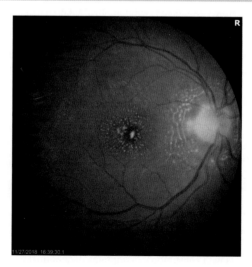

Fig. 55.1 Color fundus photograph of the right eye shows stellate exudates, an absent foveal reflex, and mild optic disc edema.

Questions to Ask

- Do you have any pets or have you had interactions with animals in the past few months?
- Have you had unprotected sex?
- Any recent injuries or scratches?
- Have you traveled outside the United States recently?

She responds that she lives with two cats, but does not recall any recent trauma. She denies unprotected sex or traveling outside the country.

Assessment

- Neuroretinitis with mild vitritis OD

Differential Diagnosis

- Syphilis
- Bartonella
- Lyme disease
- Sarcoidosis
- Leber stellate neuroretinitis
- Systemic hypertension
- Less likely: toxoplasmosis, leptospirosis, tuberculosis, anterior ischemic optic neuropathy, Rocky Mountain spotted fever

Working Diagnosis

- Infectious neuroretinitis OD, unclear organism

Testing

- Rapid plasma reagin (RPR), fluorescent treponemal antibody absorption (FTA-ABS).
- Purified protein derivative (PPD) or QuantiFERON.

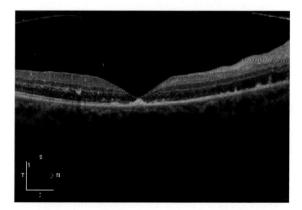

Fig. 55.2 Optical coherence tomography (OCT) of the right eye shows significant disruption of the ellipsoid zone and almost total loss of the external limiting membrane (ELM) with hyperreflective foci along the retinal pigment epithelium (RPE) and in the temporal outer plexiform layer. Left eye (not shown here) is normal.

- *Bartonella* serologies.
- Lyme serologies with reflex Western blot.
- Check systemic blood pressure. It was checked in the clinic and was 112/75.
- Check optical coherence tomography (OCT, Fig. 55.2).

Management

- Close observation. Await results of testing and see back in 1 week.

Follow-up

HPI

She notes that the level of blurriness and floaters is about the same. She has no new symptoms. All testing has been negative except for *Bartonella* serologies. *Bartonella henselae* immunoglobulin M (IgM) was positive.

Exam

	OD	OS
Vision	20/40+	20/20
IOP	17	15
Lids and lashes:	Normal	Normal
Sclera/conjunctiva:	White and quiet	White and quiet
Cornea:	Clear	Clear
AC:	Deep and quiet	Deep and quiet
Iris:	Flat	Flat
Lens:	Clear	Clear
Anterior vitreous:	1+ white cells	Clear
Dilated fundus examination (DFE):	Unchanged	Unchanged

Diagnosis

- Neuroretinitis OD secondary to cat scratch disease

Management

- Start doxycycline 100 mg by mouth (PO) twice a day (BID)

Follow-up

You have seen the patient several times, and she has been steadily improving. Now you see her 2 months later. She notes her symptoms are much improved and the vision in the right eye is almost back to normal.

Exam

	OD	OS
Vision	20/20−	20/20
IOP	14	14
Lids and lashes:	Normal	Normal
Sclera/conjunctiva:	White and quiet	White and quiet
Cornea:	Clear	Clear
AC:	Deep and quiet	Deep and quiet
Iris:	Flat	Flat
Lens:	Clear	Clear
Anterior vitreous:	1+ white cells	Clear

DFE: Unchanged

Nerve:	No disc edema
Macula:	Flat, no exudates (Fig. 55.3)
Vessels:	Normal caliber and course
Periphery:	Unremarkable

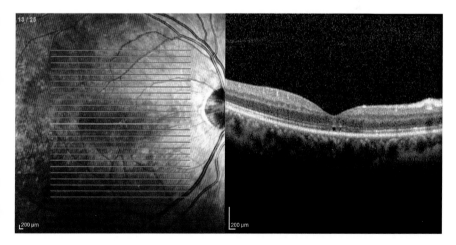

Fig. 55.3 OCT of the right eye shows resolution of the hyperreflective foci along the RPE and in the temporal outer plexiform layer and restoration of the ELM and ellipsoid layer. There remains trace disruption of the ELM and ellipsoid layers at the fovea.

Key Points

- Cat scratch disease is one of several classic causes of neuroretinitis. Although many cases are infectious, systemic hypertension (typically bilateral or bilateral asymmetric) is an underappreciated cause of a neuroretinitis presentation.
- Inflammatory causes like sarcoidosis are also in the differential, and testing for such diagnoses can be pursued if the patient does not improve as expected.
- Typical presentation involves nerve swelling and macular edema with stellate exudates or "macular star." Small neurosensory detachments are possible. Vitreal and anterior chamber (AC) inflammatory reactions are frequently absent or mild if present. Occasionally, focal or multifocal areas of punctate retinitis will develop. Rarely, vascular occlusions occur secondary to perivascular inflammation.
- The disease is typically self-limited and does not necessarily require treatment. However, doxycycline, the treatment of choice, may speed up visual recovery. Alternatives include rifampin and macrolide antibiotics, which are preferred in children.
- Serologic investigations should be pursued. Positive IgM titers are confirmatory. Positive immunoglobulin G (IgG) generally implies only remote exposure, except in cases where there is at least a fourfold increase in antibody titers, in which case it is suggestive. Polymerase chain reaction (PCR) of intraocular fluids is generally low yield but is a reasonable test in diagnostic dilemmas.

CHAPTER 56

Acute Exudative Polymorphous Vitelliform Maculopathy

Harpal S. Sandhu

History of Present Illness (HPI)

A 61-year-old woman with a remote history of laser-assisted in situ keratomileusis (LASIK) both eyes (OU) is referred to you for evaluation of posterior uveitis. She noticed a "grayish smudge" in the center, OU, starting about 2 months ago. She saw an outside ophthalmologist, who noted posterior pole lesions, started prednisolone acetate eye drops four times a day (QID), ordered basic laboratory work, and then sent her to you. She has already had a QuantiFERON, fluorescent treponemal antibody absorption (FTA-ABS), rapid plasma reagin (RPR), angiotensin-converting enzyme (ACE), lysozyme, chest x-ray, antinuclear antibodies (ANA), antineutrophil cytoplasmic antibodies (ANCA), Lyme serologies, erythrocyte sedimentation rate (ESR), C-reactive protein (CRP), complete blood count (CBC), basic metabolic panel (BMP), and urinalysis, all of which were normal.

Her symptoms have been approximately stable since onset. She denies flashes or floaters. She is extremely anxious about her condition and is worried she will go blind.

Past Medical History

- Coronary artery disease
- Hypertension
- Hypercholesterolemia

Exam

	OD	OS
Vision	20/30−	20/30
Intraocular pressure (IOP)	16	14
Lids and lashes:	Normal	Normal
Sclera/conjunctiva:	White and quiet	White and quiet
Cornea:	Clear	Clear
Anterior chamber (AC):	Deep and quiet	Deep and quiet
Iris:	Flat	Flat
Lens:	Trace nuclear sclerosis (NS)	Trace NS
Anterior vitreous:	Clear	Clear
Dilated fundus examination (DFE):	Fig. 56.1A	Fig. 56.1B

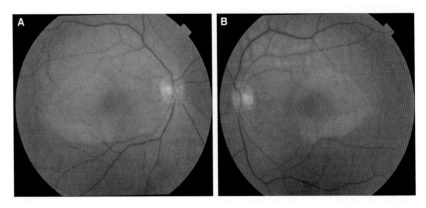

Fig. 56.1 (A) Color fundus photograph of the right eye shows a large, yellow-orange, placoid-like lesion deep to the temporal macula with several smaller, circular satellite lesions. (B) Color fundus photograph of the left eye shows remarkably similar lesions to the right eye.

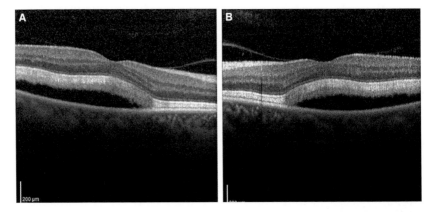

Fig. 56.2 (A) OCT of the right macula shows subretinal fluid with hyperreflective material adjacent to the outer retina. (B) OCT of the left macula shows very similar findings.

Further Questions to Ask

- Do you have any history of cancer?
- Have you felt unwell recently? Any fevers, chills, myalgias, headache, or upper respiratory symptoms?

She has no history of cancer. She had a mild viral illness about 3 months ago but nothing out of the ordinary.

Because the diagnosis was still unclear after examination, optical coherence tomography (OCT) and fluorescein angiography (FA) were pursued (Figs. 56.2 to 56.4).

Assessment

Multifocal serous macular neurosensory detachments with subretinal material OU without vitreal or anterior chamber (AC) inflammation.

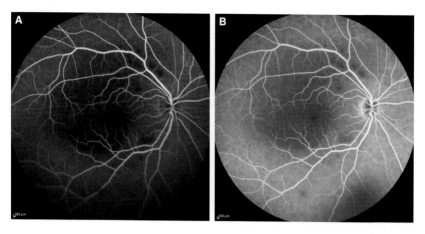

Fig. 56.3 (A) Early frame FA of the right eye shows blocking of fluorescence by subretinal material. (B) Late frame of the FA, right eye. There is no leakage or vascular inflammation.

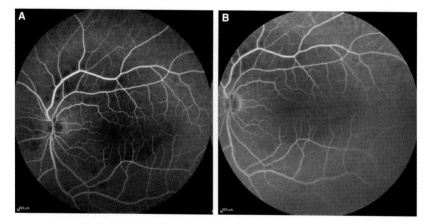

Fig. 56.4 (A) Early frame FA of the left eye shows blocking of fluorescence by subretinal material. (B) Late frame of the FA, left eye. There is no leakage or vascular inflammation.

Differential Diagnosis

- Central serous chorioretinopathy (CSR)
- Atypical melanoma-associated retinopathy (MAR)
- Syphilitic posterior placoid chorioretinopathy
- Autosomal recessive bestrophinopathy
- Acute exudative polymorphous vitelliform maculopathy (AEPVM)
- Forme fruste Vogt—Koyanagi—Harada syndrome (VKH)
- Primary vitreoretinal/subretinal lymphoma (PVRL)

Working Diagnosis

- Unclear. Syphilitic posterior placoid versus AEVPM.
- This is a very unusual and challenging case. All of the conditions on the differential diagnosis are either very rare or made unlikely by some finding. CSR is essentially ruled out by the lack of leakage on FA. MAR can present with multiple serous detachments, but the condition usually arises *after* a diagnosis of cutaneous melanoma has already been made. Although the fundus appearance is similar to autosomal recessive bestrophinopathy and AEPVM, this would be a late presentation for an inherited macular degeneration. VKH presents with multifocal detachments, but usually without this yellow-orange subretinal material and with at least some intraocular cells. PVRL is an extremely rare disease, and the distribution of fundus lesions in its "leopard spot fundus" variant is somewhat different from these. Finally, syphilitic posterior placoid is unlikely, given the negative syphilis testing. False negatives are possible and more likely in patients positive for human immunodeficiency virus (HIV).

Management

- Observe
- Check HIV and recheck RPR and FTA-ABS
- Follow up in 2 to 3 weeks

Follow-up

HPI

The patient returns 3 weeks later. HIV testing was negative, as were a repeat RPR and FTA-ABS. The patient says her symptoms are unchanged.

Exam

	OD	OS
Vision	20/30–	20/30
IOP:	13	15
Lids and lashes:	Normal	Normal
Sclera/conjunctiva:	White and quiet	White and quiet
Cornea:	Clear	Clear
AC:	Deep and quiet	Deep and quiet
Iris:	Flat	Flat
Lens:	Trace NS	Trace NS
Anterior vitreous:	Clear	Clear
DFE:	Unchanged	Unchanged

Diagnosis

- AEPVM, OU

Management

- Refer to internal medicine for a malignancy evaluation
- Observe fundus lesions

Key Points

- AEPVM is a rare condition that resembles autosomal recessive bestrophinopathy on fundus examination.
- The etiology is unclear, but most cases are presumed to be postviral. A minority of cases are paraneoplastic, which is why a thorough malignancy evaluation is indicated.
- In this case, the diagnosis was made by exclusion. If in doubt, an electro-oculogram can be ordered and frequently shows a reduced Arden ratio (light—dark ratio), just as in Best disease.
- There is no established treatment.

CHAPTER 57

MEK Inhibitor-Associated Retinopathy (MEKAR)

Harpal S. Sandhu

History of Present Illness (HPI)

A 69-year-old woman with a history of cutaneous melanoma complains of a change in her vision for the last month or so. She has difficulty describing her symptoms, but she reports that things are just a bit out of focus in both eyes (OU). She denies any other eye symptoms and has not had any recent changes to her health or recent hospitalizations.

Questions to Ask

- Have you started any new medications, either for your melanoma or anything else?
- Are you taking any steroids?

She responds that she recently started a new drug to treat melanoma based on "the DNA in the melanoma," but is unsure of its name. A review of her oncology outpatient notes shows that she is on trametinib, an inhibitor of mitogen-activated protein kinases (MEK). She denies corticosteroid use.

Exam

	OD	OS
Vision	20/25	20/20
Intraocular pressure (IOP)	14	15
Lids and lashes:	Normal	Normal
Sclera/conjunctiva:	White and quiet	White and quiet
Cornea:	Clear	Clear
Anterior chamber (AC):	Deep and quiet	Deep and quiet
Iris:	Flat	Flat
Lens:	1+ nuclear sclerosis (NS)	1+ NS
Dilated fundus examination (DFE):	See Fig. 57.1A	See Fig. 57.1B

Assessment

Serous retinal detachments, left eye greater than right eye (OS > OD)

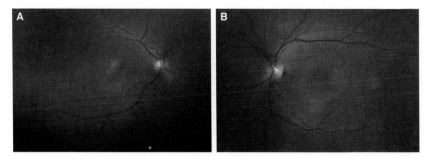

Fig. 57.1 (A) Color fundus photograph of the right eye shows clear media and a subtle, subretinal, yellow-colored lesion inferior to the fovea. (B) Color fundus photograph of the left eye shows clear media and multiple blebs of subretinal fluid in the posterior pole, including a broad foveal detachment.

Differential Diagnosis

- Central serous chorioretinopathy (CSR)
- Choroidal metastases with overlying serous detachments
- MEK inhibitor—associated retinopathy (MEKAR)
- Vogt—Koyanagi—Harada (VKH) syndrome
- Acute exudative polymorphous vitelliform maculopathy (AEPVM)
- Idiopathic exudative retinal detachment
- Less likely: serous retinal detachment secondary to an infectious process

Testing

- The funduscopic appearance of serous detachment should be confirmed and further characterized by optical coherence tomography (OCT) (Fig. 57.3).
- A fluorescein angiogram (FA) should be obtained to distinguish between various causes of serous detachment (Fig. 57.2).

Working Diagnosis

- MEK inhibitor—associated serous retinopathy OU
- Multiple shallow, serous detachments shortly after initiating a MEK inhibitor is classic for MEKAR. CSR and VKH are ruled out by the absence of leakage, and there is no evidence of choroidal metastases on funduscopic examination or OCT. AEPVM is a diagnosis of exclusion.

Management

- Observation
- Communicate with the patient's oncologist to ensure they are aware that the patient's mild visual changes are likely secondary to their cancer treatment.

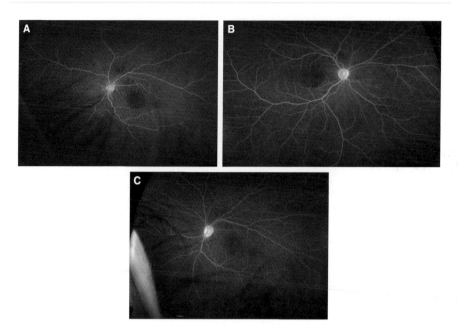

Fig. 57.2 (A) Early phase wide-field FA of the left eye shows no leakage and multiple circular areas of hypofluorescence colocalizing with the areas of serous detachment in Fig. 57.1B. (B) Late phase wide-field FA of the right eye shows no leakage and an area of hypofluorescence in the central macula larger than the typical foveal avascular zone. The margin of the disc is slightly hyperfluorescent. (C) Late phase wide-field FA of the left eye shows no late leakage or pooling and similar hypofluorescent areas to the early frames. The margin of the disc is slightly hyperfluorescent.

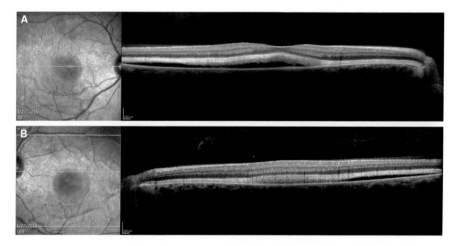

Fig. 57.3 (A) OCT of the right eye shows a broad, shallow, serous macular detachment with hyperreflective subretinal material. (B) OCT of the left eye similarly shows a broad, shallow, serous macular detachment with hyperreflective subretinal material.

Follow-up

HPI

The patient returns 4 weeks later. She notes that her vision is about the same, but she has learned to live with it, and it is not interfering with any of her activities.

Exam

	OD	OS
Vision	20/25	20/20
IOP	16	16
Lids and lashes:	Normal	Normal
Sclera/conjunctiva:	White and quiet	White and quiet
Cornea:	Clear	Clear
AC:	Deep and quiet	Deep and quiet
Iris:	Flat	Flat
Lens:	Clear	Clear
DFE:	Unchanged	Unchanged

Key Points

- MEK is a kinase in the mitogen-activated protein (MAP) kinase pathway that is important in regulating the cell cycle and cell division. Mutations in MEK and other MAP kinase proteins, such as BRAF, can lead to neoplasms, including melanoma.
- Unlike traditional chemotherapy, these patients are not immunosuppressed. However, one side effect is bilateral, multifocal, and usually shallow serous retinal detachments. Sometimes the buildup of material in the subretinal space gives them a more striking funduscopic appearance, and other times they can be subtle.
- In general, these have minimal visual significance, and given the life-extending benefits of this therapy, these drugs do not have to be discontinued simply because of the eye findings.
- Standard local therapies for macular exudation, like topical corticosteroids, nonsteroidal antiinflammatory drugs (NSAIDs), or carbonic anhydrase inhibitors, can be attempted but are generally unnecessary.

CHAPTER 58

Immune Checkpoint Inhibitor-Induced Panuveitis

Harpal S. Sandhu

History of Present Illness

A 58-year-old man complains of progressive decrease in vision in both eyes (OU) over the last month. His past medical history is notable for metastatic cutaneous melanoma. He dismissed his symptoms initially, but after his vision did not improve spontaneously—in fact, he thinks it probably worsened over that time—he presented to a local ophthalmologist who then referred him on an expedited basis to the uveitis service. The referral simply notes "inflammation" OU and notes a concern for "infection" because the patient is on "chemotherapy."

Questions to Ask

- What cancer treatments have you been on in the past and what are you on currently?
- Has your course been complicated by any recent infections or hospitalizations?

He responds that he was first diagnosed with a cutaneous melanoma on his back 10 years ago.

He underwent local excision and was stable until a little under a year ago, when he was diagnosed with metastatic disease. He has metastases to his liver and lungs. His oncologist started him on the immunotherapeutic nivolumab, a programmed death-1 inhibitor (PD-1, a T-cell immune checkpoint) about 6 months ago, and he has responded very well to it. He has had no other complications or hospitalizations since his most recent diagnosis.

Exam

	OD	OS
Vision	20/40	20/30−
Intraocular pressure (IOP)	30	28
Lids and lashes:	Normal	Normal
Sclera/conjunctiva:	White and quiet	White and quiet
Cornea:	Clear stroma, fine keratic precipitates (KP)	Clear, fine KP
Anterior chamber (AC):	2+ white cells	2+ white cells
	1+ flare	1+ flare
Iris:	Flat	Flat
Lens:	Clear	Clear
Anterior vitreous:	2+ white cells	2+ white cells
Dilated fundus examination (DFE):	See Fig. 58.1A	See Fig. 58.1B

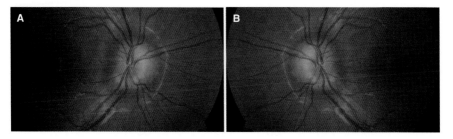

Fig. 58.1   (A) Color fundus photograph of the right eye shows moderate optic disc edema with no other fundus lesions. (B) Color fundus photograph of the left eye shows moderate optic disc edema with no other fundus lesions, very similar to the right eye.

Assessment

- Hypertensive anterior and intermediate uveitis OU
- Papillitis OU
- Note: Some clinicians might describe this presentation as panuveitis for the sake of brevity. The assessment represents the Standardization of Uveitis Nomenclature (SUN) diagnosis because there is no evidence of choroidal or retinal inflammation.

Differential Diagnosis

- Checkpoint inhibitor—induced uveitis
- Idiopathic
- Syphilitic uveitis
- Less likely: infectious causes of hypertensive uveitis (e.g., Herpesviridae, toxoplasmosis, or new diagnosis of a noninfectious uveitis syndrome, such as HLA-B27, sarcoidosis)
- Possible but highly unlikely: metastatic cutaneous melanoma with intraocular seeding

Working Diagnosis

- Checkpoint inhibitor—induced uveitis OU

Testing

- Rapid plasma reagin (RPR), fluorescent treponemal antibody absorption (FTA ABS)

Management

- Call the patient's oncologist to touch base about initiating systemic corticosteroids while on nivolumab versus discontinuing treatment. Because the patient has life-threatening disease and has responded so well to the treatment, the oncologist does not want to discontinue therapy but is amenable to an abbreviated course of systemic steroids.
- Start prednisone 60 mg by mouth (PO) daily if syphilis testing is negative
- Start prednisolone acetate 1% four times a day (QID) OU and timolol twice a day (BID) OU
- Follow up in 2 weeks.

Follow-up

Two days later, the patient's syphilis testing returned negative, so he was called at home and started on high-dose prednisone. He returns to the clinic 2 weeks later. He notes that his vision is definitely better, although it is not totally normal. He has had no problems tolerating prednisone.

Exam

	OD	OS
Vision	20/25−	20/25
IOP	24	22
Lids and lashes:	Normal	Normal
Sclera/conjunctiva:	White and quiet	White and quiet
Cornea:	Clear	Clear
AC:	Trace cells, inactive KP	Trace cells, inactive KP
Iris:	Flat	Flat
Lens:	Clear	Clear
Anterior vitreous:	2+ old cells	2+ old cells

DFE

Nerve:	Trace swelling	Trace swelling
Vitreous:	Clear	Clear
Macula:	Good foveal reflex	Good foveal reflex
Periphery:	Unremarkable	Unremarkable

Management

- Taper prednisone by 10 mg each week
- Taper prednisolone acetate 1% by 1 drop a week
- Continue timolol BID OU
- Follow up in 1 month

Key Points

- The immune checkpoint inhibitors are immunotherapies for a range of malignancies that boost the antitumor effect of T cells. Unlike traditional chemotherapy, which is cytotoxic to cells of the immune system, causing immunocompromise and rendering patients more vulnerable to infections, the immune checkpoint inhibitors do the opposite, causing immune-related adverse events 30% of the time, including uveitis.
- Checkpoint inhibitor−induced uveitis can take almost any form, including anterior, intermediate, and panuveitis; choroiditis with or without uveal effusion; exudative retinal detachment; and Vogt−Koyanagi−Harada (VKH)−like presentations.

- Other forms of ocular inflammatory disease have been described, including nonspecific orbital inflammation, myositis, cranial neuropathies, scleritis, keratitis, optic neuritis, myasthenia gravis, and even cases of corneal transplant rejection.
- Other subclasses of immune checkpoint inhibitors include programmed death ligand 1 (PD-L1) inhibitors and cytotoxic T-lymphocyte antigen 4 (CTLA-4) inhibitors, such as ipilimumab.
- It is essential to contact oncology in these cases. Depending on the oncologist and the patient's status, they may be amenable to discontinuing the drug. However, in general, these are life-extending treatments that need to be maintained. In such cases, one can treat through the immunotherapy with courses of systemic corticosteroids.
- If extended courses of systemic corticosteroids are necessary, these can interfere with the anticancer effect of the immunotherapies. In such cases, local therapy may be preferred.

CHAPTER 59

Cysticercosis

Sivakumar R. Rathinam

History of Presenting Illness

A 9-year-old healthy Indian boy presents with a complaint of blurred vision in his right eye (OD) for a week. He denied pain or floaters.

Exam

	OD	OS
Visual acuity	20/200	20/20
Intraocular pressure (IOP)	15 mm Hg	14 mm Hg
Sclera/conjunctiva	White and quiet	White and quiet
Cornea	Clear	Clear
Anterior chamber (AC)	Normal depth and quiet	Normal depth and quiet
Iris	Normal	Normal
Lens	Clear	Clear
Anterior vitreous	Clear	Clear

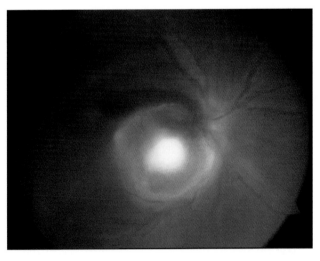

Fig. 59.1 Fundus photograph of the right eye showing clear media and a cystic lesion near the disc in the area of the macula.

Dilated fundus examination (DFE) See Fig. 59.1A

Nerve:	Cup-to-disc (c/d) 0.2, normal
Macula:	Normal
Vessels:	Normal caliber and course
Periphery:	Unremarkable

Questions to Ask

- Have you had any injury?
- Do you have a headache?
- Have you ever have any numbness, tingling, or weakness? Is there any history of prior neurologic disorders?

He answers no to all of these questions.

Assessment

- Intraocular cysticercosis with a scolex OD

Differential Diagnosis

- Intraocular cysticercosis OD
- Congenital retinal cysts OD
- Choroidal granuloma OD

Working Diagnosis

- Intraocular cysticercosis OD

Testing

- As this patient had a classic presentation of intraocular cysticercosis, namely visualization of a cyst and scolex with indirect ophthalmoscope, the diagnosis was confirmed on clinical examination. No further workup was necessary for intraocular involvement.
- However, ultrasound B scan is usually advised to rule out associated orbital lesions. No lesions were found.

Management

- Computed tomography (CT) brain to rule out central nervous system (CNS) involvement
- Pars plana vitrectomy OD to remove the intraocular cyst
  - A posterior retinotomy was made outside the inferotemporal arcade close to the subretinal cystic mass.
  - Mass was retrieved with subretinal forceps and removed *en toto* from the eye via one of the sclerotomies.
  - Fluid—air exchange was performed, followed by laser around the retinotomy.

Follow-up

The patient reported partial restoration of vision, with visual acuity (VA) improving to 20/80 OD (Figs. 59.2 and 59.3). CT brain was negative for cystic lesions.

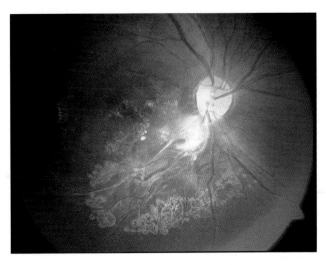

Fig. 59.2   Fundus photograph of the right eye showing clear media and surgical scar near the disc.

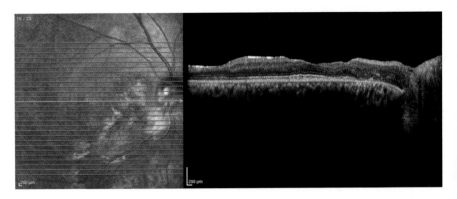

Fig. 59.3   Near-normal optical coherence tomography (OCT) approximately 2 years after surgery.

Management Algorithm

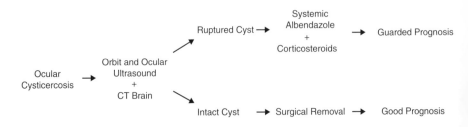

Key Points

- Involvement of the extraocular muscles is the most common manifestation of orbital cysticercosis. Orbital cysticercosis is characterized by proptosis, globe displacement, strabismus, and restricted motility.
- Intraocular cysticercosis is caused by the growth of the larvae within the vitreous or subretinal space.
- Entry of cysticercosis into the eye probably occurs via the choroidal circulation, migrating into the subretinal space and then entering the vitreous cavity through a retinal hole, which often heals by forming a chorioretinal scar.
- A translucent cyst, often with characteristic undulating movements (otherwise known as a *living pearl*), may be present in the subretinal space, vitreous cavity, conjunctiva, or anterior segment.
- Occasionally, the worm crosses the macula, causing significant vision loss.
- If the cyst ruptures, the patient may develop profound vitritis, proliferative vitreoretinopathy, uveitis, rhegmatogenous or exudative retinal detachment, retinal hemorrhages, disc edema, cyclitic membrane formation, or phthisis bulbi.
- Vitrectomy with cyst removal is the ideal treatment for intraocular cysticercosis.
- Patients should be asked to follow up periodically for a neurologic workup because of the possibility of associated CNS cysticercosis.
- When CT of the brain shows evidence of CNS cysticercosis, referral to neurology is important for addition of antiseizure treatment and systemic corticosteroids.

CHAPTER 60

Leptospirosis

Sivakumar R. Rathinam

History of Present Illness

A 33-year-old farmer from a local village in India presents for the first time to the local eye clinic complaining of blurry vision in his left eye (OS). Review of systems was positive for fever 1 month before the onset of his eye problem.

Exam

	OD	OS
Visual acuity	20/20	Hand motion
Intraocular pressure	17 mm Hg	17 mm Hg
Sclera/conjunctiva	White	Mild circumcorneal congestion
Cornea	White	Diffuse nongranulomatous keratic precipitates
Anterior chamber	Deep and quite	4+ cells/flare, see Fig. 60.1
Iris	Normal color and pattern	Normal color and pattern
Lens	Clear	Pearly white, mature cataract
Anterior vitreous	Unremarkable	Poor view due to cataract

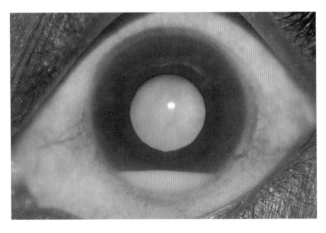

Fig. 60.1 Color external photograph of the left eye shows hypopyon anterior uveitis with nongranulomatous keratic precipitates and a mature cataract OS.

A B scan OS was performed, which showed moderate vitreous opacities and attached retina.

Questions to Ask

- Have you had any injury in your left eye?
- When was the last time your vision was close to normal?
- Have you had any similar eye problems in the past?
- Do you have close contact with cattle, pets, or other animals, such as rat bites?
- Do you have a history of fever, jaundice, or myalgias?

His vision was close to normal just a few weeks ago. He further responds that, as a farmer, he has had close association with cattle and started to have a fever after his cattle became febrile while having an abortion. He has never had anything like this before, and he denied any rat bites. He has had fever lasting for 10 days with severe myalgia and jaundice.

Assessment

- Acute, nongranulomatous, hypopyon anterior uveitis and intermediate uveitis
- Complex, rapidly progressive, white cataract OS, associated with uveitis
- Sudden-onset fever, myalgia, and jaundice suggesting systemic infection, possibly zoonotic

Differential Diagnosis

- Most likely: Leptospiral uveitis
- Traumatic cataract with lens-related uveitis
- Behçet anterior and intermediate
- Endogenous fungal endophthalmitis

Working Diagnosis

- Hypopyon uveitis OS, most likely leptospiral.
- The patient is from an area that is endemic with leptospirosis, he works in an occupation at high risk for exposure to *Leptospira*, and he has systemic symptoms consistent with the diagnosis. The rapid onset of cataract is also highly suggestive.

Testing

- Complete blood count (CBC) with differential
- Purified protein derivative (PPD)
- Rapid plasma reagin (RPR), fluorescent treponemal antibody absorption (FTA-ABS)
- Leptospirosis micro-agglutination test

Management

- Await results of testing
- Start prednisolone acetate 1% every hour (q1h) OS
- Follow up in 2 days

Follow-up

The patient follows up 2 days later. His symptoms and examination are stable. Micro-agglutination test returned positive 1:1200 for *Leptospirosis icterohaemorragica*.

Management

- Start doxycycline 100 mg by mouth (PO) twice a day (BID)
- Start prednisone 60 mg PO daily
- Continue prednisolone acetate 1% q1h OS

Further Follow-up

The patient's inflammation improved rapidly, and oral and topical corticosteroids were slowly tapered starting 2 weeks after presentation. Vision remained in the count fingers range due to mature cataract OS. After 3 months of quiescence, the patient underwent cataract extraction with intraocular lens implantation OS and ultimately regained 20/20 vision after surgery.

Key Points

- Leptospiral uveitis is one of the most common causes of hypopyon uveitis in leptospiral-endemic areas.
- Other clinical signs are retinal vasculitis, vitreous membranes, and disc hyperemia. Early onset, rapid progression, and spontaneous absorption of cataractous lens are unique features in this uveitis; however, it is seen only in 1% of leptospiral uveitis.
- Dense vitreous inflammation with the formation of veil-like membranous vitreous opacities is a pathognomonic sign seen in the posterior segment (Fig. 60.2).
- Because uveitis occurs as an immunologic response, corticosteroids are the mainstay of treatment. Leptospiral uveitis carries a good visual prognosis if treated appropriately.
- The leptospires infect a variety of animals, including rodents and cattle, which can shed leptospires in their urine throughout their life, resulting in environmental contamination.
- Systemic leptospirosis is characterized by a broad spectrum of clinical manifestations ranging from mild fever to severe and potentially fatal hepatorenal failure.

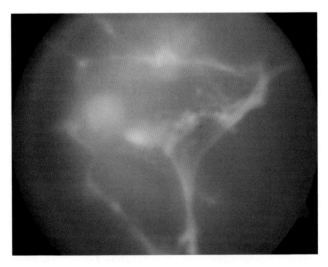

Fig. 60.2 Color fundus photograph from a separate case of leptospiral panuveitis with a clearer view of the fundus. There are dense vitreous membranes forming a veil-like configuration.

CHAPTER 61

Granulomatosis with Polyangiitis

George N. Papaliodis ■ Caroline L. Minkus

History of Present Illness

A 54-year-old woman with history of asthma and appendiceal adenocarcinoma status post-appendectomy presented to the emergency department with 3 weeks of shortness of breath, sinus congestion, cough productive of green sputum, lower extremity edema, and general malaise. She had been treated with 2 weeks of oral amoxicillin–clavulanate without improvement. She was found to be hypoxemic with oxygen saturation of 89% on room air and multiple opacities on chest x-ray. She had an elevated white blood cell count of 33,680/μL (95% neutrophils). Computed tomography (CT) scan of the chest revealed diffuse alveolar hemorrhages, which were confirmed on bronchoscopy. She was admitted to the hospital and subsequently developed oliguric acute renal failure. A renal biopsy was performed, revealing crescentic glomerulonephritis. She was given 4 days of intravenous (IV) methyl-prednisolone 1 g/day and one dose of 880 mg IV cyclophosphamide. Routine blood culture grew out yeast, and ophthalmology was consulted to evaluate for possible fungal endophthalmitis.

Exam

	OD	OS
Visual acuity	20/25	20/25
Intraocular pressure	17	18
Sclera/conjunctiva	White and quiet	White and quiet
Cornea	Clear	Clear
Anterior chamber	Deep and quiet	Deep and quiet
Iris	Unremarkable	Unremarkable
Lens	Clear	Clear
Anterior vitreous	Clear	Clear
Dilated fundus examination (DFE)	See Fig. 61.1A	See Fig. 61.1B

Fluorescein angiogram was performed to further assess the cause of blot hemorrhages and cotton wool spots (Fig. 61.2).

Questions to Ask

- Do you notice any changes in your vision? Any complaints about photopsias or floaters?
- Have you ever had any blood clots or trouble with blood pressure? Does anyone in your family have any bleeding/clotting disorders or eye problems?
- Do you have diabetes?

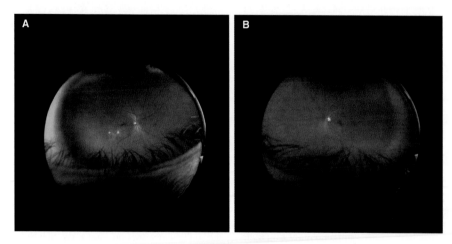

Fig. 61.1 (A) Color fundus photograph of the right eye showing clear media, healthy nerve, normal vasculature, and a few cotton wool spots. (B) Color fundus photograph of the left eye showing clear media, moderate optic nerve cupping, and rare dot blot hemorrhages in the inferior periphery.

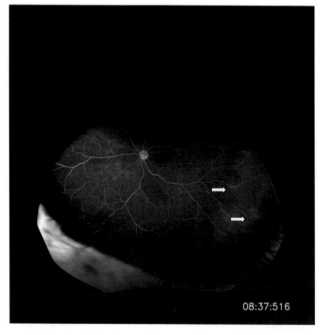

Fig. 61.2 Fluorescein angiography of the left eye with late peripheral vascular staining and leakage consistent with retinal vasculitis (see arrows).

She notes no personal or family history of eye disease, bleeding, or clotting issues. She has been noticing a "cloud" over her left eye (OS) vision inferiorly, which has been improving.

Assessment

- Retinal vasculitis OS associated with pulmonary hemorrhage and glomerulonephritis
- OS optic nerve cupping
- Improving visual, pulmonary, and renal symptoms status post IV methylprednisolone and cyclophosphamide

Differential Diagnosis

- Granulomatosis with polyangiitis (GPA)
- Sarcoid-associated retinal vasculitis with pulmonary and renal manifestations
- Occlusive vasculopathy
- Churg—Strauss syndrome
- Systemic lupus erythematosus
- Less likely: Hypertensive retinopathy, infectious retinal vasculitis in the setting of immunosuppression

Working Diagnosis

- GPA

Testing

- Given the diagnosis of bronchoscopy-confirmed diffuse alveolar hemorrhage and biopsy-confirmed crescentic glomerulonephritis, the most likely diagnosis is GPA. Check antineutrophil cytoplasmic antibodies (ANCA) to confirm.
- In the setting of retinal vasculitis and pulmonary hemorrhage, check:
  - Angiotensin-converting enzyme (ACE), lysozyme, chest imaging
  - Rapid plasma reagin (RPR) and fluorescent treponemal antibody absorption (FTA-ABS)
  - Complete blood count (CBC), coagulation profile, antinuclear antibodies (ANA), lupus anticoagulant
  - Human immunodeficiency virus (HIV)
- Optical coherence tomography retinal nerve fiber layer (OCT RNFL) and visual field testing to assess significance of optic nerve cupping OS
- Further workup (already completed in this patient) in conjunction with pulmonology and nephrology to manage respiratory and renal signs and symptoms
- With treatment, patients should be monitored for resolution of vasculitis and possible development of retinal neovascularization

The patient had confirmed C-ANCA positivity and otherwise negative testing.

Management

- Immunosuppressive therapy: IV corticosteroids first line, followed by long-term steroid-sparing immunosuppressant therapy. Treatment options include antimetabolites like mycophenolate mofetil and methotrexate (more commonly in limited disease), alkylating agents like cyclophosphamide, and biologic agents such as rituximab.
- Intravitreal anti—vascular endothelial growth factor (VEGF) injections for management of neovascularization

Follow-up

The patient noted complete resolution of all symptoms with 20/20 vision both eyes (OU). She noted a continued floater OS and was found to have development of posterior vitreal detachment OS. Visual field testing was full in each eye. She received two infusions of rituximab and has been managed subsequently on oral cyclophosphamide with undetectable C-ANCA.

Key Points

- Cotton wool spots and retinal hemorrhages can be a manifestation of retinal vasculitis, even in the absence of vascular sheathing or other intraocular inflammation.
- The differential diagnosis for retinal vasculitis is broad, but should be tailored to fit the patient's overall clinical presentation, including involvement beyond the eye.
- Retinal vasculitis requires treatment to control inflammation and prevent vision loss. Often, this entails aggressive medical management with systemic immunosuppression.
- In cases of resolved retinal vasculitis, ongoing monitoring is necessary to monitor for late-stage complications, including ocular ischemia and neovascularization.
- In cases of systemic vasculitides, a multidisciplinary approach may be necessary to address inflammatory events involving other organ systems.

CHAPTER 62

Frosted Branch Angiitis

Sruthi Arepalli ▧ Eric Suhler

History of Present Illness

A 24-year-old female presents with a known history of granulomatosis with polyangiitis (GPA), with prior laboratory tests positive for perinuclear antinuclear antineutrophil cytoplasmic antibodies (p-ANCA). Her systemic manifestations of GPA included oral ulcerations, pulmonary nodules, pericarditis, and hematuria. She had previously been treated with oral prednisone and methotrexate, although the methotrexate had been discontinued recently because of elevated transaminases. She presented to the emergency department with a headache, pain on eye movements, periocular swelling, and acute vision loss in her left eye. B scan ultrasound of the left eye confirmed a thickened posterior sclera with a positive T sign.

Exam

	OD	OS
Visual acuity	20/20	Hand motion (HM)
Intraocular pressure (IOP)	18	28
Afferent pupillary defect (APD)	No	Yes
Lids	Normal	Edema, erythema
Sclera/conjunctiva	White and quiet	Diffuse injection
Cornea	Clear	Clear
Anterior chamber (AC)	Deep and quiet	Deep and quiet
Iris	Unremarkable	Unremarkable
Lens	Clear	Clear
Anterior vitreous	Clear	Clear
Disc	Normal, 0.4	4+ edema (Fig. 62.1)
Macula	Normal	Serous neurosensory retinal detachment, diffuse intraretinal hemorrhages (Fig. 62.1)
Vessels	Normal	Extensive and severe, white-yellow perivenular sheathing throughout macula and retinal midperiphery (Fig. 62.1)
Periphery	Normal	Vasculitis extending to midperiphery with smaller white centered hemorrhages peripherally (Fig. 62.1)

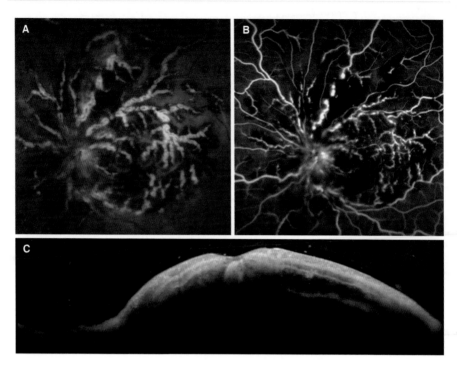

Fig. 62.1 (A) Fundus photograph of the left posterior pole shows 4+ disc edema, a serous retinal detachment in the macula, and profound vascular sheathing consistent with frosted branch angiitis. (B) Fluorescein angiogram of the left eye shows peripapillary leakage, venous beading, and predominant staining of the retinal veins. (C) Spectral domain optical coherence tomography confirms a neurosensory detachment in the macula with intraretinal fluid.

Questions to Ask

- Do you have a history of oral or genital sores?
- Do you have a history of sexually transmitted diseases or high-risk sexual behavior?
- Have you been diagnosed with human immunodeficiency virus (HIV)?
- Do you have a cough or have you been exposed to others with tuberculosis (TB)?
- Have you ever had any neurologic symptoms, including numbness, tingling, bowel or bladder changes, or trouble with your speech?

She answers no to all questions, except for the known history of oral ulcers in association with the GPA diagnosis.

Assessment

- Frosted branch angiitis primarily involving the venules and posterior scleritis of the left eye

Differential Diagnosis

- GPA
- Syphilis
- TB

- Toxoplasmosis
- Viral (cytomegalovirus [CMV], herpes simplex virus [HSV], varicella zoster virus [VZV], Epstein—Barr virus [EBV])
- Multiple sclerosis
- Sarcoidosis
- Behçet disease
- Lymphoma
- Leukemia

Working Diagnosis

- GPA-related frosted branch angiitis and scleritis

Testing

- Frosted branch angiitis is a generally rare condition but has been associated with multiple infectious, autoimmune, and neoplastic conditions
- In cases with neurologic symptoms, check the cerebrospinal fluid for protein, glucose, white blood cells, Gram stain and culture, and send for viral polymerase chain reaction (PCR)
- In the case where GPA status is unknown, test for ANCA
- Rule out infectious causes with:
  - Fluorescent treponemal antibody (FTA), rapid plasma reagin (RPR)
  - Toxoplasmosis immunoglobulin M (IgM) and immunoglobulin G (IgG) levels
  - QuantiFERON Gold
  - HIV testing
  - HSV, VZV, EBV, and CMV testing (either by IgM and IgG levels or PCR; as exposure to these viruses is quite common, a negative test may be more useful than a positive one; PCR testing of intraocular fluids may be required for difficult-to-diagnose cases)

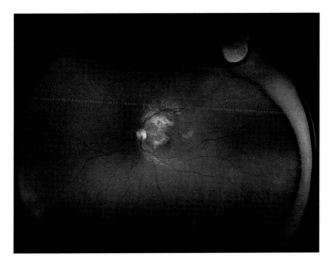

Fig. 62.2 Fundus photograph of the left eye at last follow-up shows subretinal fibrosis limiting potential visual acuity, but resolved disc edema and retinal vasculitis.

Management

- Depending on the results of the workup: If infectious, treat with appropriate antibiotics or antivirals and refer to infectious disease
- If concern for autoimmune etiology, pulse intravenous (IV) steroids (once infectious causes have been ruled out) with subsequent referral to uveitis specialist or rheumatologist for long-term immunosuppressive therapy
- In this patient, a 3-day course of high-dose IV solumedrol was administered followed by IV rituximab therapy (two infusions separated by 2 weeks, 1000 mg each)

Follow-up

- At the last follow-up, the patient had 20/400 vision in the left eye with subretinal fibrosis in the macula and resolved disc edema (Fig. 62.2)

Key Points

- Frosted branch angiitis is a rare disease entity and can be associated with a gamut of conditions, including infectious, autoimmune, and neoplastic diseases
- Frosted branch angiitis in combination with scleritis should raise suspicion for GPA
- GPA is a potentially lethal condition if untreated, so recognizing its many potential presentations is key
- Infectious differential is broad, but CMV retinitis should be ruled out and HIV status should be ascertained in the appropriate clinical context

CHAPTER 63

Susac Syndrome (Retinal Vasculitis, Hearing Loss, and Encephalopathy)

Ryan A. Shields ▓ Neil Onghanseng ▓ Muhammad Hassan ▓ Quan Dong Nguyen

History of Present Illness

A 24-year-old female with a history of polysubstance (ethanol, marijuana, tobacco) abuse presented to the emergency room at another hospital with 2 months of worsening somnolence, confusion, and new hallucinations. She became progressively encephalopathic, requiring intubation for airway protection. There was noted persistence of symptoms prompting eventual transfer to our hospital, where ophthalmology was consulted for a diagnostic examination.

Exam

	OD	OS
Visual acuity	Unable	Unable
Intraocular pressure (IOP)	15	15
Sclera/conjunctiva	White and quiet	White and quiet
Cornea	Clear	Clear
Anterior chamber (AC)	Deep and quiet	Deep and quiet
Iris	Unremarkable	Unremarkable
Lens	Clear	Clear
Anterior vitreous	Clear	Clear
Retina	Focal area of retinal whitening seen in by the inferior arcades (Fig. 63.1A)	Diffuse area of retinal whitening involving near the entirety of the inferior arcades associated with box-carring of the inferior arcade vessels (Fig. 63.1B)

Questions to Ask the Family and Management Team at the Referring Hospital

- Did the patient report any eye or vision-related concerns before the neurologic decompensation? (Pain? Blurring? Scotomas?)
- Did the patient report any other major systemic symptoms before the neurologic decompensation? (Headache? Hearing loss?)
- Did the patient have a history of head trauma? Did the patient overdose with any substance just before experiencing the neurologic symptoms?

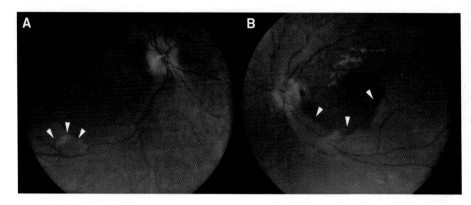

Fig. 63.1 (A) Fundus photo of the right eye demonstrating a focal area of retinal whitening (*white arrow-heads*) adjacent to the inferotemporal arcade. Vessels appear slightly tortuous, but are otherwise unremarkable. The rest of the retinal findings were unremarkable. (B) Fundus photo of the left eye demonstrating retinal whitening (*white arrowheads*) of the inferior macula with associated "box-carring" of the retinal vasculature in the inferior arcades, described as segmentation of the blood columns within the affected vessels. The rest of the retinal findings were unremarkable.

- Is there a family history of any similar problems?
- Has infection been ruled out as a possible etiology?
- What empiric treatment has been given to the patient already?

The relatives of the patient indicated that the patient had no reported changes in vision but developed migraines and reported episodic hearing loss the year prior, though hearing loss was never formally tested.

There was no history of trauma and no relevant family history of eye disease or vison loss.

The management team has ruled out infection. In terms of empiric treatment, the patient had been treated with intravenous acyclovir, multiple rounds of intravenous methylprednisolone, intravenous immunoglobulin (IVIG), and plasma exchange therapy with only temporary improvement in the neurologic status.

Assessment

- Bilateral branch retinal artery occlusions (BRAO), left eye greater than right eye (OS > OD) in the setting of white matter lesions (including the corpus callosum) on magnetic resonance imaging (MRI) and a history of episodic hearing loss

Differential Diagnosis

- Susac syndrome
- Multiple sclerosis
- Acute demyelinating encephalomyelitis (ADEM)
- Multifocal inflammatory leukoencephalopathy
- Hypercoagulable state
- Cannabis induced
- Less likely: Chronic traumatic encephalopathy, substance abuse

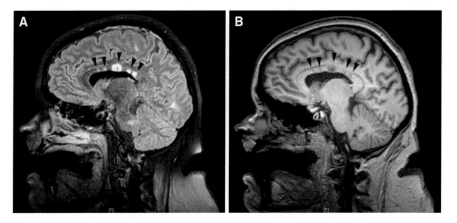

Fig. 63.2   (A) Sagittal T2 magnetic resonance imaging (MRI) of brain demonstrating hyperintensities (*black arrowheads*) in the central corpus callosum. (B) Sagittal T1 MRI showing "punched-out-holes" (*black arrowheads*) in the central corpus callosum that correspond to the T2 hyperintensities.

Working Diagnosis

- Susac syndrome

Testing

- In patients with the classic triad of Susac syndrome, including BRAOs, hearing loss, and encephalopathy such as the index patient, diagnosis is almost definite.
- Fluorescein angiography (FA) is extremely sensitive in detecting retinal vascular abnormalities, including arterial wall hyperfluorescence, Gass plaques (pseudoemboli composed of immune complex debris aggregates seen distant to bifurcation sites), and arterial collaterals. In Susac syndrome, there is a characteristic leakage of vessels distant from the site of ischemia.
- Perimetry should be done to document and assess visual field defects that may arise secondary to the BRAOs.
- MRI may show typical snowball white matter lesions, usually found at the corpus callosum; other lesions like deep gray matter involvement and leptomeningeal enhancement may also be seen (see Fig. 63.2).
- Audiogram shows sensorineural hearing loss, usually in the lower frequency ranges.

Management

- Initial treatment is with high-dose intravenous steroids (1 g methylprednisolone or equivalence per day), which may be given with IVIG to achieve disease remission. Once achieved, a slow steroid taper can be performed while transitioning to a steroid-sparing immunomodulating agent.
- Most cases of Susac syndrome are monocyclic (one episode), though a significant number of patients will present with polycyclic (relapsing) disease, which can be detected with surveillance brain MRI and FA. Flareups may happen up to many years after the initial episode.

- Tumor necrosis factor (TNF) inhibitors, such as rituximab and cyclophosphamide, have been utilized successfully for severe and refractory cases.
- The efficacy of antithrombotic agents, including aspirin, has not been demonstrated.

Follow-up

Once the formal diagnosis of Susac syndrome was made, intravenous cyclophosphamide was initiated. Despite these interventions, the patient continued to deteriorate and ultimately succumbed to her illness. A chronic, unrelenting, progressive disease course is very unusual for Susac syndrome, but fatal outcomes have been reported, especially in patients who also had a history of substance abuse.

Management Algorithm

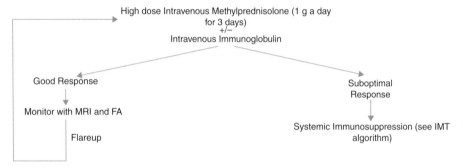

Susac Syndrome

High dose Intravenous Methylprednisolone (1 g a day for 3 days)
+/−
Intravenous Immunoglobulin

Good Response

Monitor with MRI and FA

Flareup

Suboptimal Response

Systemic Immunosuppression (see IMT algorithm)

Key Points

- Susac syndrome is an autoimmune endothelial disease leading to microvascular occlusions in the brain, retina, and inner ear, which manifests as the classic triad of encephalopathy, vision, and hearing loss.
- Young, white females are most predominantly affected.
- Three distinct clinical courses have been described, including monocyclic, polycyclic, and, rarely, a chronic-progressive course.
- FA findings in conjunction with corpus callosal lesions on brain MRI are essentially pathognomonic for Susac syndrome.
- Standard treatment includes high-dose steroids, which is usually given with IVIG, followed by a very slow and long steroid taper. Early and aggressive immunotherapy may be required in cases that are nonresponsive to steroids.
- Surveillance MRIs and FAs are helpful in following disease activity once remission has been achieved.

CHAPTER 64

IRVAN Syndrome (Idiopathic Retinal Vasculitis, Aneurysms and Neuroretinitis)

Sarah Chorfi

History of Present Illness

A 32-year-old healthy female with no past medical history presents to the eye clinic complaining of painless blurred vision, especially in the left eye (OS). She has been noticing progressive changes of vision in the past year. She has a history of retinal laser for idiopathic aneurysms in the OS a few years ago at another eye center (Figs. 64.1 and 64.2).

Exam

	OD	OS
Visual acuity	20/25	20/200
Intraocular pressure (IOP)	15	15
Sclera/conjunctiva	White and quiet	White and quiet
Cornea	Clear	Clear
Anterior chamber (AC)	Deep and quiet	Deep and quiet
Iris	Unremarkable	Unremarkable
Lens	Clear	Clear
Anterior vitreous	1+ white cells	1+ white cells
	Mild disc swelling, peripapillary flame hemorrhage	Leaking macroaneurysms surrounded by circinate exudates
	Fig. 64.1A, 64.2A	Fig 64.1B, 64.2B

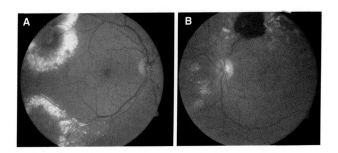

Fig. 64.1 (A) Fundus photograph of the right eye showing no haze, mild disc swelling, peripapillary flame hemorrhage, and leaking macroaneurysms surrounded by circinate exudates. (B) Fundus photograph of the left eye with no haze, exudates superior to the central macula, mild perivascular sheathing, peripapillary circinate exudates, and dilated superotemporal retinal arteriole leading to a pre-retinal hemorrhage with adjacent laser scars.

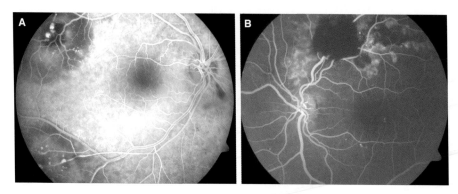

Fig. 64.2 (A) Fluorescein angiography of the right eye showing several arteriolar macroaneurysms and some leaking. No neovascularization. (B) Fluorescein angiography of the left eye showing leaking arteriolar macroaneurysms, chorioretinal atrophy post laser, subretinal exudates, dilated superotemporal retinal arteriole leading to a pre-retinal hemorrhage.

Questions to Ask

- Complete review of systems, particularly assessing for the presence of vascular disease risk factors, systemic vasculitis, and infectious etiologies.
- Were you ever diagnosed with deep venous thrombosis, stroke, miscarriage, or any other blood clotting issue?
- Is there any history of inflammatory conditions or coagulation disorders in the family?
- Were you ever treated with radiotherapy?

Assessment

- Bilateral mild optic disc edema with multiple leaking aneurysmal dilatations of retinal arterioles. Bilateral epiretinal membrane with exudation and intraretinal fluid at the macula OS. Peripheral capillary dropout bilaterally with neovascularization elsewhere (NVE) OS.

Differential Diagnosis

- Senile acquired macroaneurysms, Eales disease, Coat disease, radiation-induced retinopathy, Leber miliary aneurysm, collagen vascular disorders, antineutrophil cytoplasmic antibody (ANCA)–associated vasculitis, hypertensive retinopathy
- Idiopathic retinal vasculitis, aneurysms, and neuroretinitis (IRVAN—a diagnosis of exclusion)

Working Diagnosis

- IRVAN syndrome

Testing

- Fluorescein angiography is a useful test that can highlight several findings in IRVAN:
  - Aneurysmal arteriolar dilatations

- Late staining of the optic disc
- Areas of capillary dropout
- Neovascularization (at the optic disc or elsewhere in the retina)
- Capillary and arteriolar leakage
- Optical coherence tomography (OCT) of the optic disc and macula allows visualization of arteriolar aneurysms, macular exudation, and macular intraretinal (Fig. 64.3).
- Indocyanine green angiography (ICGA) accentuates the presence of arteriolar aneurysms.
- There is no consensus in the literature in terms of what panels should be ordered in cases of IRVAN. Systemic testing for infectious and inflammatory etiologies should be tailored according to the review of systems for each patient. There have been reports of a possible association with clotting disorders such as antiphospholipid syndrome. This association could give grounds for testing for lupus anticoagulant, antiphospholipid antibodies, and coagulation factors. Moreover, rare cases of IRVAN syndrome with concomitant presence of perinuclear antineutrophil cytoplasmic antibodies (pANCA) have been reported in the literature.
- Careful iris examination and gonioscopy to assess for the presence of neovascularization of the iris and angle.

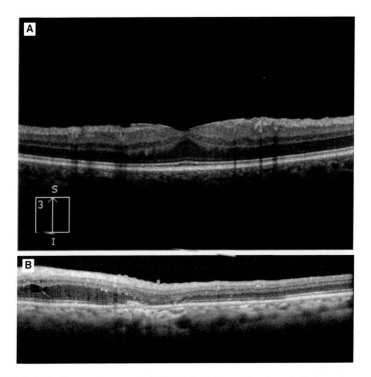

Fig. 64.3 (A) Optical coherence tomography (OCT) of the right eye showing epiretinal membrane and inner retinal hyperreflexive dots. (B) OCT of the left eye showing epiretinal membrane, subretinal, and intraretinal exudates, possible intraretinal macroaneurysm (*arrow*) surrounded by intraretinal fluid, and atrophy of the outer retinal layers.

Management

- Panretinal photocoagulation (PRP) applied to areas of peripheral nonperfusion seen on fluorescein angiography in the right eye.
- Anti–vascular endothelial growth factor (anti-VEGF) intravitreal injection in the OS.
- Follow-up in 1 month for PRP applied to areas of peripheral nonperfusion seen on fluorescein angiography in the OS.

Follow-up

The patient reports stable vision in both eyes since the last appointment 1 month ago. Vision is 20/25 OD and 20/200 OS. The ocular examination is unchanged except for resolving pre-retinal hemorrhage in the OS.

Management Algorithm

There is little consensus in the literature with regard to treatment options for IRVAN syndrome (see Management Algorithm).

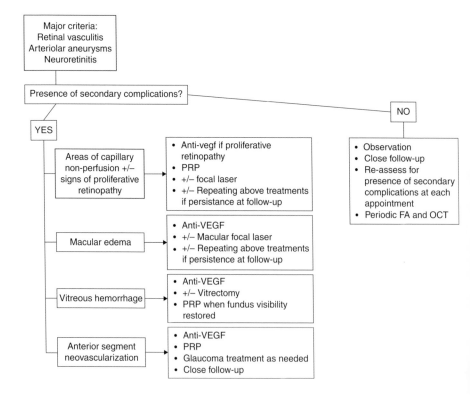

- Consider immunosuppression in the presence of severe or persisting disease, although there is limited evidence for efficacy.
- The use of corticosteroids has been reported in the literature (topical, intravitreal injection, or systemic administration), but there is a lack of consensus on this matter.

Key Points

- The major criteria of IRVAN syndrome (Chang et al.)[1]:
  - Retinal vasculitis
  - Aneurysmal dilatation at arterial bifurcations
  - Neuroretinitis (defined as optic nerve edema or leakage)
- The minor criteria of IRVAN syndrome (Chang et al.):
  - Capillary nonperfusion areas
  - Retinal neovascularization
  - Macular exudation
- Five-stage functional staging system based on ocular findings (Samuel et al.)[2]:
  - Stage 1: macroaneurysms, exudation, neuroretinitis, and retinal vasculitis
  - Stage 2: areas of capillary nonperfusion based on fluorescein angiography
  - Stage 3: posterior segment neovascularization and/or vitreous hemorrhage
  - Stage 4: anterior segment neovascularization
  - Stage 5: neovascular glaucoma
- Systemic workup should be ordered according to a complete review of systems. The literature may warrant testing for lupus anticoagulant, antiphospholipid antibodies, coagulation factors, and pANCA.
- IRVAN syndrome is a rare condition, and there is little consensus with regard to management. However, prompt treatment is important to prevent complications.

References

1. TS Chang, GW Aylward, JL Davis, WF Mieler, GL Oliver, AL Maberley, JD Gass. Idiopathic retinal vasculitis, aneursysms, and neuroretinitis. Retinal vasculitis study. Ophthalmology 1995:102(7):1089–97.
2. Samuel MA, Equi RA, Chang TS, et al. Idiopathic retinitis, vasculitis, aneurysms, and neuroretinitis (IRVAN): new observations and a proposed staging system. Ophthalmology. 2007;114:1526–1529.

CHAPTER 65

Retinal Degeneration with Coats-Like Fundus

Harpal S. Sandhu

History of Present Illness

A 22-year-old healthy man is referred to the uveitis clinic for "intermediate uveitis and macular edema unresponsive to steroids" by an outside ophthalmologist. The patient reports that he has been having vision problems for years. About 6 months ago, he presented to a local ophthalmologist complaining of progressively decreasing vision. Outside records show that he was noted to have vitreal cells and macular thickening in both eyes (OU). He was placed on prednisone 60 mg by mouth (PO) daily for nearly a month without any improvement in vision or symptoms. He was then given intravitreal injections of triamcinolone 2 mg OU. Again, there was no subjective or objective improvement. Central macular thickness and volume remained unchanged. This was followed 2 months later by injections of triamcinolone 4 mg OU. Again, there was no response. At this point, the patient was referred for a second opinion.

Exam

	OD	OS
Visual acuity	20/100	20/100
IOP	35	40
Sclera/conjunctiva	White and quiet	White and quiet
Cornea	Clear	Clear
Anterior chamber (AC)	Deep and quiet	Deep and quiet
Iris	Unremarkable	Unremarkable
Lens	Clear	Clear
Anterior vitreous	1+ cells	1+ cells
Dilated fundus examination (DFE)	See Fig. 65.1A	See Fig. 65.1B

Optical coherence tomography (OCT) was performed to assess previously documented macular thickening (Fig. 65.2).

Questions to Ask

- Do you notice floaters? If so, how long has this bothered you?
- Do you have any difficulty seeing at night or problems with peripheral vision?

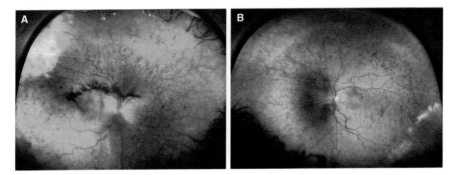

Fig. 65.1 (A) Wide-field color fundus photograph of the right eye shows diffuse pigmentary changes throughout the fundus and exudates in the superotemporal periphery. There are some pigment clumps in the posterior vitreous and a posterior vitreous detachment (PVD). (B) Wide-field color fundus photograph of the left eye shows similar findings to the right but with less exudate inferotemporally.

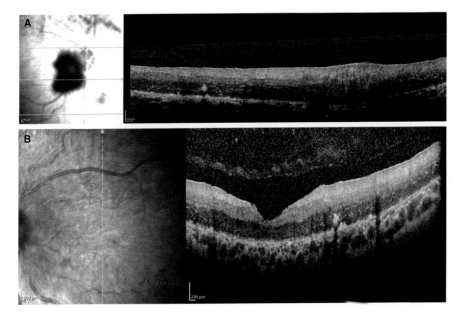

Fig. 65.2 (A) Optical coherence tomography of the right eye shows a thickened macula with abnormal retinal laminations but without frank cystoid spaces. There are also irregular, hyperreflective spots in the outer nuclear layer, as well as disruption and clumping of the RPE. (B) OCT of the left eye shows similar findings to those of the right eye. There is also severe outer retinal loss at and around the fovea and increased thickness and dilation of the choroidal vasculature.

- Is there any family history of vision problems at a young age, similar to your own problems?
- Have you been on any long-term medications?

He responds that he only sees a few floaters and is not at all bothered by them. He has had a lot of problems seeing at night. In fact, he thinks this was the first problem with his vision that he ever really noticed as a child. He has never noticed a significant problem with peripheral vision, but he is not totally sure. He is adopted and unable to provide historical information about biologic relatives. He is healthy and has never been on any medications other than the occasional antibiotic or antihistamine.

Assessment

- Retinal dystrophy OU
- Exudative retinopathy, right eye greater than left eye (OD > OS)
- Ocular hypertension OU, likely steroid response

Differential Diagnosis

- Retinitis pigmentosa (RP) with Coats-like response
- Coats disease
- Familial exudative vitreoretinopathy (FEVR)
- Other inherited retinal degeneration (IRD)
- Less likely: vitamin A deficiency

Working Diagnosis

- RP with Coats-like response
- The patient shows evidence of a retina-wide degeneration at a young age, including a highly dystrophic, thickened retina. This immediately raises suspicion for an IRD. He also has significant exudation in the temporal periphery, reminiscent of Coats disease. The single diagnosis that unifies these two striking findings is a form of RP associated with a Coats-like vasculopathy or response, typically caused by mutations in the *CRB1* gene. A few cells in the vitreous are common in RP and do not represent active uveitis.

Testing

- Visual fields: There are small islands of preserved paracentral and far temporal vision OU.
- Fluorescein angiogram (Fig. 65.3)
- Full-field electroretinogram (ERG)
- Genetic testing: RP panel

Management

- Start ocular hypotensive medications: timolol 0.5% twice a day (BID) OU, dorzolamide 2% three times a day (TID) OU, brimonidine 0.2% TID OU

Follow-up

The patient returns 1 month later. His symptoms are unchanged. Intraocular pressure (IOP) has declined to 23 OD and 25 OS. Both photopic and scotopic ERG potentials were undetectable. Genetic testing returned positive for biallelic mutations in the *CRB1* gene.

Final Diagnosis

- RP with Coats-like response

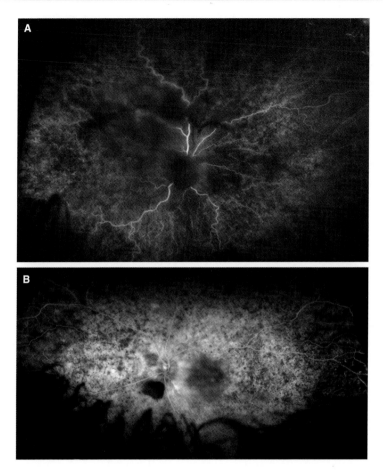

Fig. 65.3 (A) Arterial-phase fluorescein angiogram (FA) of the right eye shows alternating areas of hyperauto-fluorescence consistent with window defects adjacent to hypoautofluorescent areas throughout the fundus. There is no leakage. There is some blocking in the posterior pole due to the pigment clumps in the vitreous. (B) Late-phase FA of the left eye shows similar findings of alternating hyperfluorescent and hypofluorescent areas and absence of leakage.

Key Points

- Certain types of inherited retinal degenerations can masquerade as uveitis. Even though there is no established treatment for most IRDs at this time, it is critical to diagnose these cases correctly to provide patients with an accurate prognosis and to spare them potentially harmful treatments until proven therapeutic approaches are established.
- Macular thickening due to abnormal retinal laminations must be distinguished from cystoid spaces or diffuse thickening from epiretinal membranes or vitreomacular traction (VMT). The former is highly unusual in uveitis, whereas the latter three are common.
- Similarly, retina-wide degenerative changes are unusual in uveitis and should generate a differential based around retinal degeneration. In younger patients, IRDs would be most likely, whereas cancer-associated retinopathy and nonparaneoplastic retinopathies are more

likely in older or middle-aged patients. Toxic/metabolic causes, such as vitamin A deficiency or medications associated with retinal degenerations, can usually be ruled out by history.

- RP due to *CRB1* mutations has a wide phenotypic range and does not always present with Coats-like vasculopathy and prominent pigment clumping. Other presentations include preservation of the para-arteriolar RPE and profound, early-onset retinal degeneration (also called *Leber congenital amaurosis*). Hyperopia and a thickened, dystrophic macula, as in this case, are classic findings.

- It is ideal not to treat the areas of exudation with retino-ablative procedures (e.g., cryotherapy or thermal laser) because these patients already suffer from widespread photoreceptor dysfunction. However, if the exudation is extensive enough that it is contributing to further vision loss, it is amenable to the same treatment modalities as classic Coats disease.

CHAPTER 66

Congenital Zika Syndrome

Camila V. Ventura ▓ Liana O. Ventura ▓ Rubens Belfort Jr.

History of Present Illness

A 4-month-old female baby was referred for an ophthalmologic evaluation. The baby was delivered via C-section at 36 weeks in a public maternity hospital in Recife, the capital of Pernambuco state, in the northeast of Brazil. Physical examination at birth revealed severe microcephaly with partially collapsed skull (head circumference: 27 cm and birth weight: 2324 grams).

Initial Examination at 4 Months

Exam

	OD	OS
Visual acuity (Teller visual acuity cards)	0.32 cy/cm at 38 cm	0.43 cy/cm at 38 cm
Pupillary reflexes	Sluggish	Sluggish
Extraocular muscles (EOM)	Normal	Normal
Nystagmus	Absent	Absent
Anterior segment	Unremarkable	Unremarkable
Retina	Figs. 66.1, 66.2, and 66.3	Figs. 66.1, 66.2, and 66.3

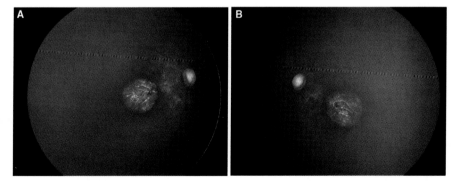

Fig. 66.1 (A and B) Fundus photograph of both eyes showing optic nerve hypoplasia, pallor, and increased disc cupping and a chorioretinal scar with gross pigment mottling in the macular region.

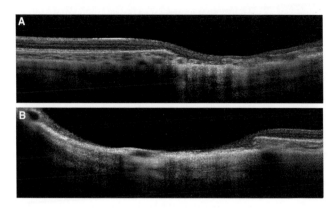

Fig. 66.2 (A and B) Spectral domain optical coherence tomography images of both eyes showed severe neurosensory retina loss with discontinuation of the ellipsoid zone (IS/OS junction), a hyperreflectivity underlying the retinal pigment epithelium (RPE), and choroidal thinning. A colobomatous-like excavation was observed in the affected retina, RPE, and choroid.

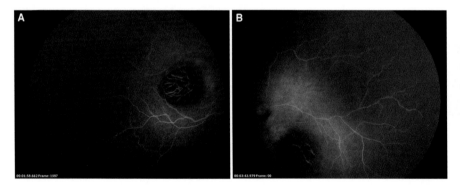

Fig. 66.3 (A and B) Fluorescein angiography enhanced the optic nerve hypoplasia, chorioretinal scars, pigment mottling and revealed diffuse avascularity of the peripheral retina in both eyes.

Questions to Ask

- Is there any family history of neurologic or genetic diseases?
- Did the mother feel any symptoms during pregnancy such as rash, itchiness, fever, and joint pain? If so, what trimester?

The mother denied previous neurologic and genetic diseases in the family. She developed fever, rash, itchiness, and joint pain during the second trimester of pregnancy.

Assessment

- Bilateral chorioretinal scar and optic nerve hypoplasia associated with severe microcephaly

Differential Diagnosis

- Genetic etiologies (Chromosomal and metabolic disorders)
- Nongenetic etiologies

- Congenital infections
  - Toxoplasmosis, rubella, cytomegalovirus, herpes, syphilis, varicella zoster virus, parvovirus B19, and human immunodeficiency virus (HIV)
- Maternal alcoholism
- Exposure to ionizing radiation
- Prenatal injuries such as hypoxia and trauma
- Severe malnutrition

Working Diagnosis

- Bilateral macular chorioretinal scar both eyes (OU) at birth, presumably secondary to congenital Zika virus infection

Testing

- Check mother's prenatal examinations: no history of such examinations
- Serology
  - Toxoplasmosis, rubella, cytomegalovirus, herpesviruses, syphilis (TORCHS), dengue virus, chikungunya virus, and HIV (negative)
  - Zika virus: immunoglobulin M (IgM) testing for Zika antibodies (Zika IgM enzyme-linked immunosorbent assay [MAC-ELISA]) positive in infant cerebrospinal fluid (CSF).
  - Computed tomography (CT) scan central nervous system (CNS): demonstrated cortical malformations, cerebral calcifications (cortical, subcortical, periventricular, and thalamus), parenchymal volume reduction, and ventriculomegaly.

Management

- Initiate early intervention with a multidisciplinary team, including a physiotherapist, speech and language therapist, and occupational therapist.
- Patient referrals to:
  - Pediatric neurology for comprehensive neurologic examination and follow-up
  - Infectious diseases to rule out other congenital infections
  - Clinical geneticist to rule out genetic diseases
  - Orthopedist for limb anomalies evaluation and management (e.g., clubfoot, hip subluxation, and arthrogryposis)
  - Gastroenterologist for dysphagia evaluation and management
  - Otolaryngologist for diagnosis and management of hearing loss

Specific recommendations for ophthalmologic management:

- Referral for initial fundus evaluation and follow-up every 6 months.
- Referral to pediatric ophthalmologist for diagnosis and management of strabismus, refractive error, hypoaccommodation, and visual impairment.

Follow-up

The patient developed esotropia (ET) = 35D at 8 months of age and subsequently underwent strabismus surgery (Fig. 66.4).

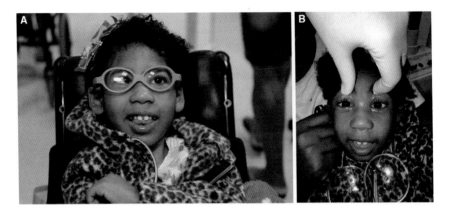

Fig. 66.4 (A and B) Photography showing patient's esotropia before and after strabismus surgery.

Management Algorithm

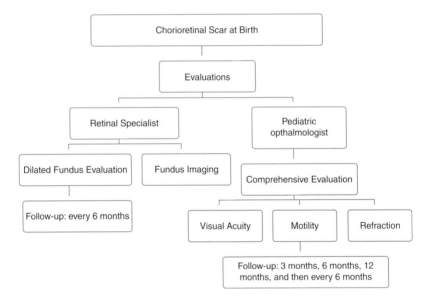

Key Points

- Ocular complications of Zika virus infection can involve the retina and retinal vasculature, as well as the optic nerve, making retinal examination mandatory with this diagnosis.
- Central chorioretinal atrophy does not increase in size with time. Fluorescein angiography may reveal peripheral avascularity of the retina.
- Close follow-up with pediatric ophthalmology for diagnosis and management of hypoaccommodation, refractive errors, and strabismus; surgery may be an option to treat stable strabismus cases.

CHAPTER 67

West Nile Retinopathy

Kareem Moussa ▨ Dean Eliott

History of Present Illness

A 60-year-old man with a history of prediabetes presents to the emergency department with 2 days of increasing floaters and blurry vision in both eyes, as well as 4 days of malaise, body aches, and chills. He denied fevers, neck stiffness, dysarthria, or focal weakness. Two days before presentation, his primary care physician prescribed oral doxycycline for a presumed tick-borne illness, but the patient's symptoms continued to worsen.

Exam

	OD	OS
Visual acuity	20/100	20/100
Intraocular pressure (IOP)	13	13
Sclera/conjunctiva	White and quiet	White and quiet
Cornea	Clear	Clear
Anterior chamber (AC)	2+ white cells	2+ white cells
Iris	Unremarkable	Unremarkable
Lens	Clear	Clear
Anterior vitreous	2+ cells	2+ cells
Dilated fundus examination (DFE)	See Fig. 67.1A	See Fig. 67.1B

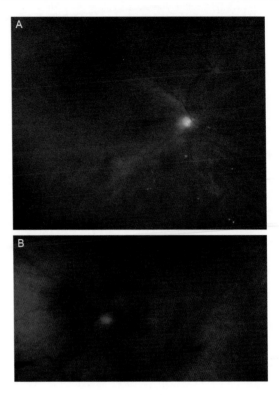

Fig. 67.1 (A) Fundus photograph of the right eye showing hazy media due to vitritis and multiple round chorioretinal lesions in a curvilinear pattern in the nasal periphery. (B) Fundus photograph of the left eye showing hazy media due to vitritis and an unremarkable periphery.

Questions to Ask

- Have you had recent exposure to mosquitoes?
- Have you traveled abroad recently?
- Do you engage in unsafe sex practices?

He reported recent exposure to mosquitoes. He denied recent travel or participation in unsafe sex practices.

Assessment

- Bilateral acute nongranulomatous panuveitis with chorioretinal lesions

Differential Diagnosis

- West Nile virus (WNV)—associated panuveitis
- Less likely: tuberculosis-, syphilis-, or sarcoid-associated panuveitis or lymphoma

Working Diagnosis

- WNV-associated panuveitis

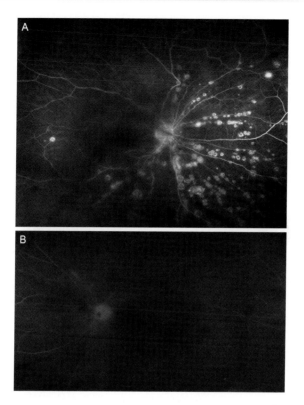

Fig. 67.2 (A) Fluorescein angiogram of the right eye showing multiple round "target" lesions with hypofluorescent centers and hyperfluorescent edges arranged in a curvilinear pattern in the nasal periphery. (B) Fluorescein angiogram of the left eye showing a few "target" lesions nasally.

Testing

- Serology (immunoglobulin M [IgM] and immunoglobulin G [IgG] WNV antibodies) should be obtained from blood to confirm the diagnosis. Polymerase chain reaction (PCR) testing from blood is less likely to yield a positive result after the first week of illness. In cases with mental status changes, headache, and/or stiff neck, serology and PCR testing can be performed on cerebrospinal fluid (CSF).
- Fluorescein angiography highlights the "target" lesions with hypofluorescent centers and hyperfluorescent edges, which may be challenging to visualize on examination (Fig. 67.2).
- Optical coherence tomography demonstrates loss of the retinal pigment epithelium and ellipsoid zone in the "target" lesions.
- For atypical cases, check:
  - Fluorescent treponemal antibody absorption (FTA-ABS), rapid plasma reagin (RPR)
  - QuantiFERON Gold or purified protein derivative (PPD)
  - Angiotensin-converting enzyme (ACE), lysozyme, and chest x-ray (CXR)
- A neurology consult should be obtained to evaluate neurologic symptoms

Management

- Topical corticosteroid (prednisolone acetate 1% four times a day [QID] both eyes [OU]) and cycloplegia (atropine 1% every day OU) drops
- Follow up in 1 week

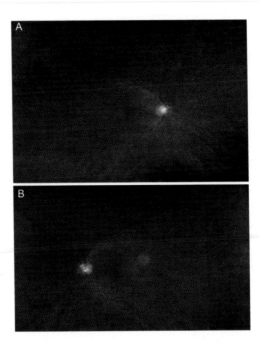

Fig. 67.3 (A) Fundus photograph of the right eye showing relatively clear media and stable target lesions nasally 3 weeks after presentation. (B) Fundus photograph of the left eye showing relatively clear media and an unremarkable periphery.

Follow-up

The patient follows up a week later. He reports improvement in vision and reduced floaters. Visual acuity was 20/50 in each eye. Serology obtained the day of presentation revealed positive IgM (4.77, positive > 0.9) and IgG (2.85, positive >1.3) WNV antibodies, confirming the diagnosis.

Three weeks after presentation, the patient reports continued improvement in vision, and visual acuity was 20/40 in the right eye and 20/25 in the left eye (Fig. 67.3).

Key Points

- A history of blurry vision and/or floaters in the setting of flulike symptoms or neurologic symptoms should raise concern for WNV infection.
- Fluorescein angiography highlights the "target" lesions, which are highly suggestive of WNV chorioretinitis, especially when arranged in a linear or curvilinear pattern, and may be challenging to visualize on examination.
- Serology is more likely to yield a positive diagnostic result than PCR testing after the first week of illness. Blood testing is performed on all patients, whereas CSF testing is performed on patients with neurologic manifestations.
- Tuberculosis, syphilis, sarcoidosis, and lymphoma should always be considered as possible etiologies in patients with unexplained ocular inflammation.
- A neurology consult should be obtained for patients with suspected WNV infection, as neurologic involvement indicates severe disease, which can be fatal.
- Treatment is supportive.
- Patients should be monitored for the development of cystoid macular edema, a rare complication that may respond to treatment with intravitreal anti−vascular endothelial growth factor (VEGF) injections.

CHAPTER 68

Dengue Retinopathy

Sivakumar R. Rathinam

History of Present Illness

A 25 yo male presented with painless blurring of vision OU for 2 days. One month prior he presented with adult respiratory distress syndrome (RDS) and thrombocytopenia diagnosed as dengue fever for which he was hospitalized and symptomatic treatment was given.

Ocular Examination

Exam

	OD	OS
Snellen visual acuity	20/40	CF 4′
Intraocular pressure (IOP)	14 mm Hg	12 mm Hg
Sclera/conjunctiva	Normal	Normal
Cornea	Clear	Clear
Anterior chamber (AC)	Flare 1+ , cells 1+	Flare 1+ , cells 1+
Iris	Normal	Normal
Lens	Clear	Clear
Vitreous cells	Vitritis 1+	Vitritis 1+
Fundus	Fig. 68.1	Fig. 68.2

Questions Asked

- Did he have any visual acuity (VA) problems at the time of diagnosis of dengue fever?
  - No.
- What symptoms of dengue fever did he have on presentation, and how was his RDS managed?
  - He presented with fever, skin rashes, and difficulty in breathing for which he was hospitalized.
- How did he catch the disease—namely, was there any activity he was participating in that would have increased his likelihood of having the disease?
  - No.
- How was dengue fever diagnosed?
  - Dengue fever was diagnosed based on positive serology.

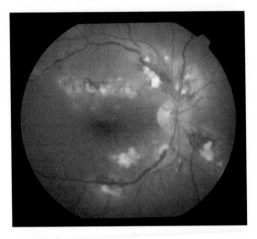

Fig. 68.1 Hyperemic disc, yellowish-white retinal lesions with intraretinal hemorrhages and macular edema with internal limiting membrane folds OD.

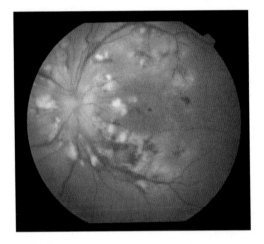

Fig. 68.2 Hyperemic disc, multiple cotton-wool spots, and intraretinal hemorrhages in the peripapillary region with macular edema OS.

Assessment

- Infectious multifocal retinitis both eyes (OU) with macular edema, left eye (OS).

Differential Diagnosis

- Chikungunya
- Cytomegalovirus (CMV) retinitis
- Acute leukemia
- Human immunodeficiency virus (HIV)

Working Diagnosis

Dengue retinopathy and associated panuveitis, OU, with macular edema OS

Testing

- Complete blood count (CBC): normal
- Serology
  - Positive: dengue immunoglobulin G (IgG) and immunoglobulin M (IgM) antibodies
  - Negative: HIV I/II and Chikungunya
- Chest x-ray: normal
- Mantoux test: negative

Fundus Fluorescein Angiography

Figs. 68.3 and 68.4 showed early hypofluorescence and late hyperfluorescence of chorioretinal lesions with disc leakage and diffuse perivascular leakage.

Spectral Domain Optical Coherence Tomography

Fig. 68.5 showed hyperreflective dots (inflammatory cells) in the posterior vitreous cavity, hyper-reflectivity in the inner retinal layers, loss of foveal contour, and neurosensory detachment, including the fovea.

Management

Topical corticosteroids and cycloplegia, OU, as well as systemic corticosteroids.

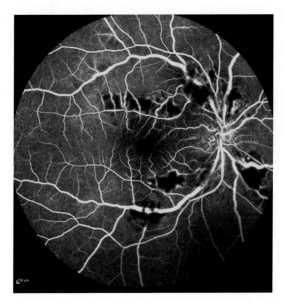

Fig. 68.3   Early hypofluorescent lesions secondary to intraretinal and inner retinal edema and blood.

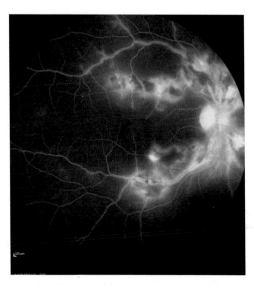

Fig. 68.4 Late hyperflourescence of chorioretinal lesions, with fluorescein leakage from the optic disc and retinal veins.

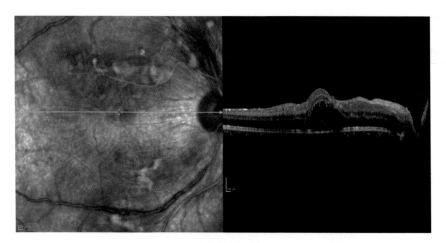

Fig. 68.5 Hyperreflective dots (inflammatory cells) in the posterior vitreous cavity, hyperreflectivity in the inner retinal layers, loss of foveal contour, and neurosensory detachment, including the fovea.

Follow-up

After 4 weeks, retinitis and panuveitis started to resolve OU. Topical and systemic medications were slowly tapered.

Key Points

- Dengue virus is a flavivirus, transmitted by the *Aedes aegypti* and *Aedes albopictus* mosquitos. There are four closely related serotypes: dengue 1 to 4. Infection with one serotype does not protect against the others.

- The virus causes dengue fever in humans. In addition to fever, infection can cause severe headaches, myalgia, and thrombocytopenia, resulting in bleeding manifestations such as a purpuric rash and conjunctival hemorrhage as dengue hemorrhagic fever (DHF). Hypotension may also occur in the dengue shock syndrome (DSS), which carries a high mortality.
- Symptoms of infection usually begin 4 to 7 days after a bite and last for 3 to 10 days.
- The mosquito can transmit the infection to others by feeding on infected individuals, even before the person becomes symptomatic. Some people remain asymptomatic but can still infect mosquitoes.
- The mosquito remains infected for the remainder of its life, which might be days or a few weeks.

CHAPTER 69

Primary Vitreoretinal Lymphoma (PVRL)

Madison E. Kerley ■ George Magrath ■ Aparna Ramasubramanian

History of Present Illness

A 72-year-old Caucasian male with a 6-year history of primary central nervous system (CNS) lymphoma, confirmed on histopathology of tissue acquired by brain biopsy of the left hemisphere to be diffuse large B-cell lymphoma, presents to the eye clinic with blurred vision of the right eye (OD).

Exam

	OD	OS
Visual acuity	20/60	20/20
Intraocular pressure (IOP)	16	18
Sclera/conjunctiva	White and quiet	White and quiet
Cornea	Clear	Clear
Anterior chamber (AC)	Trace cells	Deep and quiet
Iris	Unremarkable	Unremarkable
Lens	Clear	Clear
Anterior vitreous	Vitreous seeding	Clear

Dilated Fundus Examination (DFE) (See Fig. 69.1)

Nerve:	Pink, sharp
Macula:	Flat
Vessels	Normal caliber and course
Periphery:	Unremarkable

Questions to Ask

- Do you have any symptoms in the left eye (OS)?
- Have you had any symptoms of shortness of breath, weight loss, neurologic symptoms lymph node enlargement, or any gastrointestinal (GI) symptoms?
- What previous history of lymphoma treatment have you had?

The patient denied any change in vision in the OS. He had neurologic symptoms like headache and seizure that were controlled on medication. He also had a history of significant weight loss and complained of nausea and vomiting. He denied any shortness of breath and did not have any lymph

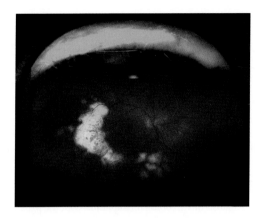

Fig. 69.1   Color fundus photograph of the right eye shows vitritis and multiple sub-RPE infiltrates.

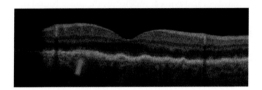

Fig. 69.2   Optical coherence tomography of the right eye confirms the infiltrate at the level of the subretinal and sub-RPE space.

node enlargement. He added that he has had an extensive history of previous management of lymphoma, but did not remember all the details.

Differential Diagnosis

- Secondary vitreoretinal lymphoma
- Infectious vitritis

Working Diagnosis

- Secondary vitreoretinal lymphoma OD

Testing

- With the presence of vitritis, pars plana vitrectomy can be diagnostic. As large a vitreous sample as possible (0.5+ cc) should be sent for polymerase chain reaction (PCR), culture, cytology, and flow cytometry.
- Flow cytometry can be performed to detect clonal B-cell populations.
- To test for infiltrates and retinal detachment, fluorescein angiography and optical coherence tomography (OCT) should be performed (Fig. 69.2).
- Ultrasound can be used to determine the degree of choroid thickening.

Follow-up

PCR and culture were negative for microbes. Flow cytometry and cytology were positive for a clonal population of CD20+ B cells, consistent with vitreoretinal lymphoma.

Management

- 20 Gray (Gy) external beam radiation (EBR) with 10 fractions
- Systemic methotrexate (eight doses) and rituximab with temozolomide
- Consolidation therapy with cytarabine and etoposide

Further Follow-up

Eighteen months after diagnosis of vitreoretinal lymphoma OD, the patient developed vitritis and sub—retinal pigment epithelium (RPE) infiltrates in the left eye. He was started on 20 Gy EBR in 10 fractions to the OS.

Twelve months after treatment of the OS, there was bilateral recurrence of both vitritis and infiltrates, confirmed by bilateral vitrectomy. The patient received 11 more fractions of radiation to the left eye, as well as 8 rounds of intravitreal methotrexate and 1 round of intravitreal rituximab to the right eye.

The right eye developed severe corneal edema and neovascular glaucoma, managed by anti—vascular endothelial growth factor (VEGF) and cyclophotocoagulation. Vision at last follow-up was light perception OD and 20/50 OS.

He has had no recurrence of CNS lymphoma since initiating treatment of vitreoretinal lymphoma OD.

Key Points

- Primary vitreoretinal lymphoma presents on slit lamp examination as vitritis with an "aurora borealis" appearance resulting from a build-up of lymphocytes.
- If vitritis is present and vitreoretinal lymphoma is suspected, a diagnosis can be attained through pars plana vitrectomy. Without vitritis, a chorioretinal biopsy can be obtained.
- MYD88, an oncogene that encodes a protein involved in signal transduction of innate immune responses, is mutated in a high proportion of cases and is a further confirmatory test that can be performed on surgical specimens.
- After a diagnosis is confirmed, screening for CNS lymphoma should be performed if the patient does not already carry the diagnosis, along with testing for neurologic deficits due to the high comorbidity of CNS lymphoma and vitreoretinal lymphoma.
- If there is no CNS involvement, local therapy with EBR or intravitreal chemotherapy with rituximab and methotrexate can be considered.
- If there is CNS involvement, management must be coordinated with oncology and involves a combination of chemotherapy, immunotherapy, and radiation. Because of the rarity of the disease, randomized controlled trials of these different treatment modalities are lacking.

CHAPTER 70

Leukemia Metastatic to the Retina

Harpal S. Sandhu ▓ Albert M. Maguire

History of Present Illness (HPI)

A 51-year-old man with a history of cutaneous T-cell lymphoma (mycosis fungoides) complains of severe loss of vision in his right eye (OD). It is difficult for him to speak and provide a history because of significant pain in his mouth. He has ulcers on his tongue and is being treated for oral candidiasis with fluconazole (Fig. 70.1). Details are limited, but he is able to communicate that it has been getting worse over the course of the last 3 weeks or so. He denies eye pain (Fig. 70.2).

Exam

	OD	OS
Vision	Count fingers 3′	20/25
Intraocular pressure (IOP)	20	16
Lids and lashes:	Normal	Normal
Sclera/conjunctiva:	White and quiet	White and quiet
Cornea:	Clear	Clear
AC:	2+ white cells	Deep and quiet
Iris:	Flat	Flat
Lens:	Clear	Clear
Anterior vitreous:	2+ white cells	Clear

Dilated Fundus Examination (DFE) (See Fig. 70.1)

Nerve:	Cup-to-disc (c/d) 0.3, pink, sharp
Macula:	Flat
Vessels:	Normal caliber and course
Periphery:	Unremarkable

Further Questions to Ask

- Besides oral candidiasis, have you been treated for any other infections lately?
- Any recent hospitalizations? How do you feel right now? Any malaise, night sweats, or chills?
- Do you have any indwelling hardware?
- What treatment have you had for your cancer?

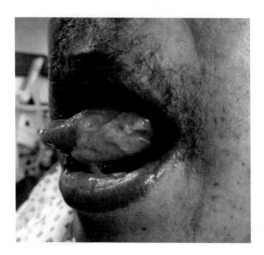

Fig. 70.1 Color external photograph of the patient's tongue, left lateral view. There is an obvious white discoloration and probable ulceration. (From Sandhu H, Kim E, Maguire A. Cutaneous T-cell lymphoma metastatic to the retina. *Ophthalmology* 2016;123[4]:736.)

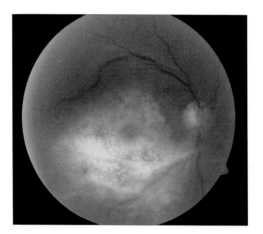

Fig. 70.2 Color fundus photograph of the right eye shows hazy media consistent with vitreal inflammation and a dense white preretinal infiltrate. Left eye (not shown here) is normal. (From Sandhu H, Kim E, Maguire A. Cutaneous T-cell lymphoma metastatic to the retina. *Ophthalmology* 2016;123[4]:736.)

- Are you on medications that suppress your immune system, like steroids or chemotherapy?

The patient answers no to all of the questions. He has generally had an increased level of fatigue and depressed mood since his cancer diagnosis, but no recent changes. He denies any recent steroids but knows he has been treated with them in the past. The only specific treatment he recalls for his cancer is interferon-alpha, but he is otherwise unsure.

Optical coherence tomography was performed to better characterize the extent of retinal involvement (Fig. 70.3).

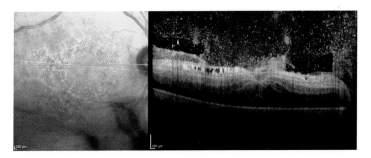

Fig. 70.3 Optical coherence tomography (OCT) of the right eye shows extensive posterior vitreous cells, including a hyperreflective subhyaloid infiltrate, a hyperreflective streak through the inner retina with disruption of the nerve fiber layer, and diffuse retinal thickening with a small foveal detachment. Left eye (not shown) is normal.

Assessment

- Panuveitis OD with macular retinitis

Differential Diagnosis

- Endogenous endophthalmitis
- Infectious retinitis
  - Herpetic retinitis/progressive outer retinal necrosis (PORN)
  - Severe atypical toxoplasmosis
  - Syphilis
- Behçet disease
- Least likely: metastatic cutaneous T-cell lymphoma

Working Diagnosis

- Endogenous endophthalmitis, likely fungal

Further Testing

- The patient has a systemic malignancy and is currently being treated for an infection. Although oral fungal diseases are generally noninvasive, the status of this patient's immune system is unknown, and it is unclear if he has been on chemotherapy in the past. The safest course of action is to treat this as an endogenous endophthalmitis and take a culture of the vitreous for bacterial and fungal testing and polymerase chain reaction (PCR) for viruses, bacteria, and fungi.
- Check complete blood count (CBC) and CD4 count
- Check rapid plasma reagin (RPR), fluorescent treponemal antibody absorption (FTA-ABS), and toxoplasma serologies

Management

- Tap the vitreous and inject broad-spectrum antimicrobials, including antifungals
  - Vancomycin 1 mg/0.1 mL
  - Ceftazidime 2.25 mg/0.1 mL
  - Voriconazole 100 μg/0.1 mL
- Follow up the next day

Follow-up #1

HPI

The patient is seen on postprocedure day 1. Besides a subconjunctival hemorrhage at the site of intravitreal injection, he notes no changes. CBC showed a normal white count, no neutropenia, and CD4 count of 805.

Exam

	OD	OS
Vision	Count fingers 3′	20/20
IOP	17	15
Lids and lashes:	Normal	Normal
Sclera/conjunctiva:	temporal subconjunctival hemorrhage	White and Quiet
Cornea:	Clear	Clear
AC:	2+ white cells	Deep and quiet
Iris:	Flat	Flat
Lens:	Clear	Clear
Anterior vitreous:	2+ white cells	Clear
DFE:	Unchanged	Unchanged

Management

- It is postprocedure day 1 after a tap and injection procedure. No change in examination is common.
- Start prednisolone acetate 1% four times a day (QID), moxifloxacin QID, and atropine twice a day (BID) OD

Follow-up #2

The patient returns on postprocedure day 3. He again notes no changes. Vision, pressure, anterior chamber (AC) cell, and fundus examination are identical to preprocedure. Vitreous culture was negative for organisms. PCR, including viral PCR, was negative. Syphilis and *Toxoplasma* serologies returned negative.

Management

- An infectious endophthalmitis would be expected to show some improvement by now. Thus one must question the original diagnosis and return to the original differential diagnosis. Viral PCR, which is quite sensitive, was also normal. Moreover, the presentation with numerous intraocular cells and a dense premacular infiltrate is inconsistent with PORN, which features no cells and smaller infiltrates. He is also not immunosuppressed sufficiently to develop PORN or a severe, atypical toxoplasmosis. Syphilis and *Toxoplasma* serologies were also negative.
- Perform diagnostic vitrectomy and send vitreous sample for flow cytometry and cytology. The infiltrate is in too visually significant an area to be amenable to chorioretinal biopsy.

Follow-up #3

The patient presents a week after uncomplicated vitrectomy. He notes his vision is the same, although he has fewer floaters. Examination is unchanged aside from decreased vitreous haze and cell. Cytology and flow cytometry revealed a clonal population of T cells.

Diagnosis

- Cutaneous T-cell lymphoma metastatic to the vitreous and retina OD

Management

- The patient was referred back to oncology and radiation oncology to arrange external beam radiotherapy.
- The patient underwent fractionated radiotherapy for a total of 30 Gy treatment to OD.

Follow-up #4

HPI

The patient returns a week after finishing radiotherapy. He notes that his vision is about the same but that his eye feels dry and frequently irritated.

Exam

	OD	OS
Vision	Hand motions	20/25
IOP	17	16
Lids and lashes:	Normal	Normal
Sclera/conjunctiva:	Trace injection	White and quiet
Cornea:	Clear	Clear
	2+ superficial keratopathy	
AC:	Deep and quiet	Deep and quiet
Iris:	Flat	Flat
Lens:	Clear	Clear
DFE:	See Figs. 70.4 and 70.5	Unchanged

Key Points

- Systemic malignancies metastatic to the retina are extremely rare. Intraocular metastasis more commonly involves the uveal tract, which is richly vascularized.
- T-cell lymphomas in general are rare. Most lymphomas, including those that affect the eye, are B-cell lymphomas.
- When cutaneous T-cell lymphoma does affect the eye, it usually metastasizes to the ocular adnexa. Intraocular metastasis is very rare.

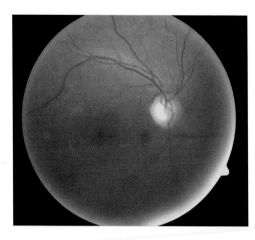

Fig. 70.4 Color fundus photo of the right eye shows improved media quality and a completely resolved macular infiltrate.

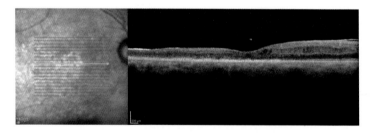

Fig. 70.5 OCT of the right eye shows significant macular thinning, with intraretinal cysts, OD, and rare posterior vitreous cells.

- A high suspicion for infectious etiologies is important in cancer patients, who are frequently immunosuppressed. Recent or current treatment for infection is a red flag that there may indicate hematogenous spread of infection to the eye. Because of the potentially devastating consequences of not treating endophthalmitis immediately, the safer course of action in a case like this is to treat for infection first and then reconsider the diagnosis later if the patient's course is inconsistent with infection.
- External beam radiotherapy can be effective for leukemia/lymphoma with intraocular metastasis, but adverse effects to the eye are myriad. In this case, the patient ultimately developed radiation optic neuropathy, which limited his vision in combination with macular atrophy, as well as mild radiation keratopathy.

CHAPTER 71

New-Onset Macular Edema

Harpal S. Sandhu

History of Present Illness

A 38-year-old man with a history of idiopathic recurrent anterior uveitis both eyes (OU) and no significant past medical history complains of blurred vision in his left eye (OS). He noticed some change about 2 or 3 weeks ago but did not think anything of it. It has been getting worse, and he says images look misshapen and smaller out of his left eye than out of the right. He has never experienced something like this before, and it is unlike his usual flares, which present with intense photophobia and mild blurring of vision.

Exam

	OD	OS
Visual acuity	20/20	20/40+
IOP	12	14
Sclera/conjunctiva	White and quiet	White and quiet
Cornea	Clear	Clear
Anterior chamber (AC)	Deep and quiet	Deep and quiet
Iris	Unremarkable	Unremarkable
Lens	Clear	Clear
Anterior vitreous	Clear	1+ old cells

Dilated Fundus Examination (DFE)

Nerve:	Cup-to-disc (c/d) 0.2, pink, sharp	c/d 0.2, pink, sharp
Macula:	Normal	Blunted foveal reflex
Vessels:	Normal caliber and course	Normal caliber, sheathing temporally
Periphery:	Unremarkable	Unremarkable

Questions to Ask

- Before being treated at this clinic, were you ever told you had swelling in the retina?
- Have you been treated with injections directly into the eye or around the eye in the past?
- Have there been any changes in your general health since you last came to the eye clinic?
  The patient answers "no" to all questions.
  Because of the suspicion of macular edema in the left eye, optical coherence tomography (OCT) and fluorescein angiography (FA) were performed (Figs. 71.1 and 71.2).

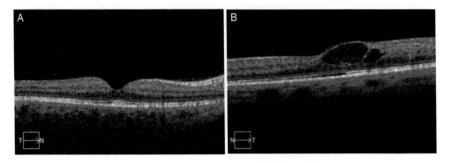

Fig. 71.1   (A) OCT of the right eye is normal. (B) OCT of the left eye shows moderate cystoid macular edema.

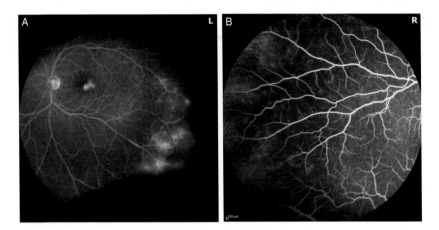

Fig. 71.2   (A) A late-phase FA of the left eye shows leakage in the macula consistent with macular edema and peripheral vessel staining with leakage. Similar vessel staining was seen in the right eye (not shown here). (B) A late-phase FA of the right eye shows diffuse, deep leakage in the temporal periphery.

Assessment

- Uveitic cystoid macular edema (CME) OS
- Active retinal vasculitis OU

Differential Diagnosis

- The patient has no significant past medical history and has had an extensive evaluation for infectious and inflammatory etiologies, including cytoplasmic antineutrophil cytoplasmic antibodies (cANCA) and perinuclear antineutrophil cytoplasmic antibodies (pANCA). It is reasonable to assume for now that the vasculitis is a manifestation of his idiopathic uveitis.

Working Diagnosis

- Idiopathic retinal vasculitis OU complicated by CME OS

Testing

- None

Management

- Prednisone 60 mg by mouth (PO) daily

Follow-up

Over the course of the following weeks, the vasculitis improves, cystoid macular edema resolves, and the patient's vision returns to 20/20 OU. However, over the next 3 months, the prednisone dose cannot be reduced to below 15 mg PO daily without recurrence of active retinal vasculitis and CME OS.

Management

- Start immunomodulatory therapy. Methotrexate was initiated and titrated up to 20 mg PO every week.

Follow-up #2

After 4 months of methotrexate therapy, the prednisone dose has been reduced to 7.5 mg PO daily while the vasculitis remains inactive. However, the patient presents again with recurrent CME OS and vision has declined to 20/40 OS.

Management

- Intravitreal triamcinolone 2 mg/0.05 cc OS

Follow-up #3

The patient returns a month later. He is pleased and reports he is seeing much better. His vision has improved to 20/20 OS, but intraocular pressure (IOP) is 40 (Fig. 71.3).

Management

- Start multiple ocular hypotensive agents: timolol twice a day (BID), dorzolamide three times a day (TID), and brimonidine OS TID

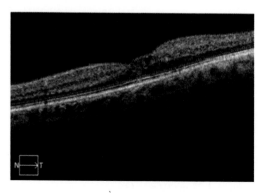

Fig. 71.3 OCT of the left eye shows resolution of the majority of the macular edema and restoration of the normal foveal contour.

Follow-up #4

The patient returns 6 weeks later. He reports he has been taking the drops diligently, but again his vision has begun to decline.

Eye-Related Medications

- Prednisone 7.5 mg PO daily
- Methotrexate 20 mg PO every week
- Timolol BID OS
- Dorzolamide TID OS
- Brimonidine TID OS

Exam

	OD	OS
Visual acuity	20/20	20/30−
IOP	12	29
Sclera/conjunctiva	White and quiet	White and quiet
Cornea	Clear	Clear
AC	Deep and quiet	Deep and quiet
Iris	Unremarkable	Unremarkable
Lens	Clear	Clear
Anterior vitreous	Clear	1+ old cells

DFE

Nerve:	c/d 0.2, pink, sharp	c/d 0.2, pink, sharp
Macula:	Normal	Blunted foveal reflex
Vessels:	Normal caliber and course	Normal caliber
Periphery:	Unremarkable	Unremarkable

FA: No active vasculitis OU

Assessment

- Inactive uveitis and retinal vasculitis OU
- Ocular hypertension OS secondary to corticosteroid response, on three topical ocular hypotensive agents
- Recurrent cystoid macular edema (Fig. 71.4)

Management

- Intravitreal bevacizumab 1.25 mg/0.05 cc OS
- Continue all ocular hypotensive drops

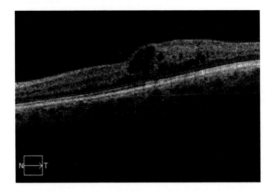

Fig. 71.4 OCT of the left eye shows recurrent cystoid macular edema.

Follow-up #5

The patient returns 1 month later. He reports his vision has returned to normal and that he continues to take all his medications as prescribed. Vision has returned to 20/20 OU, IOP is 24 OS, and OCT shows resolution of macular edema.

Management Algorithm

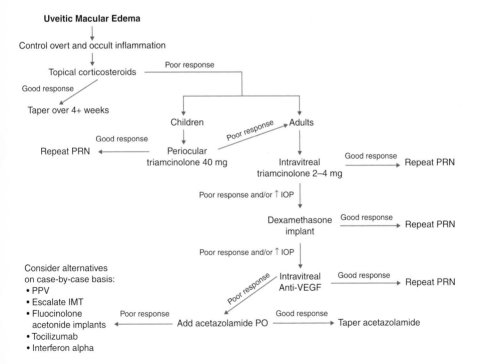

Key Points

- Macular edema is a major structural complication of uveitis and a common cause of vision loss.
- Macular edema often accompanies active intraocular inflammation. Refractory CME in an apparently quiet eye is sometimes due to occult inflammation, such as occult retinal vasculitis or choroiditis. Hence fluorescein and indocyanine green angiograms are an important part of the evaluation of refractory or frequently recurrent uveitic macular edema.
- Control of active inflammation is the first step in controlling uveitic macular edema. However, it can still occur in quiet eyes. In that case, a stepwise approach is warranted (see management algorithm).
- The author prefers a trial of periocular corticosteroid in children before intravitreal therapy as they are more prone to excessive elevations in IOP in response to corticosteroids.
- Based on recent data from a phase 4 trial (POINT Trial), the respective efficacies and IOP profiles of intravitreal triamcinolone and the dexamethasone implant are comparable. However, in vitrectomized eyes, an intravitreal bolus of triamcinolone is cleared from the eye more quickly, and thus the dexamethasone implants, which elutes corticosteroid at a steady rate, have theoretical advantages. Unfortunately, vitrectomized eyes are also more prone to wound leak from the 22-gauge instrument that injects the dexamethasone implant.
- Although anti-VEGF agents have no role in controlling inflammation, in quiet eyes with macular edema, they can be effective. They are particularly advantageous in patients with corticosteroid response. A series of multiple injections every 4 weeks may be necessary to cause complete resorption of edema.
- Patients with refractory edema may benefit from pars plana vitrectomy with induction of a posterior vitreous detachment and peeling of any epiretinal membranes. Other treatments include fluocinolone acetonide implants (either the in-office or surgically implanted device), escalation of immunomodulatory therapy, oral acetazolamide, and interferon alpha. As in any complex case, appropriate management is highly dependent on the individual case.
- The efficacy and role of other agents like intravitreal methotrexate, intravitreal sirolimus, and suprachoroidal corticosteroids are still unclear.

CHAPTER 72

Cystoid Macular Edema After Infectious Uveitis

Harpal S. Sandhu

History of Present Illness (HPI)

A 64-year-old woman with a history of moderate amblyopia right eye (OD) and herpetic keratitis with anterior uveitis left eye (OS) presents to your office complaining of decreased vision in the OS for the last few weeks. The last time she was seen was 6 months ago, when the uveitis and keratitis were both inactive. An episode of herpetic keratouveitis had left her with a paracentral corneal scar in the left eye and mildly decreased vision to about 20/40. Vision was correctable to 20/30 OS at her last visit with a hard contact lens, but she does not like to wear it. She notes that although the vision is decreased, she does not have the pain, tearing, redness, or light sensitivity that she has had with her previous flare-ups in that eye.

Exam

	OD	OS
Vision	20/125	20/60
Intraocular pressure (IOP)	14	13
Lids and lashes:	Normal	Normal
Sclera/conjunctiva:	White and quiet	White and quiet
Cornea:	See photo	Paracentral scar
Anterior chamber (AC):	Deep and quiet	Deep and quiet
Iris:	Transillumination defect (TIDs) superonasally	Flat
Lens:	Posterior chamber intraocular lens (PCIOL)	PCIOL
Anterior vitreous:	Clear	Clear

Dilated Fundus Examination (DFE)

Nerve:	Cup-to-disc (c/d) 0.3, pink, sharp	c/d 0.3, pink, sharp
Macula:	Flat	Blunted foveal reflex
Vessels:	Normal caliber and course	Normal caliber and course
Periphery:	Unremarkable	Unremarkable

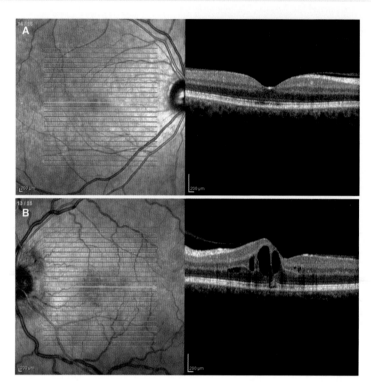

Fig. 72.1 (A) Spectral domain OCT (SD-OCT) of the right eye is normal. (B) SD-OCT of the left eye shows cystoid macular edema with a vitreomacular adhesion.

Because of the decreased vision in the left eye and blunted foveal reflex on examination, optical coherence tomography (OCT) was ordered (Fig. 72.1).

Questions to Ask

- Have you had any flares in the last 6 months before this current episode of decreased vision in the OS?
- Have you started any new medications, or have there been any other changes to the rest of your health?

The patient answers no to all of these questions.

Assessment

- Uveitic cystoid macular edema (CME) OS

Differential Diagnosis

- Postinfectious uveitic CME OS
- Vitreomacular traction OS
- Less likely: pseudophakic CME OS

Working Diagnosis

- Postinfectious uveitic CME OS

Management

- Intravitreal bevacizumab 1.25 mg/0.05 cc OS number one in a series of 3 injections, administered every 4 weeks

Follow-up

HPI

Twelve weeks later, the patient has received three monthly injections of bevacizumab in the left eye. She says that her vision is a little bit better.

Exam

	OD	OS
Vision	20/125	20/40
IOP	12	12
Lids and lashes:	Normal	Normal
Sclera/conjunctiva:	White and quiet	White and quiet
Cornea:	See photo	Paracentral scar
AC:	Deep and quiet	Deep and quiet
Iris:	TIDs superonasally	Flat
Lens:	PCIOL	PCIOL
Anterior vitreous:	Clear	Clear

DFE

Nerve:	c/d 0.3, pink, sharp	c/d 0.3, pink, sharp
Macula:	Flat	Flat (see Fig. 72.2)
Vessels:	Normal caliber and course	Normal caliber and course
Periphery.	Unremarkable	Unremarkable

Management

- Observe
- Repeat intravitreal bevacizumab OS as needed

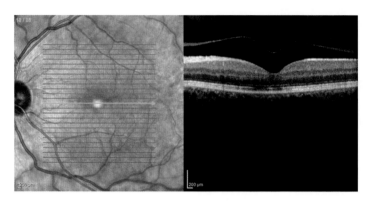

Fig. 72.2   OCT of the left eye shows that the cystoid macular edema has resolved and that the posterior hyaloid has separated from the macula.

Key Points

- Macular edema (ME) can complicate both infectious and noninfectious uveitis.
- Herpes simplex and varicella zoster viruses can reactivate with the use of local corticosteroids, including topical ones, which are first-line agents for mild uveitic CME (see chapter on uveitic CME). Thus the author prefers intravitreal anti–vascular endothelial growth factor (VEGF) agents in these cases.
- Toxoplasmosis and tuberculosis are other important infectious causes of uveitis that can reactivate with periocular or intravitreal corticosteroids.
- An alternative management option is to begin appropriate antimicrobial therapy to cover the patient and then treat the ME with local corticosteroids. Simultaneous antimicrobial therapy decreases the risk of reactivation with local corticosteroid treatment.
- Much like noninfectious ME, epiretinal membranes and vitreomacular traction can secondarily exacerbate ME or even be the primary cause.

CHAPTER 73

Polypoidal Choroidal Vasculopathy (PCV) in SLE

Henry J. Kaplan

History of Present Illness

A 42-year-old African American gentleman returned for routine follow-up, without any new visual complaints. He was diagnosed with systemic lupus erythematosus (SLE) in his 20s and had several episodes of "uveitis" in both eyes (OU) that required treatment with oral and topical medications. Nevertheless, he slowly had gradual progression of visual loss, OU, right eye greater than left eye (OD > OS). He received previous sector panretinal photocoagulation for ischemic retinal disease OD.

Exam

	OD	OS
Visual acuity	20/80	20/30
Intraocular pressure (IOP)	12	12
Sclera/conjunctiva	Within normal limits (WNL)	WNL
Cornea	Clear	Clear
Anterior chamber (AC)	No cell or flare	No cell or flare
Iris	No iris neovascularization (NV)	No iris NV
Lens	Mild nuclear sclerosis	Mild nuclear sclerosis
Vitreous cavity	No cells	No cells
Retina/optic nerve	Normal optic disc. Fibrosed retinal NV frond along superotemporal (ST) arcade. Light laser photocoagulation scars in superotemporal quadrant (STQ) of retina	Marked attenuation of retina arterial vasculature with arteriovenous (AV) nicking.

Questions to Ask

- What complications have you had because of SLE?
- Did you receive laser treatment to both eyes?
- Are you on medication for your SLE and/or complications from the disease?

He responds that he had been told that he developed occlusive retinal vasculitis with retinal neovascularization (NV) in the OD that required laser treatment. He denied laser treatment to the OS. He added that he was on chronic dialysis because of lupus nephritis and taking azathioprine 100 mg every morning.

Assessment

- Retina vascular ischemia OU in a patient with SLE

Differential Diagnosis

- Behçet disease
- Syphilis
- Polyarteritis nodosa
- Takayasu disease
- Granulomatosis with polyangiitis
- Severe hypertensive retinopathy
- Proliferative diabetic retinopathy

Working Diagnosis

- SLE occlusive retinal vasculopathy OU (OD > OS)

Although the patient's retinopathy may also show changes of systemic hypertension secondary to chronic renal disease, it is not the primary cause of his retinal occlusive disease and NV. Additionally, he experienced medication-induced diabetes mellitus because he was maintained on systemic prednisone before other immunomodulatory therapy (IMT) for his SLE, and his retina does not show the hallmark changes of diabetic retinopathy.

Testing

- Consultation with nephrology for evaluation of his lupus nephritis and current systemic evaluation of SLE. Appropriate laboratory tests will be ordered by that service.
  - Fundus autofluorescence (FAF) (Fig. 73.1)

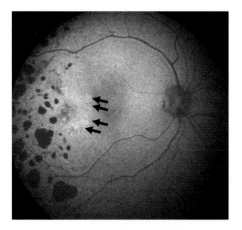

Fig. 73.1 Fundus autofluorescence (FAF) OD demonstrating multiple hypofluorescent foci from prior laser treatment. Notice the curvilinear line temporal to the fovea, which represents fibrotic traction from involutional retinal NV following laser (*black arrows*). Polypoidal Choroidal Vasculopathy Complicating Retinal Laser in Quiescent Uveitis. DOI: 10.1155/2019/6147063 (Picture courtesy: Burke TR, Lightman SL. *Case Rep Ophthalmol Med*. 2019;2019.)

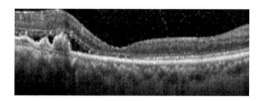

Fig. 73.2 SD OCT OD demonstrating multiple pigment epithelial detachments temporal to the fovea associated with subretinal fluid. Polypoidal Choroidal Vasculopathy Complicating Retinal Laser in Quiescent Uveitis. DOI: 10.1155/2019/6147063 (Picture courtesy: Burke TR, Lightman SL. *Case Rep Ophthalmol Med.* 2019; 2019.)

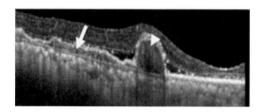

Fig. 73.3 EDI (enhanced depth imaging) SD OCT OD demonstrating hyperreflective area between retinal pigment epithelium (RPE) and Bruchs membrane suggestive of branching vascular network (*white arrow*). The hyperreflectivity within the PED is likely related to a vascular polyp (*arrowhead*). Polypoidal Choroidal Vasculopathy Complicating Retinal Laser in Quiescent Uveitis. DOI: 10.1155/2019/6147063 (Picture courtesy: Burke TR, Lightman SL. *Case Rep Ophthalmol Med.* 2019; 2019.)

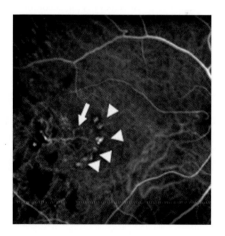

Fig. 73.4 ICGA OD demonstrating a branching choroidal vascular network (*white arrow*) and terminal hypercyanescent polyps (*white arrowheads*). Polypoidal Choroidal Vasculopathy Complicating Retinal Laser in Quiescent Uveitis. DOI: 10.1155/2019/6147063 (Picture courtesy: Burke TR, Lightman SL. *Case Rep Ophthalmol Med.* 2019; 2019.)

- Spectral domain optical coherence tomography (SD OCT) (Fig. 73.2)
- Enhanced depth imaging (EDI): Fig. 73.3
- Indocyanine green chorioangiography (ICGA): Fig. 73.4

Management

- Imaging studies identify polypoidal choroidal vasculopathy (PCV) as a cause of central visual loss in this patient, in addition to perifoveal retinal vascular ischemia. The disease is characterized by polyp-shaped vascular networks most often in individuals over 60, but it may occur in those much younger. African Americans and Asians are affected more often than Caucasians.
- Treatment of PCV involves either photodynamic therapy with verteporfin (a laser-absorbent dye) and/or anti–vascular endothelial growth factor (VEGF) medications. Response to treatment is variable.
- Follow up in 1 month.

Follow-up

On follow-up at 1 month his examination is unchanged except that visual acuity (VA) OD has improved from 20/80 to 20/60. Limited central VA is most likely related to associated macular ischemia. ICGA and optical coherence tomography angiography (OCTA) imaging suggest regression of the PCV. However, the patient will have to be followed closely because of the danger of subsequent neovascular complications.

Key Points

- Multifocal retinal vascular occlusive disease and NV can be observed in several uveitic autoimmune diseases: Behçet disease, polyarteritis nodosa, Takayasu disease, and granulomatosis with polyangiitis and syphilis.
- Although choroidal neovascularization (CNV) is an uncommon complication of uveitis, it is more frequent in posterior uveitides such as polypoidal choroidal vasculopathy (PIC), multifocal choroiditis (MFC), serpiginous choroidopathy, and Vogt–Koyanagi–Harada (VKH) disease.
- CNV and retinal NV arise from release of angiogenic factors, like VEGF and stroma cell–derived factor 1-alpha (SDF-1a), as a result of ischemic hypoxia. Thus any uveitic disease that produces ischemia either from compromised blood flow or destruction of retinal tissue can cause NV (e.g., toxoplasma retinochoroiditis, presumed ocular histoplasmosis syndrome [POHS], etc.).
- Current methods of treatment for SLE are very effective, with a 10-year survival rate >90%. However, poor visual outcomes can occur with complications such as vaso-occlusive disease, retinal vasculitis, central retina artery occlusion, and central retinal vein occlusion.
- It is important to recognize that severe retinal vascular disease in SLE has a strong correlation with central nervous system (CNS) disease, more so than with nephritis or hematologic abnormalities.

CHAPTER 74

Chronic Hypotony with Metastatic Melanoma and Checkpoint Inhibitor

Henry J. Kaplan

History of Present Illness

A 73-year-old Caucasian man was diagnosed with cutaneous melanoma 10 months ago and underwent resection of the tumor, sentinel lymph node biopsy, and regional lymph node dissection. Three months ago he was diagnosed with metastatic melanoma and started on an immune checkpoint inhibitor, pembrolizumab (Keytruda), 2 mg/kg intravenously (IV) every 3 weeks. Within the past 3 weeks he has noted bilateral red, painful eyes with marked photophobia and was referred for evaluation and treatment.

Exam

	OD	OS
Visual acuity	20/60	20/80
IOP (mm Hg)	2	8
Lids/brows	Poliosis lashes and brows	Poliosis lashes and brows
Sclera/conjunctiva	Moderate perilimbal injection	Moderate perilimbal injection
Cornea	Multiple folds in Descemet membrane. (Fig. 74.1A and B). Diffuse nongranulomatous (NG) keratic precipitate (KP)	Diffuse NG KP
Anterior chamber (AC)	2+ cell/3+ flare	2+ cell/ 3+ flare
Iris	No posterior synechiae (PS)	Extensive PS
Lens	Pseudophakic	Phakic/clear
Vitreous cavity	2+ vitreous cell, ciliary body (CB) detachment (Fig. 74.2A and B)	2+ vitreous cell, CB detachment
Retina/optic nerve	Choroidal thickening/folds, macula swelling (see Fig. 74.2C) and optic disc edema (see Fig. 74.2D)	Choroidal thickening/folds macula swelling and optic disc edema

Questions to Ask

- Why did you have surgery in your right eye (OD)?
- How was metastatic disease detected? Are you symptomatic?
- Have you noticed any neck stiffness, changes in your hearing, or changes in the color of your skin or hair?
- Do you have Native American ancestry?

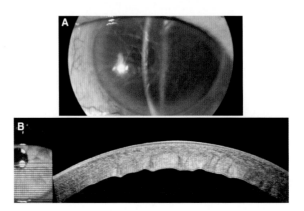

Fig. 74.1 (A) Descemet folds in the cornea. (B) Anterior segment optical coherence tomography (OCT) demonstrating Descemet folds. (Picture courtesy: Hossein Asghari, MD.)

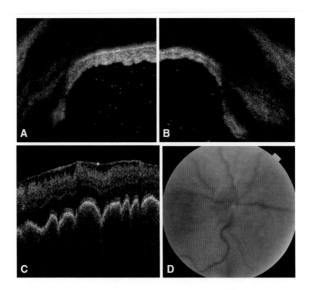

Fig. 74.2 (A and B) Anterior segment OCT demonstrating ciliary body detachment OU and anterior vitreous cells. (C) Spectral domain optical coherence tomography (SD OCT) retina demonstrating multiple choroidal folds in hypotonus maculopathy. (D) Optic nerve swelling secondary to hypotony. (Picture credit: G Reid, P Loirgan, H Heimann, M Hovan. Management of Chronic Hypotony Following Bilateral Uveitis in a Patient Treated with Pembrolizumab for Cutaneous Metastatic Melanoma. *Ocul Immunol Inflamm.* 2019;27 [6]:1012−1015.)

Ten years ago he developed a rhegmatogenous retinal detachment (RRD) OD and underwent phacoemulsification and pars plana vitrectomy (PPV) for repair of his retinal detachment, with best-corrected visual acuity (VA) 20/40. Routine testing with positron emission tomography/computed tomography (PET/CT) imaging after diagnosis of cutaneous melanoma detected metastasis in the abdominal lymph nodes, lung and liver. He noticed increased shortness of breath recently. He has not noticed any neck stiffness or issues with hearing, but his eyelid lashes and brows have recently turned white. None of his grandparents were of Cherokee descent.

Assessment

- Panuveitis with severe hypotony, ciliary body detachments, and choroidal effusions, OU, right eye greater than left eye (OD > OS)

Differential Diagnosis

- Adverse reaction to checkpoint inhibitor
- Vogt–Koyanagi–Harada (VKH) syndrome
- Sympathetic ophthalmia
- Rare: systemic leukemia/lymphoma

Working Diagnosis

- Adverse reaction to checkpoint inhibitor

Testing

- The presentation of bilateral, nongranulomatous panuveitis with severe hypotony, ciliary body detachment, and optic nerve swelling are consistent with an adverse reaction to checkpoint inhibitors; hypotonus maculopathy explains the central posterior segment changes. Poliosis can be associated with this diagnosis, as well as VKH (or simply Harada syndrome if there is no systemic involvement). However, the absence of multifocal large serous neurosensory detachments would exclude that diagnosis. The history of surgery to the OD raises the possibility of sympathetic ophthalmia, although severe hypotony with bilateral ciliary body detachments at onset is most unusual.
- Laboratory data: normal complete blood count (CBC) with differential.
- Fundus fluorescein angiography (FFA): late frames of the OD did not demonstrate leakage from multiple hyperfluorescent spots and pooling of fluorescein into multiple areas of serous retinal detachment, excluding a diagnosis of VKH.
- Indocyanine green chorioangiography (ICGA): no leakage or hypoperfusion from choroidal vasculature.

Management

- Discontinuation of pembrolizumab
- Admit to the hospital or infusion center and begin methylprednisolone 1000 mg IV daily for 3 to 5 days
- Discharge on prednisone 100 mg by mouth (PO) daily
- Continue prednisone 0.75 mg/kg/day with taper after 2 weeks
- Topical prednisolone acetate 1% every 2 hours (q2h) and 1% Cyclogyl twice a day (BID) to treat anterior uveitis
- Follow up in 2 weeks

Follow-up Evaluation

The patient returns 2 weeks later with further decrease in vision and profound bilateral hypotony (0 to 2 mm Hg), even though his panuveitis is slowly resolving.

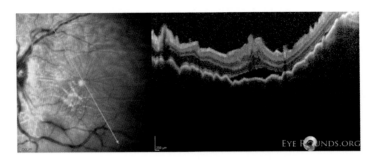

Fig. 74.3 Worsening of hypotonus maculopathy with multiple choroidal folds and neurosensory detachment OS. (Picture credit: Jeffrey Welder. University of Iowa Department of Ophthalmology & Visual Sciences and EyeRounds.org websites.)

Follow-up Assessment

Intraocular pressure (IOP) has not responded despite discontinuation of checkpoint inhibitor and continued high-dose prednisone. Although panuveitis is decreased, VA is worse because of a hypermetropic shift (R +10.5, L 8.0) and severe hypotonus maculopathy OU (Fig. 74.3).

Management

Patient continued on high-dose prednisone (7.5 mg/kg/day), with calcium and vitamin D; topical treatment for anterior uveitis tapered; return appointments every 2 weeks for another month. In general, lack of response in such a situation suggests a severe autoimmune disease refractory to typical oral antiinflammatory treatment.

Working Diagnosis #2

- Severe panuveitis and chronic hypotony, OU, with IOP refractory to standard oral therapy

Management

- After 3 months of therapy a trial of an ophthalmic viscoelastic device (OVD) Healon GV (1.4% sodium hyaluronate) and periocular triamcinolone acetate was initiated, OU. Over the next 3 months repeat monthly injections were performed.
- Topical therapy was tapered and ultimately discontinued. Immunomodulatory therapy (IMT) with mycophenolate mofetil (CellCept) was started and prednisone tapered and eventually discontinued.

Follow-up

Patient had only transient increases in IOP (up to 4 mm Hg) after OVD injections, with no significant change in VA; additionally, he developed a cataract OS. Phacoemulsification and cataract extraction (PCE) with PPV and SiO injection was performed OS; SiO injection only was performed OD, because he had a previous PPV to repair his RRD. His IOP improved OU ($\approx$ 8 to 10 mm Hg) with VA of 20/80 OU.

Key Points

- Hypotony is an uncommon complication of chronic uveitis and usually appears in patients with uveitis onset at a young age, in non-Caucasian races, and in those with long-standing disease. It is one of the most devastating complications of chronic uveitis and may ultimately result in phthisis bulbi.

- Ultrasound biomicroscopy may reveal cyclitic membranes leading to ciliary body detachment. Ciliary body atrophy is not treatable, and there is no proven medical therapy to restore IOP. Results with ibopamine are inconclusive, and the drug is not available in the United States.

- A surgical approach to relieve chronic hypotony includes lensectomy, PPV with removal of ciliary membranes and traction, and SiO tamponade. In eyes with normal ciliary processes, removal of ciliary membranes alone may be sufficient to restore IOP. The goal of surgery is to prevent phthisis bulbi.

- Case reports of uveitis after pembrolizumab are uncommon and usually resolve with cessation of drug therapy. Ciliary body shutdown, choroidal effusions, and chronic hypotony after resolution of inflammation are extremely rare.

- Immunotherapy for cancer, such as metastatic melanoma, involves monoclonal antibodies blocking PD-1 (e.g., pembrolizumab and nivolumab) and CTLA-4 (e.g., ipilimumab). They block the interaction of these T-cell surface receptors with ligands on the cancer cell surface and enhance the cytotoxic immune response. Blockade of the PD-1/PD-L1 axis may have fewer immune-related adverse events than CTLA-4 blockade.

- Clinical distinction of panuveitis from checkpoint inhibitors from VKH and sympathetic ophthalmia should be considered. VKH is an autoimmune, multisystem disease characterized by poliosis, vitiligo, hearing loss, meningismus, and bilateral panuveitis. American Indian ancestry is associated with susceptibility to VKH. Sympathetic ophthalmia resembles both of these diseases but only occurs after ocular trauma or surgical ocular procedures.

- Rarely, systemic leukemia metastatic to the choroid can simulate these diseases and should be suspected in patients with constitutional symptoms or abnormal white blood cell counts.

CHAPTER 75

Uveitic Cataract

Henry J. Kaplan

History of Present Illness (HPI)

A 40-year-old woman with a history of chronic idiopathic anterior uveitis in the right eye (OD) complains of progressively decreasing vision in this eye for the last 6 months. She was diagnosed with uveitis almost a decade ago and has required many rounds of intensive topical steroid therapy and even a few courses of oral prednisone. She has been stable on methotrexate 15 mg by mouth (PO) every week for the last year.

Exam

	OD	OS
Vision	20/100	20/20
Intraocular pressure (IOP)	16	17
Lids and lashes:	Normal	Normal
Sclera/conjunctiva:	White and quiet	White and quiet
Cornea:	Clear	Clear
Anterior chamber (AC):	Quiet, 1+ flare	Deep and quiet
Iris:	Flat	Flat
Lens:	See Fig. 75.1	Clear
Anterior vitreous:	Clear	Clear

Dilated fundus examination (DFE)

Nerve:	Cup-to-disc (c/d) 0.3, pink, sharp	c/d 0.3, pink, sharp
Macula:	Flat	Flat (poor view)
Vessels:	Normal caliber and course	Normal caliber and course
Periphery:	Attached	Attached

Further Questions to Ask

- When was the last time you had a flare-up in this eye?
- Have you ever had trauma or radiation exposure to this eye?

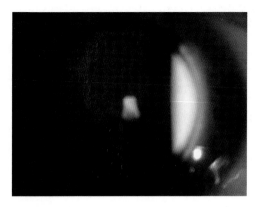

Fig. 75.1 Color slit lamp photograph of the right eye under retroillumination shows a large, centrally located, posterior subcapsular cataract (PSC). The cataract was graded as trace nuclear sclerosis (NS), 3+ PSC. (From Liu A, Manche EE. Bilateral posterior subcapsular cataracts associated with long-term intranasal steroid use. *J Cataract Refract Surg* 2011;37[8]:1555–1558.)

She confirms that her last flare-up was almost 1 year ago. She denies trauma or radiation to either eye.

Assessment

- Visually significant posterior subcapsular cataract OD

Management

- Schedule cataract extraction/intraocular lens implantation (CE/IOL) OD
- Continue methotrexate 15 mg PO every week
- Start prednisone 60 mg PO daily starting 3 days before surgery

Follow-up

The patient returns on postoperative day (POD) #1 after an uneventful cataract surgery. Iris hooks were used to dilate the pupil intraoperatively. Phacoemulsification energy was not particularly high, as the lens was relatively soft. She has foreign body sensation but no pain. After taking off the eye shield, she says her vision has not improved.

Exam

	OD	OS
Vision	20/400	20/20
IOP	7	15
Lids and lashes:	Normal	
Sclera/conjunctiva:	Trace injection	
Cornea:	2+ stromal edema	
AC:	3+ cell, 2+ flare	
Iris:	Flat	
Lens:	Posterior chamber intraocular lens (PCIOL)	

Assessment

- Expected anterior chamber (AC) reaction and corneal stromal edema on POD #1 status post–CE/IOL OD

Management

- Continue prednisone 60 mg PO daily for 3 more days
- Start prednisolone acetate 1% every hour (q1h) or difluprednate 0.05% every 1 to 2 hours (q1–2h) OD, moxifloxacin (or other broad-spectrum antibiotic) four times a day (QID) OD, and topical nonsteroidal antiinflammatory drug (NSAID)
- Continue methotrexate 15 mg PO every week
- Follow up in 3 to 4 days, and anticipate taper of prednisone by 10 mg every 2 to 3 days (q2–3 days) thereafter

Further Follow-up

The patient was tapered off prednisone over 3 weeks. The AC reaction resolved over this time, and visual acuity (VA) improved to 20/20 OD.

Management Algorithm

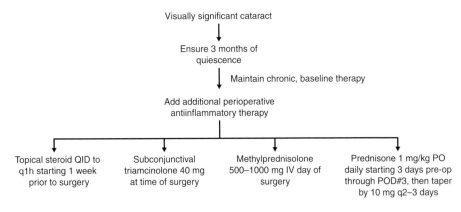

Key Points

- Cataract is a common structural complication of uveitis, as both intraocular inflammation and corticosteroid therapy are cataractogenic.
- By convention, one should ensure at least 3 months of quiescence before any intraocular surgery in uveitic patients.
- Aggressive perioperative antiinflammatory therapy in addition to the patient's usual chronic therapy is critical to minimize the risk of uveitis flare-ups from surgery. The author favors pretreatment with prednisone, as noted earlier, combined with intensive postoperative topical steroids, but there are multiple other options (see "Management Algorithm"). High-quality data comparing these different treatment options are limited.

- Besides uveitis flare-ups, other complications of uveitic cataract surgery include hypotony, ocular hypertension, iris atrophy, macular edema, and serous retinal detachments.
- Cataract surgery in uveitis patients demands good surgical technique with minimal manipulation of the iris, limitation of phacoemulsification energy, and an IOL in the capsular bag, if possible. A thorough discussion of these points is beyond the scope of this book.

CHAPTER 76

Advanced, Undetected Steroid-Induced Glaucoma

Judith Mohay

History of Present Illness

A 41-year-old woman with a past ocular history significant of redness and "inflammation" of both eyes (OU) treated by an optometrist in town presents for the first time to the clinic complaining of blurred vision and severe headaches for the last 6 weeks. The headaches are more intense lately, and the last 2 days she has associated emesis and photophobia.

She also has a history of high myopia and wears soft contact lenses. Her optometrist started her on corticosteroid eye drops for the redness and discomfort about 1 year ago. The prescription of corticosteroid eye drops was refilled continuously by her primary care physician. Her last eye examination was 1 year before her current presentation.

Exam

	OD	OS
Visual acuity	Count fingers (CF) 4′	20/30
Intraocular pressure (IOP)	47	40
Sclera/conjunctiva	White and quiet	White and quiet
Cornea	Clear	Clear
Anterior chamber (AC)	Deep and quiet	Deep and quiet
Iris	Normal, no transillumination defects (TID)	Normal, no TID
Lens	+ PSC cataract	+ PSC cataract
Anterior vitreous	Clear	Clear

Dilated Fundus Examination (DFE)

	OD	OS
Optic nerve (cup-to-disc [C/D])	1.0	0.9
Macula	Pigmented scar	Normal
Vessels	Normal	Normal
Periphery	Multiple chorioretinal (CR) scars and lattice (Fig. 76.1A)	Multiple CR scars and lattice (Fig. 76.1B)

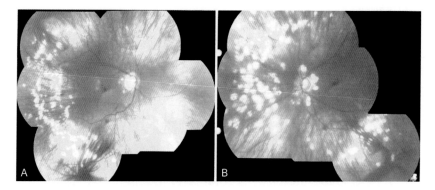

Fig. 76.1 (A) Color fundus photograph of the right eye shows an optic nerve with complete loss of the neuroretinal rim with peripapillary atrophy; a macular scar; lattice degeneration; and scattered inactive, punched-out chorioretinal scars in the periphery. (B) Color fundus photograph of the left eye shows an optic nerve with advanced loss of the neuroretinal rim, with peripapillary atrophy; normal macula; lattice degeneration; and scattered inactive, punched-out spots of the periphery.

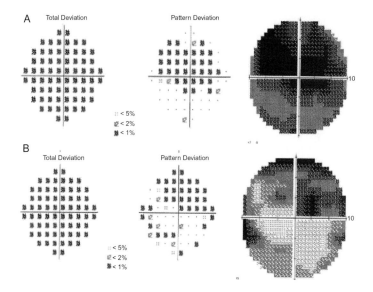

Fig. 76.2 (A) 10-2 Humphrey visual field test of the right eye shows a near-complete loss of peripheral vision with a central scotoma. (B) 10-2 Humphrey visual field test of the left eye shows a severe loss of peripheral vision with a dense superior and inferior arcuate defect.

Questions to Ask

- Have you ever been diagnosed or checked for glaucoma?
- Do you have a family history of glaucoma?
- Have you had any injury of your eyes or head recently?
- What kind of steroid medications/eye drops have you been using and for how long?

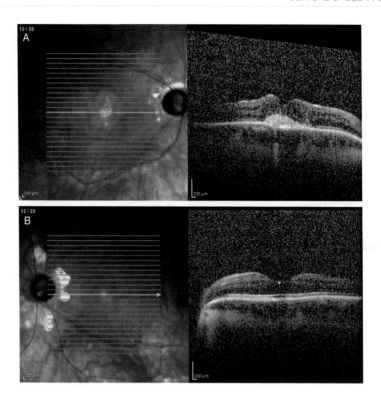

Fig. 76.3 (A) Spectral domain optical coherence tomography (SD OCT) of the right macula shows a subretinal scar consistent with an old subretinal neovascular membrane. (B) SD OCT of the left macula is grossly normal.

The patient responds that she has never been diagnosed or treated for glaucoma (former records from the optometrist office documented normal intraocular pressure [IOP] and normal appearance of both optic nerves about 1 year ago). She has no family history of glaucoma and has had no eye injuries. She was on loteprednol, fluorometholone (FML), and prednisolone acetate 1% eye drops three times a day on and off for about 1 year for inflammation of both eyes.

Assessment

- Multifocal choroiditis OU, inactive
- Severe glaucomatous optic neuropathy, right eye greater than left eye (OD > OS)
- Involuted subretinal neovascular membrane with severe vision loss OD
- Posterior subcapsular cataracts (PSCs) OU

Differential Diagnosis

- Advanced corticosteroid-induced open angle glaucoma
- Pigmentary glaucoma
- Uveitic glaucoma
- Angle-closure glaucoma

Working Diagnosis

- Advanced corticosteroid-induced open angle glaucoma with uncontrolled IOP
- The presence of PSC cataracts and the lack of clinical signs of other types of secondary glaucoma (pigmentary, uveitic, or traumatic) are key points in suggesting this diagnosis, as well as the history of chronic topical corticosteroid use without IOP monitoring.

Testing

- Gonioscopy: wide open angle with no peripheral anterior synechiae, no neovascularization, no evidence of heavy pigmentation or angle recession
- Humphrey visual field test 24-2 (Fig. 76.2)
- Optical coherence tomography (OCT) of the macula (Fig. 76.3)
- Fundus and optic nerve photo for baseline documentation (see Fig. 76.1)

Management

- Stop corticosteroid eye drops
- Start topical glaucoma medications: travoprost at bedtime OU, brimonidine 0.15% twice a day (BID) OU
- Monitor IOP, visual fields, and optic nerve
- Monitor macula

Follow-up

IOP was normalized within a period of 2 weeks on two glaucoma medications. The glaucomatous optic neuropathy and visual field remained remarkably stable over 8 years of follow-up. Her clinical course was complicated by a rhegmatogenous retinal detachment/repair and cataract surgery of the OS 2 years after presentation. Both procedures have resulted in complete recovery of baseline vision.

Key Points

- Every patient on topical corticosteroid medications should be carefully monitored for elevated IOP and glaucoma.
- Incidence of corticosteroid-induced glaucoma is 8% in the general population, but it is 90% in patients with open-angle glaucoma.
- Every week of corticosteroid eye drop use will increase the chance of developing glaucoma by approximately 4% per week.
- Gradually increasing IOP typically will not result in the usual clinical signs of acute glaucoma, even if IOP is extremely high. The vision will remain at baseline, the cornea will remain clear, and symptoms can be misleading.
- Prostaglandin analogues are relatively contraindicated in cases of herpetic uveitis with ocular hypertension/glaucoma, but can be used with caution in other cases of uveitis.

CHAPTER 77

Corneal Decompensation After Dexamethasone Implant

Harpal S. Sandhu

History of Present Illness (HPI)

A 64-year-old man complains of a relatively sudden decrease in vision in his left eye (OS). He has a history of idiopathic anterior uveitis OS complicated by recurrent macular edema. He was last here 3 weeks ago, when he saw one of your colleagues, who injected an intravitreal steroid implant into the eye.

Exam

	OD	OS
Vision	20/20	20/70
Intraocular pressure (IOP)	19	21
Lids and lashes:	Normal	Normal
Sclera/conjunctiva:	White and quiet	1–2+ injection
Cornea:	Clear	2+ stromal edema
Anterior chamber (AC):	Deep and quiet	See Fig. 77.1
Iris:	Flat	Flat
Lens:	Posterior capsule intraocular lens (PCIOL)	Sulcus IOL, open posterior capsule

Dilated Fundus Examination (DFE) Deferred

Nerve:	Normal, cup-to-disc (c/d) 0.4
Macula:	Flat
Vessels:	Normal caliber and course
Periphery:	Unremarkable

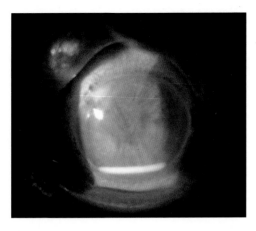

Fig. 77.1 Color external photograph of the left eye shows significant corneal edema and a thin, long, white foreign body consistent with the dexamethasone intravitreal implant in the inferior anterior chamber. (From Bernal L, Estevez B. Corneal toxicity after Ozurdex migration into anterior chamber. *Arch Soc Esp Oftalmol.* 2016;91[6]:292–294.)

Questions to Ask

- When did you first notice a decrease in vision?
He responds that he first noticed blurred vision yesterday.

Assessment

- Migration of dexamethasone intravitreal implant (Ozurdex) into the anterior chamber (AC) OS

Management

- Dilate the left eye maximally by adding phenylephrine 10%, and position the patient in a supine position. If the implant migrates posteriorly, constrict the pupil with pilocarpine.

One-Hour Follow-up

The implant fails to migrate posteriorly.

Management

- Arrange for urgent surgical evacuation of the implant in the operating room.
- Start prednisolone acetate 1% every 2 hours (q2h) and NaCl 5% OS postoperatively.

Further Follow-up

HPI

The patient returns postoperative week one and reports that his vision is improving, but not back to where it usually is. The surgery was uneventful.

Exam

	OD	OS
Vision	20/20˙	20/30–
IOP	20	17
Lids and lashes:	Normal	Normal
Sclera/conjunctiva:	White and quiet	White and quiet
Cornea:	Clear	Trace stromal edema
AC:	Deep and quiet	Deep and quiet
Iris:	Flat	Flat
Lens:	PCIOL	Sulcus IOL
DFE:	Deferred	Deferred

Management

- Continue present management
- Avoid dexamethasone implant injections in the future

Key Points

- Dexamethasone intravitreal implants migrating into the AC are an ophthalmic emergency. Without urgent treatment, there is significant risk of corneal decompensation. Although less studied, this remains a potential problem with fluocinolone acetonide intravitreal implants as well.
- Pseudophakes with open posterior capsules, prior vitrectomy, and zonular loss are major risk factors for this complication. The implant is contraindicated in aphakes.
- Conservative maneuvers as detailed earlier can be sufficient in some cases. Repeat migration remains a risk until the implant biodegrades.
- Definitive management involves surgical removal of the implant in the operating room and is indicated if conservative measures fail.
- Although a detailed discussion of surgical technique is beyond the scope of this book, it is helpful to grasp the implant lengthwise, as it is prone to fracturing if grasped along its short axis.

CHAPTER 78

Epiretinal Membrane and Panuveitis

Harpal S. Sandhu

History of Present Illness

A 47-year-old man with a history of idiopathic panuveitis in the left eye (OS) presents for a routine follow-up visit. His disease has been quiet for almost a year and never required systemic therapy. Follow-up was gradually extended out because his clinical course had stabilized. He denies any episodes akin to a flare in the intervening time, but does report that his vision is more distorted than it used to be. He has no complaints in the right eye (OD), which has never been involved. Baseline vision in the left eye has been in the 20/25 to 20/30 range.

Exam

	OD	OS
Visual acuity	20/20	20/50+
Intraocular pressure (IOP)	14	14
Sclera/conjunctiva	White and quiet	White and quiet
Cornea	Clear	Clear
Anterior chamber (AC)	Deep and quiet	Deep and quiet
Iris	Flat	Flat
Lens	Clear	Posterior chamber intraocular lens (PCIOL)
Vitreous	Clear	1+ old vitreous cell 0 haze + Weiss ring

Dilated Fundus Examination (DFE)

Nerve	Pink, sharp	See Fig. 78.1
Macula	flat	
Vessels	Normal caliber and course	
Periphery	Unremarkable	

Epiretinal membrane (ERM) was noted on his prior examination but not thought to be visually significant. Optical coherence tomography (OCT) was pursued to further evaluate the ERM and vision loss (Fig. 78.2).

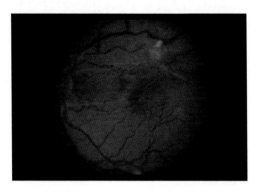

Fig. 78.1 Color fundus photograph of the left eye shows clear media and an epiretinal membrane overlying the macula. Periphery (not shown here) was stable with scattered old chorioretinal scars inferiorly.

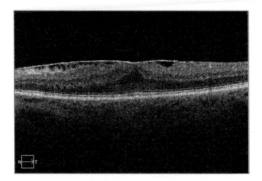

Fig. 78.2 Spectral domain optical coherence tomography of the left eye shows a thickened macula without frank cystoid spaces and an epiretinal membrane. Central macular thickness (CMT) is 448 μm. The ellipsoid and external limiting membrane layers are intact.

Questions to Ask

- How long has it been since you noticed the distortion?
- Has it been getting worse?
- How is your vision with both eyes open? Are you having trouble with any activities you do on a regular basis?

He has noticed the vision in the left eye becoming more distorted in the last 3 months. It has been gradual, but he feels it is getting worse. With both eyes open, his vision is fine for seeing most things at distance. However, he reads "all the time" in his work as a professional historian and finds that he is closing his left eye when he reads to see words clearly.

Assessment

- Idiopathic panuveitis OS, inactive
- ERM OS, progressive and visually significant

Management

- Pars plana vitrectomy with membrane peel OS.
- Pretreat with prednisone 60 mg by mouth (PO) daily for 3 days before surgery and methylprednisolone 50 mg intravenously (IV) on the day of surgery.

Follow-up

The surgery was uneventful. Prednisone was continued at 60 mg PO daily for 3 days postoperatively, then tapered by 10 mg every 2 days down to zero. There was mild anterior chamber (AC) reaction in the first week postoperatively but no recurrence of vitreal or chorioretinal inflammation. After 6 months, the patient's vision improved to 20/30−, central macular thickness (CMT) improved to 361 μm, and metamorphopsia had improved enough that he could read with both eyes open (Fig. 78.3).

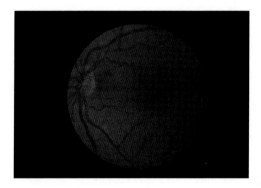

Fig. 78.3 Color fundus photograph of the left eye 6 months postoperatively. The ERM is no longer funduscopically visible, and the media remain clear.

Key Points

- ERM is a common structural complication of intermediate, posterior, and panuveitis.
- Most ERMs have little visual significance and can simply be observed. Indications for surgical intervention include significant vision loss due to progressive macular thickening, disabling metamorphopsia, and uveitic macular edema associated with ERM that has become resistant to medical therapy.
- In uveitis patients, it is critical to ensure that the ERM is in fact the true cause of any change in vision. Just because there is an absence of clinically apparent cellular infiltrate or inflammatory chorioretinal lesions does not necessarily mean that the ERM is the cause of vision loss. Other possible causes of vision loss such as optic neuropathy or photoreceptor disruption must be ruled out.
- Intact ellipsoid and external limiting membrane layers on spectral domain optical coherence tomography (SD OCT) are predictive of a good response to surgery.
- The clinician should ensure at least 3 months of disease quiescence before elective surgery in uveitis patients. Aggressive perioperative antiinflammatory therapy is recommended. See chapter 75 for more details.

CHAPTER 79

Globe Perforation After Sub-Tenon's Injection

Harpal S. Sandhu

History of Present Illness (HPI)

A 57-year-old man with a history of anterior uveitis both eyes (OU) associated with sarcoidosis presents for a scheduled sub-Tenon's triamcinolone injection left eye (OS). The left eye was noted to be quiet 1 week ago at his last visit, but vision had declined due to recurrent cystoid macular edema (CME). He could not stay for an injection last visit so he returns today for the procedure.

Past Ocular History (POH)

- Anterior uveitis OU, as noted earlier, associated with sarcoidosis
- Uveitic glaucoma OU
- Phthisical right eye (OD) secondary to poorly controlled uveitis and uveitic glaucoma OD
- Medications:
  - Mycophenolate mofetil 1000 mg by mouth (PO) twice a day (BID)
  - Prednisolone acetate 1% daily OD
  - Atropine 1% at bedtime daily OD
  - Dorzolamide/timolol three times a day (TID) OS

Exam

	OD	OS
Vision	Count fingers (CF) 3′	20/70
Intraocular pressure (IOP):	8	19
Lids and lashes:	Normal	Normal
Sclera/conjunctiva:	Trace injection	White and quiet
Cornea:	Band keratopathy	Clear
	2+ stromal edema	
Anterior chamber (AC):	Deep, no cells	Deep, no cells
	2+ flare	1+ flare
Iris:	Flat	Flat
Lens:	Posterior chamber intraocular lens (PCIOL)	PCIOL

Dilated Fundus Examination (DFE)

Nerve:	No view	Cup-to-disc (c/d) 0.7, pink, sharp
Macula:		+CME
Vessels:		Normal caliber and course
Periphery:		Attached, no chorioretinal lesions

Further Questions to Ask

- None. Patient is well known to you and has already consented to a sub-Tenon's triamcinolone injection, which has worked well for his CME OS in the past (Fig. 79.1).

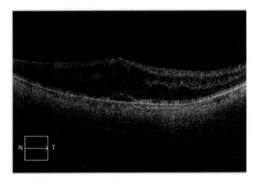

Fig. 79.1 Optical coherence tomography (OCT) of the left eye demonstrates large cystoid spaces, a small amount of subfoveal fluid, and a thin epiretinal membrane.

Assessment

Uveitic CME OS consistent with moderately subnormal vision OS

Management

- Sub-Tenon's triamcinolone 40 mg/0.1 cc transconjunctivally in the inferotemporal fornix

Follow-up

You begin to inject but feel resistance early in the injection. The patient begins to complain of intense pressure in the eye and immediately sees floaters. You stop injecting, withdraw the needle, and examine the left eye.

Exam

	OD	OS
Vision		Hand motion (HM)
IOP		Unrecordably high

	OD	OS
Lids and lashes:		Normal
Sclera/conjunctiva:		White and quiet
Cornea:		Clear
AC:		Deep and quiet, 1+ flare
Iris:		Flat
Lens:		Clear
Anterior vitreous:		Clear
DFE:		No view of the fundus. Dense white particles throughout the vitreous

Assessment

- Globe perforation OS secondary to sub-Tenon's injection
- The rock-hard eye and intravitreal white steroid particles confirm that the needle has penetrated the globe and inadvertently entered the eye.

Management

- Immediate AC paracentesis to relieve pressure.
- There is no view of the fundus and no ability to visualize and thus safely treat the retinal defect at the perforation site to prevent retinal detachment. Follow up tomorrow.

Follow-up #2

HPI

The patient complains that he cannot see anything. He is very concerned and anxious.

B scan OS: retina attached. Dense vitreous opacities.

Exam

	OD	OS
Vision		HM
IOP		20
Lids and lashes:		Normal
Sclera/conjunctiva:		White and quiet
Cornea:		Clear
AC:		Deep and quiet, 1+ flare
Iris:		Flat
Lens:		Clear
Anterior vitreous:		Clear
DFE:		No view of the fundus. Dense white particles admixed with red vitreous hemorrhage throughout the vitreous cavity.

Management

- Urgent pars plana vitrectomy with laser of retinal defect and intraocular gas tamponade, if necessary.
- The examination is unchanged. The patient has by definition an untreated retinal defect that cannot be treated in the office. He is at high risk of rhegmatogenous retinal detachment and is monocular. Aggressive treatment is indicated.

Follow-up #3

HPI

The surgery was uncomplicated. The retina was attached intraoperatively and laser was placed around the defect in the inferotemporal retina. Air was left in the vitreous cavity at the end of the surgery. After an uneventful postoperative day (POD) #1 visit, he is seen a week later. Vision has improved to 20/30−, IOP is normal, and the retina is attached with laser scars inferotemporally around a white focus (Fig. 79.2).

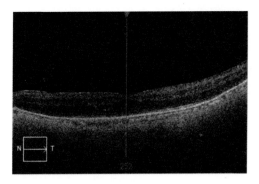

Fig. 79.2 OCT of the left eye shows complete resolution of the cystoid macular edema and small neurosensory detachment.

Key Points

- Globe perforation after sub-Tenon's injection is a vision-threatening complication that requires emergent management to control IOP and urgent measures to treat the underlying retinal defect. The penetration site itself is usually self-sealing, given the size of needles used to perform sub-Tenon injections (27 or 25 gauge).
- Periocular steroids can be administered through various approaches: an inferior transconjunctival approach (as in this case), a superior transconjunctival approach (Nozick technique), and a transseptal/orbital floor approach. The inferior transconjunctival approach has poorer visualization of the sclera than the superior transconjunctival approach, and the transseptal approach keeps the needle farthest from the globe.
- All approaches are safe in trained hands and with a cooperative patient, but transseptal may be the safest in a poorly cooperative patient.

- High doses of intraocular triamcinolone (whether preserved, as in Kenalog, or preservative-free, as in Triesence) are better tolerated than dexamethasone (Depo-Medrol), which is a major reason why the author prefers to use the former in periocular/peribulbar injections in case of inadvertent perforation. This patient suffered no retinal toxicity from a massive dose of Kenalog in the eye.
- It is important to treat the underlying retinal defect in a time-sensitive fashion. Cryotherapy and laser retinopexy are preferable, noninvasive approaches if the retinal defect can be adequately visualized.

CHAPTER 80

Sterile Endophthalmitis

Harpal S. Sandhu

History of Present Illness

A 44-year-old man with a history of sarcoidosis-associated panuveitis both eyes (OU) controlled on mycophenolate mofetil 1000 mg by mouth (PO) twice a day (BID) presents urgently to your office 2 days after an intravitreal injection. At the previous appointment earlier in the week, the uveitis was quiescent but he had cystoid macular edema in the left eye (OS) with visual acuity (VA) decreased to 20/60 from his baseline of 20/40. Intravitreal triamcinolone 2 mg/0.05 cc was injected. Today, he states that his vision has become much cloudier. He is accustomed to seeing many large floaters after the injection, which clear after a few days, but this is different. His vision is totally blurred and has been getting worse over the last day.

Exam

	OD	OS
Vision	20/30	20/400
Intraocular pressure (IOP)	16	15
Lids and lashes:	Normal	Normal
Sclera/conjunctiva:	White and quiet	White and quiet
Cornea:	Clear	Clear
Anterior chamber (AC):	Deep and quiet	See Fig. 80.1
Iris:	Flat	Flat
Lens:	Posterior chamber intraocular lens (PCIOL)	PCIOL
Anterior vitreous:	Clear	Poor view, +cells
Dilated fundus examination (DFE):	Deferred	Poor view

B scan OS: 3+ vitreous opacities, retina attached.

Questions to Ask

- Are you in pain? If so, how much?
- Have you had any discharge from the eye?

The patient denies any pain or discharge. He says the eye feels fine, but he simply cannot see out of it.

351

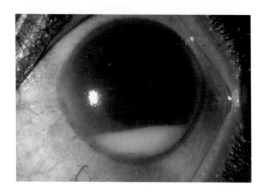

Fig. 80.1 Color slit lamp photograph shows the unusual combination of white and quiet conjunctiva with a hypopyon in the anterior chamber.

Assessment

- Severe, acute inflammation with hypopyon OS after intravitreal injection of triamcinolone

Differential Diagnosis

- Infectious endophthalmitis
- Noninfectious, postinjection inflammation ("sterile endophthalmitis")
- Less likely: flare of sarcoid panuveitis, migration of triamcinolone into the anterior chamber (AC)

Working Diagnosis

- Infectious endophthalmitis OS

Management

- Vitreous tap and injection of vancomycin 1 mg/0.1 cc and ceftazidime 2.25 mg/0.1 cc

Follow-up

The patient returns the following day. He notes the vision is no different. Gram stain of the vitreous sample was negative for organisms, and polymerase chain reaction (PCR) showed no bacterial or fungal deoxyribonucleic acid (DNA).

Exam

	OD	OS
Vision	20/30	20/400
IOP	15	17
Lids and lashes:		Normal
Sclera/conjunctiva:		Small subconjunctival hemorrhage temporally
Cornea:		Clear
AC:		2-mm hypopyon (unchanged)
Iris:		Flat
Lens:		Clear
Anterior vitreous:		Poor view, + cells
DFE:		Poor view

Working Diagnosis

- Noninfectious inflammation ("sterile endophthalmitis") postinjection

Management

- Start prednisolone acetate 1% drops every hour left eye (OS) and cycloplegia
- Observe closely

Further Follow-up

The patient is seen multiple times over the course of the next month. One month after presentation, the patient's inflammation has finally cleared while on frequent topical steroids. Vision improved to 20/50−, a slight decline from baseline.

Key Points

- "Sterile endophthalmitis" is somewhat of a misnomer. The term describes noninfectious intraocular inflammation that occurs after intravitreal injection of a variety of different drugs inside the eye.
- The presentation can be similar to infectious endophthalmitis; therefore initial management is typically to tap the eye and inject broad-spectrum antibiotics.
- Differences in presentation from acute infectious endophthalmitis include less pain and little to no conjunctival injection or chemosis. However, there is a range of presentations, and thus distinguishing the entity from infectious endophthalmitis on initial presentation can sometimes be difficult.
- There is some evidence that the risk of this complication is higher with preserved triamcinolone formulations (e.g., Kenalog) compared with preservative-free formulations of triamcinolone (e.g., Triesence).

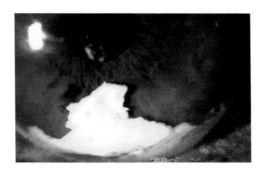

Fig. 80.2 An example of "pseudohypopyon" caused by migration of triamcinolone into the anterior chamber. Note the particulate appearance of the white material. (From Lee SJ, Kim YD, Kyung H. Pseudohypopyon after management of posterior capsule rupture using intracameral triamcinolone injection in cataract surgery. *Korean J Ophthalmol.* 2014;28[4]:356–357.)

- This entity is distinct from "pseudoendophthalmitis," which refers to the anterior migration of triamcinolone particles into the AC, which layer in the inferior AC to form a pseudohypopyon. It can be diagnosed by the particulate appearance of white material within the pseudohypopyon (Fig. 80.2).
- Acute noninfectious inflammation has been described after injections of the anti–vascular endothelial growth factor (VEGF) agents bevacizumab, ranibizumab, and aflibercept, as well as the corticosteroid triamcinolone. Severe noninfectious inflammation after aflibercept characteristically presents as predominantly vitreal inflammation with less AC reaction.
- Extended courses of topical corticosteroids are generally sufficient to resolve the inflammation. Prognosis is fair to good. Many patients will eventually (i.e., over the course of a month or more) regain their baseline vision, but some may experience a permanent decrement in vision.
- The etiology of the inflammation is unknown. Some have suggested contaminants of lipopolysaccharide or other immunogenic antigens within the drug are the culprits. Others have suggested that preservatives themselves are the problem, but it is still unclear.

CHAPTER 81

Contralateral Retinitis in a Patient on Systemic Immunomodulatory Therapy

Kathryn Pepple ■ Russell Neil Van Gelder

History of Present Illness

A 70-year-old woman was referred 4 years prior for scotomas left eye (OS) with associated photopsias and difficulty on light–dark transition. Electroretinography (ERG) at that time was markedly reduced OS, and a presumptive diagnosis of acute zonal occult outer retinopathy (AZOOR) OS was made. After significant discussion with the patient that minimal data on efficacy of treatment were available, she opted for a short course of oral corticosteroids, resulting in subjective improvement in symptoms and objective improvement on visual fields. The patient was then transitioned to mycophenolate mofetil 1000 mg by mouth (PO) twice a day (BID). She was stable on this regimen until 2 weeks prior to presentation, when she noted decreasing vision right eye (OD) with associated malaise and fever.

Exam

	OD	OS
Visual acuity	20/20 −	20/40 −
Intraocular pressure (IOP)	15	20
Sclera/conjunctiva	White and quiet	White and quiet
Cornea	Clear	Clear
Anterior chamber (AC)	Deep and quiet	Deep and quiet
Iris	Unremarkable	Unremarkable
Lens	Clear	Posterior chamber intraocular lens (PCIOL) with 1+ posterior capsular opacification (PCO)
Anterior vitreous	Debric	Debris
DFE	See Fig. 81.1	unremarkable

Questions to Ask

- Has there been any redness or pain in either eye?
- Any risk factors for new infection, particularly sexually transmitted diseases such as human immunodeficiency virus (HIV) or syphilis?
- Have you traveled outside of the country recently?

She answers no to all of these questions.

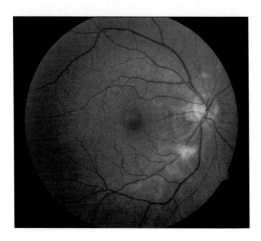

Fig. 81.1 Color fundus photo of right eye shows retinal swelling with mild, associated hemorrhage inferotemporal to the disc and with smaller associated spots of possible retinitis or cotton-wool spots.

Assessment

- New retinitis vs. cotton-wool spot OD in a patient on chronic immunomodulatory therapy

Differential Diagnosis

- Cytomegalovirus (CMV) retinitis
- Hypercoagulable state
- Early acute retinal necrosis syndrome (ARN)
- HIV retinopathy
- Syphilis or tuberculosis

Working Diagnosis

- CMV retinitis

Testing

- Complete blood count (CBC)/complete metabolic panel (CMP): white blood cell (WBC) 4.15, absolute lymphocyte count (ALC) 1.27K, aspartate aminotransferase (AST) 52, alanine transaminase (ALT) 56
- HIV and syphilis: both negative
- Serum CMV polymerase chain reaction (PCR): positive at 3×10^5 copies/mL

Management

- Discontinue mycophenolate
- Valganciclovir load 900 mg BID for 3 weeks, followed by 900 mg daily for 3 months

Follow-up

One month into antiviral treatment, the patient reports complete resolution of symptoms OD.

Repeat color fundus photo of right eye 3 months after initiation of treatment shows resolution of cotton-wool spots and a small residual retinal scar in the area of previous retinitis after treatment with valganciclovir (Fig. 81.2).

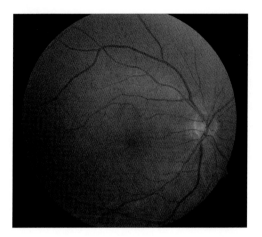

Fig. 81.2 Repeat color fundus photo of right eye 3 months after initiation of treatment shows resolution of cotton-wool spots and a small residual retinal scar in the area of previous retinitis after treatment with valganciclovir.

Management Algorithm

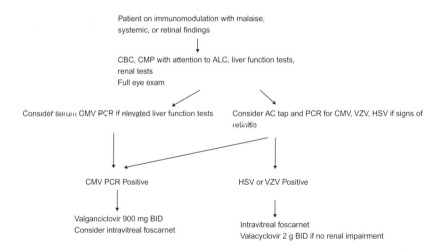

Patient on immunomodulation with malaise, systemic, or retinal findings

↓

CBC, CMP with attention to ALC, liver function tests, renal tests
Full eye exam

Consider serum CMV PCR if elevated liver function tests

Consider AC tap and PCR for CMV, VZV, HSV if signs of retinitis

CMV PCR Positive

HSV or VZV Positive

Valganciclovir 900 mg BID
Consider intravitreal foscarnet

Intravitreal foscarnet
Valacyclovir 2 g BID if no renal impairment

Key Points

- Immunomodulation for uveitic disease can rarely give rise to systemic and/or ocular opportunistic infection, including CMV retinitis and ARN.
- Disease may manifest as CMV viremia with associated organ dysfunction, particularly hepatic.
- Diagnosis relies on detection of virus either systemically or from anterior chamber (AC) tap.
- Discontinue immunomodulation if possible.
- Treat with appropriate antiviral (valganciclovir for CMV and valacyclovir for herpes simplex virus [HSV] or varicella zoster virus [VZV]).
- Use adjunctive intravitreal antivirals (i.e., foscarnet) as indicated for active retinitis.
- Patients with noninfectious uveitis who develop systemic infections need to be monitored carefully for uveitic flares while off immunomodulatory therapy (IMT). If they flare while off IMT, local therapies should be used or escalated (see Chapter 3).

CHAPTER 82

Rhegmatogenous Retinal Detachment in Intermediate Uveitis

Henry J. Kaplan

History of Present Illness

A 20-year-old woman had a sudden loss of vision left eye (OS), which was noticed on awakening this morning. She has a history of pars planitis (intermediate uveitis) both eyes (OU) since age 8 that has recently been quiescent. She is currently on no medication for treatment of her ocular disease.

Exam

	OD	OS
Visual acuity	20/20	20/400
Intraocular pressure (IOP)	14	8
Sclera/conjunctiva	Quite without inflammation	Quiet without inflammation
Cornea	Clear	Clear with nongranulomatous (NG) keratic precipitate (KP) in inferior one-third
Anterior chamber (AC)	No cell or flare	1+ flare, 1+ cell
Iris	Within normal limits (WNL)	WNL. No posterior synechiae.
Lens	Clear	Clear with trace posterior subcapsular cataract (PSC) haze
Vitreous cavity	1+ vitreous cells with few snowballs in inferior vitreous	3+ vitritis with partial posterior vitreous detachment (PVD), vitreous traction to inferotemporal retina (Fig. 82.1)
Retina/optic nerve	Normal optic nerve and retina. No CME. No traction on peripheral retina inferiorly but there is a persistent small snow bank inferiorly.	Retinal detachment with large horseshoe tear at 7:00 in periphery resulting in macula-off detachment (Fig. 82.2)

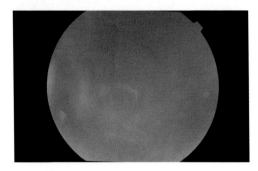

Fig. 82.1 Fundus photograph of the left eye showing significant vitritis with snowballs. Notice vitreous bands extending to the inferior/inferotemporal retina. (This image was originally published in the Retina Image Bank website. Author: Mallika Goyal. Title: Retinal detachment with uveitis. Retina Image Bank. Year 2014; Image Number 13232. © the American Society of Retina Specialists.)

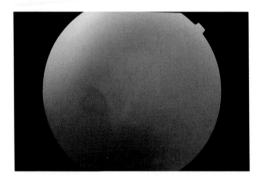

Fig. 82.2 A rhegmatogenous retinal detachment OS with involvement of macula. A large horseshoe tear of the retina caused by vitreous contraction and traction on peripheral retina. (This image was originally published in the Retina Image Bank website. Author: Mallika Goyal. Title: Retinal detachment with uveitis. Retina Image Bank. Year 2014; Image Number 13231. © the American Society of Retina Specialists.)

Questions to Ask

- Have you had trauma to your left eye?
- Were you treated for complications of pars planitis previously and, if so, what treatments?
- Have you been diagnosed with any systemic disease?
- Do you have numbness, tingling, or weakness on one side of the body? Is there any history of neurologic disorders in your family?

She denies any history of trauma to either eye. Shortly after presenting with pars planitis as an 8-year-old, she developed decreased visual acuity (VA) OU secondary to cystoid macular edema (CME). She was given periocular injections of triamcinolone acetonide in OU on several occasions, and her CME resolved. Her vision returned to 20/20 OU, but she has noticed increased floaters OS over the past 3 months. She is otherwise healthy and has no symptoms of neurologic disease, nor does anyone in her family.

Assessment

- Macula-off rhegmatogenous retinal detachment (RRD), OS, secondary to retinal tear

Differential Diagnosis

- Pars planitis (intermediate uveitis without systemic disease)

Working Diagnosis

- Macula-off RRD, OS, secondary to pars planitis
- Bilateral pars planitis, OS > OD (right eye)

Testing

- In patients with a retinal detachment and classic history of pars planitis, such as this one, no further workup is necessary. Because the disease can be a presenting symptom of multiple sclerosis, a workup should be pursued if the patient has neurologic symptoms or signs. Infectious retinitis has classical features that are not seen in this patient (e.g., acute retinal necrosis, chronic progression of retinitis, etc.). Therefore no specific testing is required.

Management

- Surgical repair of retinal detachment OS, within 24 to 48 hours, involving a pars plana vitrectomy, transretinal drainage of subretinal fluid with pneumatic air tamponade, endolaser photocoagulation around the flap tear, and an encircling scleral band to relieve peripheral retinal traction by an organized vitreous. Intravitreal 20% sulfur hexafluoride would be considered for prolonged retinal hole retinal tamponade if the encircling band did not support the flap tear.
- Routine topical drops (corticosteroid, cycloplegic, antibiotic) after retinal surgery.
- Tapering course of oral prednisone, starting with 0.75 mg/kg/day, over 2 weeks to prevent postsurgical reactivation of intraocular inflammation.
- Routine postsurgical follow-up on days 1, 7, and 14.

Follow-up

The patient had an uncomplicated postoperative course with resolution of intravitreal air in 7 days and no recurrence of intraocular inflammation. At 1 month postoperatively, VA was 20/20 OD and 20/25 OS.

Key Points

- Many patients with pars planitis can have asymmetric disease, so that continued follow-up of both eyes is necessary. CME is the most common cause of vision loss in these patients. Retinal tears and RRD are infrequent but possible complications of pars planitis.
- RRDs are caused by a hole or tear in the retina, in contrast to traction retinal detachment (RD) caused by epiretinal fibrotic proliferation or serous RD associated with posterior segment diseases, such as Vogt—Koyanagi—Harada (VKH).
- Posterior segment uveitis is most frequently associated with RRD because of vitreous traction on the retina causing a retinal tear(s), or necrotic infectious retinitis resulting in

multiple retinal holes or a large retinal tear. The incidence of RRD among uveitis patients ($\approx 3\%$) is higher than RRD in the general population and is frequently bilateral in patients with viral retinitis.

- Visual outcome in patients with RRD and uveitis is worse than in the general population with RRD. Reasons for worse visual outcome may be severe CME, necrotic retina (e.g., herpetic retinitis—cytomegalovirus [CMV], varicella zoster virus [VZV], herpes simplex virus [HSV]), epiretinal proliferation, organized vitreous with tractional bands to the peripheral vitreous base, ongoing intraocular inflammation, and chronic hypotony.
- Surgical correction of RRD in uveitis depends on the clinical presentation. For example, in pars planitis there is frequently traction on the inferior retina with one or more horseshoe tears that can be repaired by PPV, endolaser photocoagulation, and an encircling scleral buckle to support the peripheral vitreous base. However, in CMV retinitis where there are many small holes in the necrotic retina, PPV must be accompanied by silicone oil tamponade.
- Surgery in the presence of active intraocular inflammation is associated with a worse prognosis. Thus intravenous Solu-Cortef (hydrocortisone sodium succinate) during the operative procedure followed by oral prednisone for 7 to 14 days should be considered depending on the severity of intraocular inflammation.

INDEX

Page numbers followed by "*f*" indicate figures, "*t*" indicate tables, and "*b*" indicate boxes.

P

R